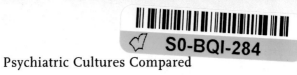

Psychiatric Cultures Compared

PSYCHIATRIC CULTURES COMPARED

Psychiatry and Mental Health Care
in the Twentieth Century:
Comparisons and Approaches

Edited by
Marijke Gijswijt-Hofstra
Harry Oosterhuis
Joost Vijselaar
Hugh Freeman

AMSTERDAM UNIVERSITY PRESS

The publication of this book has been made possible by a grant from
the Netherlands Organisation for Scientific Research (NWO)
and the Huizinga Institute

Lay out Hanneke Kossen, Amsterdam
Cover design Geert de Koning, Kampen
Cover illustration © Charley Toorop, *Vrouw uit Zwakzinnigengesticht*,
c/o Beeldrecht Amsterdam 2005

ISBN 90 5356 799 2
NUR 875

Contents

Acknowledgements

This volume is based on papers presented at the international workshop 'Cultures of Psychiatry and Mental Health Care in the Twentieth Century: Comparisons and Approaches', held at the Royal Netherlands Academy of Arts and Sciences (KNAW) and the University of Amsterdam, 18-20 September 2003. We would like to acknowledge the Board of the Humanities Division of the Netherlands Organisation for Scientific Research (NWO) and the Huizinga Institute for their generous funding of the conference. We would also like to warmly thank for their assistance the Huizinga Institute Manager, Paul Koopman, the (former) Assistant Manager, Francien Petiet, and a student at the University of Maastricht, Leonieke Verhoeven, who contributed enormously to the smooth running of the workshop.

The articles presented here owe a great deal to the comments and intellectual feedback of the participants at the workshop. They have contributed much to the content of this book. We are also very much endebted to our co-editor, Hugh Freeman, who has been of inestimable help in assisting with the correction of the English and much more than that.

The Dutch editors

Introduction

Comparing National Cultures of Psychiatry

Marijke Gijswijt-Hofstra and Harry Oosterhuis[*]

When in 1905 the Budapest asylum doctor Kárlmán Pándy published his 'comparative study' of the care for the insane in Europe, he was by no means the first one to do so, nor would he be the last.[1] The history of psychiatry and mental health care offers numerous examples of cross-national inquiries by doctors and others who wished to learn about psychiatry in other parts of the Western world, and perhaps seek models to adopt in their home country. International study trips were – and still are – a favourite way to collect information firsthand.[2] Correspondence with foreign colleagues and international conferences on psychiatry and mental health and hygiene provided other opportunities to become informed. After the Second World War, the World Health Organization (WHO) played an active part in generating information about the state of mental health care in various countries, largely in order to set international standards for it.[3] The European Community has also functioned as a framework for reporting on mental health policies in the member states.[4] The reports and publications resulting from these various internationally orientated, fact-finding and policy-orientated reports, however different in scope, depth, and method, all bear witness to attempts to learn about and from each other for practical purposes.

While mental health professionals and policymakers have time and again reported on different countries, historians of psychiatry have only hesitantly followed suit, focused as most of them were on their home-countries. An early exception was *Bürger und Irre: Zur Sozialgeschichte und Wissenschaftssoziologie der Psychiatry* (1969) by the German psychiatrist Klaus Dörner about the development of institutional psychiatry in Britain, France, and Germany in the eighteenth and nineteenth centuries. The French psychiatrist J. Postel and historian C. Quetel, in their *Nouvelle Histoire de la Psychiatrie* (1983), also followed an international perspective.[5] In recent years, other attempts have been made at comparative history. Some monographs and collections address the way in which insanity or mental problems were defined and treated in a range of different countries and societies, including a volume which brings together studies from all the continents.[6] Although not aiming to present systematic and fully fledged comparative studies, these works reveal and also, to a certain extent, analyse and contextualise differences and similarities between national psychiatric cultures.[7] Next to Edward Shorter's *History of Psychiatry: From the Era of the Asylum to the Age of Prozac* (1997) about the USA and several European countries, and Mark Micale's and Roy Porter's historiographic collection *Discovering the History of Psychiatry* (1994), collections have appeared – to mention some recent examples – on the 'confinement of the insane' in the nineteenth and early twentieth centuries worldwide, in the UK and some of its former colonies; on neurasthenia around 1900 in Great Britain, Germany, and the Netherlands; on social psychiatry and psychotherapy in the twentieth century in these same three countries; and on post-war psychiatry and mental health care in the UK and the Netherlands.[8] Some conferences of the European Society for the History of Psychiatry, founded in 1990, have resulted in collections of papers about several European countries – albeit without any systematic comparison.[9] Whereas most comparative historical studies on psychiatry are about the nineteenth and early twentieth centuries, this volume focuses on the twentieth century.

Comparing national psychiatric cultures or aspects of these cultures has proved to be rewarding but also difficult, for at least two different reasons. Firstly, we are faced with the problem of the availability of historical research with a sufficiently similar focus, especially when relating to fairly recently developed research interests such as the patient's view, the role of the family, the different options for care and treatment, the way patients were admitted to and discharged from mental institutions, psychiatric nursing, psychopharmacology, social psychiatry, outpatient services, and the financial aspects of mental health care. Secondly, we are confronted with methodological problems relating to the availability of sources, and the translation and comparability of terminology and data from different countries and periods.[10] The term 'mental health care', for example, does not have the same meaning in various national cultures. In some, it refers to a wide sphere of activity, including the care for the mentally handicapped and demented elderly as well as outpatient facilities and counseling centres for psychological and social problems. In others, it mainly concerns psychiatry in a narrower sense: the care and treatment of the mentally ill. The way the boundaries of the mental health domain were and are drawn as well as its relation to adjacent fields, such as poor relief, general health care, social work, pastoral care, education, and justice, vary from nation to nation. Concepts like 'social psychiatry', 'psychotherapy', and 'de-institutionalisation' may give rise to confusion. In some countries, psychotherapy and counseling were part and parcel of psychiatry and (public) mental health care, but in others they developed in the context of private practice, psychosomatic medicine, or social work. In general, comparative research seems to be most rewarding when it is problem-orientated and focuses on a particular subject.

The present volume is the result of an international workshop entitled *Cultures of Psychiatry and Mental Health Care in the Twentieth Century: Comparisons and Approaches*, which took place in September 2003 in Amsterdam.[11] This workshop was inspired by the research project *The Disordered Mind: Theory and Practice of Mental Health Care in the Netherlands during the Twentieth Century*. This project started in 1998 under the aegis of the Huizinga Institute for Cultural History, the Netherlands Organisation for Scientific Research (NWO), the University of Amsterdam, and the University of Maastricht. The concrete goal of this project is to write a history of mental health care in the Netherlands in which its cognitive content, intervention practices, organisation, and institutional, social, and cultural settings are analysed in their mutual interconnections. The research team consisted of eight scholars doing research on patients' files in Dutch mental hospitals, the history of the psychiatric profession, the history of 'anti-psychiatry', the history of psychiatric nursing, and the financing of mental health care. Also, other scholars working on various topics have participated in the team's meetings. In addition to monographs and articles by the participants, the directors of the project will publish a synthesis, offering a general overview of the history of psychiatry and mental health care in the Netherlands from the late nineteenth to the early twenty-first century. It will attempt to understand the development of Dutch psychiatry and mental health care from a social and cultural angle and to situate it in an international context.[12]

This volume has two aims. The first is to compare Dutch developments in psychiatry and mental health care in the twentieth century with those in some other Western countries. Which similarities and differences can be discovered? To what extent is the Dutch case exceptional? Both the Netherlands and the countries that have influenced it in this field – Germany, France, the UK, and the USA – are covered by national overviews. The second objective is to present some new approaches and promising research topics in the twentieth-century history of mental health care. For this reason, some other countries – Italy, Japan, and Sweden – have been selected. Studies on patterns of institutional admission and discharge and the practice of family care in the first two countries demand comparison with new Dutch research on the various ways mental patients were cared for. A fairly new topic of research concerns psychiatric nursing, and here Sweden is the counterpart of the Netherlands.

The essays in this volume have been organised into three parts. The first includes the national overviews of developments in psychiatry and mental health care and a comparative overview of the outpatient sector and de-institutionalisation in the Netherlands, the UK, Germany, France, Italy, and the USA. As a point of reference, this section starts with three articles on the Netherlands, the first focusing on intramural psychiatry, the second on extramural mental health care, and the third on 'anti-psychiatry' in the 1960s and 1970s. These contributions are followed by chapters on the surrounding countries and the United States, of which the former West and East Germany are covered most extensively. In the second part, some new and promising topics and approaches are presented: the care of patients in the context of the interaction between asylums and the family in the Netherlands, Italy and Japan; psychiatric nursing in the Netherlands and Sweden; and psychotropic drugs, mainly in the Netherlands. Two reflective reviews, one historiographic by a specialist in medical history and the other contextual and comparative by two specialists in political and cultural history, form the third and final part of the volume.

This collection of essays offers one of the first attempts in the history of psychiatry towards a more systematic comparison of national developments in a number of major Western countries during the twentieth century – a period that is only beginning to be the object of historical research. By making Dutch mental health care the point of reference and confronting it with developments abroad, the volume highlights contrasts and analogies which were partly unexpected. Like the professionals and policymakers mentioned above, historians of psychiatry, including the authors of this volume, show an increasing eagerness to learn about and from each other. Though practical purposes may not be their primary concern, the search for historical knowledge and understanding certainly is.

General Trends, Themes and Issues

To ensure that the overviews of the various countries would more or less cover a similar range of topics, the authors were invited to deal with crucial trends and developments, major features and turning points, as well as significant discussions and controversies in their home countries. Other points of special interest that we suggested were: the external and internal boundaries of mental health care domains; the organisation and funding of care (public or voluntary; centralised or on a regional or local basis); legislation and policies in this field; the role of various professions (doctors, nurses, psychologists, social workers, etc.) and the demarcation of their fields of work; the broader social and cultural context, the impact of two World Wars and, in some countries, of totalitarian regimes. Last but not least, we asked questions about patients: their profile, complaints, and the diagnoses of their mental disorders; their differentiation into new categories of care (such as in- and outpatients, chronic and acute, the mentally handicapped and demented elderly); self-organisation and influence of patients; and patients' rights. The authors were thus confronted with an ambitious list of queries and issues as a heuristic framework. For the individual author, it was impossible to answer all of these, simply because of lack of space or of relevant research. Covering a whole century and the whole range of intramural and outpatient mental health care is quite a challenge. The Dutch authors had the advantage of participating in the running research project *The Disordered Mind*. Yet, as will become clear, both the national overviews and the contributions on special topics are very helpful in understanding the way in which Dutch psychiatry and mental health care resembled and differed from those in other countries.

Some common trends in twentieth-century psychiatry and mental health care can be hypothesised. As far as intramural psychiatry is concerned, this period witnessed a gradual transformation of more or less closed asylums, where patients were admitted only or mainly with legal certification and more often than not for social rather than medical reasons, into more open mental hospitals, with increasing numbers admitted on a voluntary basis and according to medical criteria. This is not to say that in the past asylums were by definition institutions of social control and that there was something like a great confinement. Such a view, propagated by revisionist authors, has been convincingly refuted.[13] Some of the contributions in this volume, focusing on actual patients, show how complicated and divergent patterns of care and of institutional admission and discharge actually were. However, the revisionists were to some extent right in that medical criteria were often less crucial than social, political, administrative, and financial considerations as well as family interests and gender and class relations.

It was only in the course of the twentieth century that the main function of mental institutions shifted from shelter and care to treatment and cure. Distant, isolated mental institutions were to an increasing extent considered outdated, the more so if they were huge, overcrowded and in poor condition. In many countries, the 1950s appear to mark a turning point: more and more patients were actually being treated instead of just sheltered and cared for; from then on, the average time-periods in which they were hospitalised steadily decreased. At the same time, patients were differentiated and segregated according to medical criteria: mentally handicapped and psycho-geriatric people, for example, moved to specialised institutions, thus leaving behind those with 'pure' psychiatric disorders. Of crucial importance were the changes in the way mental institutions were financed and administered. Until far into the twentieth century, they were largely dependent in many countries on poor relief, while their social and medical status was low. Sooner or later, in the context of a welfare state, collective medical insurance and social security schemes replaced poor relief. More money and the growing involvement of national governments often contributed to the improvement of the quality of care and living conditions for the mentally ill. Also, the accessibility of care, both in terms of legal or financial regulations and of geographical distance, was considerably broadened.

Probably the most drastic changes concern the expansion of the psychiatric domain and, closely connected to that, the development of mental health care outside mental institutions. Whereas in the nineteenth century psychiatry was predominantly confined to asylums and, in certain places, sanatoria and spas, in the course of the twentieth century, it also gained ground in newly established facilities such as psychiatric wards in general hospitals, outpatient clinics, private practice, social-psychiatric services, and counseling centres. Psychiatry became part of the more-embracing field of mental health care and mental hygiene. Its expansion was accompanied by a growing number of professionals and an increasingly professional diversity. Until the 1950s, psychiatrists and nurses or attendants still dominated the field. Afterwards, they began to be confronted with growing numbers of psychologists, social workers, and other, often new professions. This institutional and professional expansion and diversification reflected an increasingly wider spectrum of patients and clients. The development of the psychiatric domain since the late nineteenth century appears to have been driven by an internal dynamic to include new groups: in addition to the insane, feeble-minded, and neurological patients, this included a diversity of nervous sufferers, psychosomatic patients, psychopathological criminals, sexual perverts, alcoholics, problem children, traumatised war victims, and others. Some psychiatrists began to present themselves as social-hygiene experts, focusing on the mental health of society at large. Not only mental illnesses, but also an increasing variety of milder nervous, psychosomatic and psychological disorders and complaints, personality problems, and a diversity of more or less common problems in modern life became part of the mental health system's sphere of action.[14]

The idea that psychiatric patients should preferably be discharged from a mental institution as soon as possible, or even that it was better to keep them as much as possible outside it, can be traced back to the late nineteenth and early twentieth centuries. Officially sanctioned family care was then practised on a small scale in most Western countries and on a larger scale in some, like Belgium (Gheel), Italy, Norway, and Japan.[15] Also, the first social-psychiatric facilities, outpatient clinics, and prevention-orientated counseling centres were set up before the Second World War. The two World Wars, especially the last, promoted a number of psychiatric innovations in the Anglo-Saxon world: new principles of in- and outpatient treatment along social and psychological lines, like brief psychotherapy, group therapy, and the therapeutic community were then picked up by innovative psychiatrists in other Western countries. In most, however, it was not until the 1960s and 1970s that the role of extramural mental health care really grew more prominently and that the scope of outpatient facilities was enlarged. This was largely a consequence of the policy of de-institutionalisation, implemented in all Western countries, although its form, scale, and timing varied substantially. Outpatient facilities were no longer conceived as merely complementing psychiatric hospitals, but as replacing them to a large extent. The shift from intra- to extramural care was advanced by a diversity of factors which included practical considerations or necessities as well as ideological and ethical principles. These included: the introduction of psychotropic drugs from the 1950s; nationally designed plans to integrate psychiatry into the overall health and social care-providing system of the welfare state; the anti-psychiatric criticism of institutional and medical psychiatry; the striving for humanistic reform of the care and treatment of psychiatric patients and enhancement of their social integration and civil rights; and last but not least, financial and political considerations.

The dynamic of modern psychiatry suggests that to some extent supply increasingly created demand. However, next to this push factor, some external pull factors such as social developments in modern society should be taken into account to explain the expansion of mental health care. The Western world in the twentieth century witnessed a growing dependence of laypeople on scientific knowledge. According to the British sociologist Anthony Giddens, this is part of the 'reflexivity of modernity': the regularised use of expert knowledge, often in popularised forms, about personal and social life as a constitutive element in its organisation and transformation.[16] In this connection, the Dutch sociologist Abraham de Swaan coined the term 'proto-professionalisation' to indicate the growing tendency of laypeople to adopt professional language and modes of interpretation.[17] Rising levels of education and heightened communication among the general population play an important role in this process. To a much lesser extent than in the past, people in Western societies are willing to accept individual shortcomings or unhappiness as an inevitable part of life, as God's will, or as simply a matter of bad luck. People's rising expectations about their ability to treat and solve personal problems, to fashion their individual lives by free choice, and to create or recreate their self have furthered the demand for mental health services, although their expansion and organisation – public or private – differ substantially between countries.

The strong growth of mental health care, especially in the second half of the last century, reflected a more general process of psychologisation – a change of mentality combining growing individualisation, internalisation, and self-guidance, related to changing social manners and relationships. The psychological interpretation of the self and of other people's motives and behaviour can be traced back to the late eighteenth century, but until far into the twentieth it was largely restricted to intellectual and bourgeois circles and mental health professionals themselves. In general, it was not until the 1950s and 1960s, when economic, social and political developments enabled the definitive breakthrough of individualisation on a massive scale and with a focus on authenticity, self-determination and self-expression, that the psychological way of thinking gradually spread among the populations of Western societies.[18]

Political developments should also be taken into account. From the late eighteenth century, psychiatry, as a product of the bourgeois society that emerged during the era of the Enlightenment and the French Revolution, had developed in a dynamic between humanization and disciplining, emancipation and coercion, social integration and exclusion, and democratic citizenry and political control.[19] Until far into the twentieth century, institutional psychiatry fulfilled two functions: a medical one (care and cure), which gave priority to the interests of the individual patients or their relatives, and a social-political one (segregation), which was geared toward freeing society of the nuisance, danger or harmful influence associated with the insane. How these two functions related to each other and which was most prominent varied over time and from place to place, and was also closely linked with a country's political constellation. In countries where a liberal constitutional state was realised, there were constraints on the possibility of admitting people involuntarily to a mental asylum. From around 1840, various West-European countries and American states adopted measures to regulate the institutionalisation of the insane. Within the margins of the constitutional state, these regulations served to protect citizens against the random deprivation of freedom and to allow effective admission procedures to ensure timely medical treatment for those who needed it, as well as the security of public order. The basic tenet of this regulation was that the insane – within and, on occasion, outside institutions – fell under a special jurisdiction and state supervision, based on their mental incapacitation. This meant that their civil rights were suspended for either a shorter or longer period of time. To this extent, mental illness was at odds with citizenship, as articulated in the ideals of freedom and equality since the American and French Revolutions.

Despite the constitutional state's juridical safeguards built into this arrangement, in the course of the last two centuries, it was not uncommon for these safeguards and the medical-humanitarian motives to lose out against the view of mental disease as a social order, public health or financial-economic problem. This happened in part on account of larger historical processes, notably growth in size, bureaucratisation and increasing state intervention. Collective and state interests might thereby outweigh the well-being of the individual patient, while the boundaries of acceptable coercion became stretched little by little. These trends were at work in many countries, albeit to different degrees, but went the furthest in Germany. There, since about 1900, eugenics gained more following among psychiatrists, who let themselves be used as a tool by the Nazi regime in large-scale mandatory sterilisation and euthanasia programmes. In liberal-democratic countries, psychiatry was also involved in social-hygienic policies, which subordinated individual civil rights to what was regarded as public health and national strength. For example, several American states and social-democratic Scandinavian countries enforced eugenic intervention. This was almost entirely for mental retardation. In the Soviet Union, psychiatry was used to confine dissidents and subject them to medical treatment for their 'mental disorders' in order to discredit their political opposition.[20]

In the nineteenth and early twentieth centuries, the relationship between institutional psychiatry and citizenship was 'negative' or 'exclusive' in the sense that hospitalisation in an asylum – apart from the voluntary admission that was made possible in many countries – generally implied legal certification and therefore the potentially serious infringement of basic civil rights. Later, however, a more 'positive' or 'inclusive' connection between psychiatry and liberal-democratic citizenship was established in two ways. Firstly, from about 1970, there was a growing attention to and recognition of the civil rights of the mentally ill. In many Western countries, the legislation on insanity was amended, reflecting a shift from values associated with maintaining law and order and protecting citizens against arbitrary detention or the insane against themselves, for their own benefit, to values associated with patients' autonomy, responsibility and consent, as well as their right to adequate care and treatment.[21] Secondly, from the early years of the twentieth century, in psychiatry as well as in the broader field of mental hygiene and mental health care, socio-psychological definitions of citizenship were advanced. Expressing views about the position of individuals in modern society and their possibilities for self-development, psychiatrists, psycho-hygienists and other mental health workers connected mental health to ideals of democratic citizenship and civic virtue. Thus, they were clearly involved in the modern liberal-democratic project of promoting not only virtuous, productive, responsible and adaptive citizens, but also autonomous, self-conscious, assertive and emancipated individuals as members of an open society.[22]

Whilst the history of psychiatry and mental health care can only be understood in its social, political, economic and cultural contexts, it was not possible to cover these systematically in this volume. The format of the chapters hardly allowed that – although many authors refer or allude to these contexts. One of the other important topics discussed during our workshop was to what extent continuity and discontinuity, ruptures or watersheds can be discerned in the different countries in the course of the twentieth century. If, for example, the 1950s were to be characterised as a watershed, what exactly would this refer to? To the introduction of new psychotropic drugs, referred to by some as the 'psychopharmacological revolution'?[23] Or to the more or less gradual realization of more differentiated options for treatment and care, both within and outside mental hospitals? Or to both, the first creating the conditions that were favourable for the second? And to what extent could these developments in the 1950s be considered as the foreboding for what was presented as 'anti-psychiatry' in the late 1960s and after? Or should that period itself, rather than the 1950s, be marked as a watershed? If so, in which respects was it important: in rejecting the 'medical model'; in setting a different 'moral agenda'; in 'emancipating' both patients and psychiatric nurses; or in enhancing the accessibility of mental health care?[24] How did these developments relate to what came to be called 'de-institutionalisation'?[25] Perhaps the clearest yet at the same time much more localised example of a rupture is presented by Nazi psychiatry and its 'euthanasia' programme.[26]

Another issue raised during the workshop concerned the assessment of the quality of institutional or other types of care of the mentally ill, as they developed in the course of the twentieth century. On the one hand, everybody seemed to agree that it is quite legitimate or even imperative for a historian to look into the quality of care according to the standards of the period itself and of the different parties concerned.[27] On the other hand, there was less consensus about whether or not historians should themselves attempt to strike a balance and make evaluative judgements, e.g. in terms of the degree of 'humanity' or therapeutic effectiveness of psychiatric cultures or regimes over time. The risk of finding oneself on the slippery slope of Whiggish thinking in terms of 'progress' is indeed far from imaginary.[28] Yet this risk can be considerably contained. First, by making explicit how and according to which criteria the quality of mental health care is being assessed. And second, by making a clear distinction between the quality of mental health care as it was actually realised, and the way in which this came about – whether or not it was planned or intended as such is but one important aspect of this question. Both issues will be discussed at some length in the final chapter of this volume.

Contributions to This Volume

The first part of this volume, the national overviews, opens with three Dutch contributions. The first one, by Marijke Gijswijt-Hofstra, provides an overview of Dutch institutional psychiatry between the late nineteenth century and 2000. The central themes in her overview include: the development from closed asylums to their gradual opening up from around the 1920s, and the recent integration and mergers of mental hospitals with half-way or community care facilities; the development of private, voluntary or charitable versus public involvement in institutional care of the mentally ill; processes of differentiation of mental institutions, both internally through allocating separate wards for different kinds of patients and externally by building separate institutions for mentally handicapped, epileptic, alcoholic or psycho-geriatric patients; the development of hospital versus asylum functions, including the tension between medical aspirations and what was actually realised; and, finally, the development of the quality of care. Interesting results include the relatively early opening up of asylum wards for 'voluntary', uncertified admissions, and the relatively late and cautious introduction of 'socialisation', as the Dutch variant of de-institutionalisation was called.

The second chapter, by Harry Oosterhuis, maps the various Dutch extramural organisations, facilities and practices in which psychiatrists and other professional groups have played a role during the twentieth century. He discusses the institutional development of outpatient mental health care, the professional groups that shaped it and the approaches and treatments they adopted, their various groups of patients and clients and, finally, the larger socio-cultural context. Especially notable is that the Netherlands acquired an extensive network of extramural services in the course of the twentieth century, ranging from pre- and aftercare for the core group of severely mentally ill people to a broad psycho-social and psychotherapeutic mental health sector that, particularly from the 1960s, attracted a large clientele. It is emphasized that the growing supply of professional care created, as it were, its own demand. It is also suggested that the cultural revolution of the 1960s, in combination with rapid secularisation and the erosion of 'pillarisation' – the far-reaching Dutch social and political compartmentalisation along denominational and ideological lines – resulted in a spiritual vacuum that was partially filled by 'the new psychotherapeutic ethos'.

The third chapter on the Netherlands, by Gemma Blok, is about the impact of anti-psychiatry on the actual practice of clinical psychiatry during the 1970s. She attempts to explain its popularity in the context of the situation in clinical psychiatry at that time, as well as of broader cultural changes. Interestingly, it was not the abolition of psychiatry as such, but rather an intensification of psychiatric treatment – especially in the form of psychotherapy, the therapeutic community, or family therapy – that Dutch critical psychiatry stood for. Much was expected from the new 'social model' – in fact a psychotherapeutic model – with its emphasis on self-determination and the personal responsibility of the 'clients'.

From the Netherlands we cross the North Sea. The central theme of Hugh Freeman's overview of British psychiatry is the relationship between the state and the care of the mentally ill. Before the establishment of the National Health Service (NHS) in 1948 – a watershed according to Freeman – the mainly public British asylum system was, like in many countries, closely intertwined with poor relief. The NHS placed the 'mental hospitals' together with general hospitals in one nationalised system of health care. From the late 1950s onwards, the emphasis of British psychiatry gradually shifted from mental hospitals to 'community care'. It was only from the mid-1970s onwards, however, that de-institutionalisation was officially stated as government policy, although financial support was inadequate. Indeed, financial limitations and dictates cropped up time and again, especially during the Thatcher regime, when the NHS withdrew from providing long-term care, and the social security system began to pay for transferring patients with chronic mental illness to privately run nursing homes.

Gerald Grob's chapter on the USA focuses on the origins, goals and outcomes of de-institutionalisation, including the different meanings of this term over time and the reasons why it did not benefit all patients. The emergence of de-institutionalisation was facilitated by the growing role of the federal government in social welfare and health policies soon after the war, together with the impaired authority of state governments that were responsible for the public mental hospitals. With the Community Mental Health Centres Act of 1963, the federal government advanced a radically new policy. Community Mental Health Centres (CMHCS) were meant to facilitate social support for mental patients as well as early identification of symptoms and preventive treatments, and thereby make (long-term) hospitalisation superfluous. However, the outcome did not meet expectations. Due to the financial incentive of the enactment of Medicare and Medicaid in 1965, long-term, primarily elderly patients were moved from state mental hospitals to nursing homes, resulting in trans-institutionalisation rather than de-institutionalisation. Also, it soon become clear that the CMHCS attracted a clientele with less serious problems, rather than assuming responsibility for the aftercare and rehabilitation of chronic patients with serious mental disorders.

Germany is discussed in the next three chapters. Volker Roelcke questions the conventional tripartite periodisation of twentieth-century German psychiatry, parallel to German political history, with the Third Reich as the obvious second period. He does so by considering three dimensions of psychiatry from the early twentieth century up to the 1970s: the professional policies, the organisation of mental health care, and scientific research. Apart from notable discontinuities, Roelcke signals considerable continuities extending from 1933 to 1945. The Weimar period, for example, already contained strong eugenicist tendencies. Without denying that the ruthless way the Nazis put eugenics and racial hygiene into practice was unparalleled in history, Roelcke argues that Hitler's regime represented not so much a rupture as continuity. Moreover, he points out that, certainly as far as personnel and the strong medical focus were concerned, 1945 represented no clear break, although eugenically inspired genetic research programmes almost disappeared. If all three dimensions of psychiatric activity are taken into consideration, it was only much later, around 1970, that we can speak of a clear rupture. There was then a shift away from large-scale mental hospitals; other professional groups, such as psychologists and social workers, were integrated into mental health care settings; and a more open attitude emerged towards social psychiatry and psychotherapy.

Greg Eghigian's contribution is about the German Democratic Republic (GDR), and he focuses on the role of politics there. Was there something particularly 'communist' about East German psychiatry? Or, more generally, do totalitarian or authoritarian regimes necessarily imply that psychiatry is also repressive? He argues that the connection between politics and psychiatry is by no means straightforward, and that liberal, fascist and communist societies alike have tended to give mental health care an increasingly important role in the management of (ab)normality. With respect to the regime of the GDR, Eghigian demonstrates how, after an initial period of reticence, party officials and the government increasingly accepted psychiatric expertise. From the 1960s onwards, during the period of de-Stalinisation, psychiatrists and psychologists played a prominent role in certain social reform projects. In the 1970s and 1980s, East German psychiatry experienced a phase of 'openness', including more international professional contacts.

Focusing on the federal state of North Rhine-Westphalia, Franz-Werner Kersting examines asylum psychiatry from 1940 to 1975. More particularly, he explores how the acknowledgement of the fate of psychiatric patients in the Third Reich affected the reform process of German psychiatry. For the West German reform movement in psychiatry, advocating a shift from a medical to a social approach, the Nazi past served as a warning example to show that an exclusive biomedical and institutional focus easily entailed the danger of an inhuman, repressive psychiatry, possibly with deadly consequences. The reform effort started in the 1950s as an internal debate in the psychiatric world. It was the interaction between the aims of innovative psychiatrists and those of the broader protest movement of the 1960s that made it into a public issue, resulting in the Psychiatry Commission of the German parliament in the early 1970s. There was reason enough for Kersting to conclude that '1968' was a turning point, thereby agreeing with Roelcke.

From Germany, we cross the Rhine to arrive in France. Jean-Christophe Coffin outlines the development of the French public mental health care system between 1920 and 1980, paying special attention to the debates that inspired its transformation. Coffin examines the innovative ideas of a group of psychiatrists around Henri Ey in Paris, who were active after the Second World War. They pleaded for radical innovation in psychiatric thinking and practice: hospitalisation should only be the ultimate solution in a whole range of options to be made available for mental patients, such as open care services, social re-adaptation facilities and care at home. However, reform plans launched by the government in the early 1950s and 1960s failed to materialise, although local experiments with 'therapeutic communities' and outpatient projects were indeed started around 1950. It was only in the 1970s that the sector model was finally implemented, meaning the integration of various in- and outpatient mental health provisions within geographical districts so as to make them more accessible to the population. However, at the same time, psychiatry was strongly criticized, so that Ey and his colleagues concluded that the more radical reform of psychiatry which they advocated – its demedicalisation and a push back of mental hospitals – had not been realised.

The national overviews, most of which focus especially on institutional psychiatry, are followed by a comparative essay in which Harry Oosterhuis explores the development of outpatient mental health care and de-institutionalisation in the five countries discussed in the previous chapters, as well as Italy. He shows that there is no simple relation between the growth of outpatient services and community care on the one hand and de-institutionalisation on the other, in the sense that more or less de-institutionalisation was paralleled by the creation of more or fewer outpatient services. In countries with relatively highly developed outpatient facilities and community services – France and the Netherlands – de-institutionalisation was introduced rather late and cautiously, compared with other nations. Germany, with considerably fewer outpatient services, likewise pursued de-institutionalisation in a gradual and moderate way. In Italy, the USA and the UK, on the other hand, de-institutionalisation was implemented earlier and more drastically, whereas outpatient facilities or community care lagged behind.

The second part of the volume includes six chapters in which some recent and promising approaches and research topics are discussed: the history of the psychiatric patient, of psychiatric nursing and of psychotropic drugs. The three chapters on patients demonstrate in different ways what can be gained by analysing medical records and other written sources on the practice of psychiatric care. 'Doing medical history from below' fixes attention not only on the patient, but also on their relatives and, perhaps, their friends and neighbours.[29] How were the mentally ill cared for? What were the options, and which options were successively used and why? What was the role of the family in this whole process? Joost Vijselaar's chapter is about the patterns of admission and discharge in three Dutch mental institutions between 1890 and 1950. His detailed study of patients' records sheds light on a number of the social mechanisms that surrounded admission and discharge, in particular the interaction between asylum and family. Vijselaar demonstrates that for families with a relative suffering from mental illness, the asylum was often far from being the first option, and that asylums were not bent on keeping patients hospitalised at all costs and, depending on the social situation, rather encouraged their (early) return to society.

The next chapter, by Akihito Suzuki, explains the excess – between three-fifths and two-thirds – of male patients in the Japanese asylum population: numbers that were not equalled in the Western world before the Second World War. Against the background of the mental health care system in Japan, which was characterised by relatively few asylums and widespread family care, and focusing on the diagnosis of schizophrenia, Suzuki explores the reasons for the over-representation of men in asylums. Analysing statistical materials and patients' records, Suzuki concludes that since psychiatric beds were rather scarce, priority was given to the hospitalisation of male patients, because their symptoms were perceived to be of a more public nature and more threatening to others. Female patients were more frequently cared for at home, while their symptoms tended to be regarded as more private and more directed against themselves, while the traditional extended family was able to 'absorb privately troublesome cases'.

Patrizia Guarnieri's contribution on subsidised home care of mental patients by their relatives in Italy in the early twentieth century focuses on the province of Florence, where the provincial administration bore the costs of asylum care for the poor. In 1866, the province started a family-care programme, which was cheaper and alleviated the overcrowding of the asylums. Initially, home care was only subsidised for those patients who had first been admitted to an asylum. Soon, however, support was extended to patients who had not been institutionalised before and who were already cared for by their indigent families. In the last two decades of the nineteenth century, the number of mentally ill people entrusted to family care rose from around 200 to 700. Guarnieri examines the different roles and often conflicting interests of provincial and local authorities, the attitude of psychiatrists, and finally, what actually went on in the small homes of the families concerned. It appears that relatives did not keep their patients at home for the money – the subsidy was much too low for that – but that they often preferred to care for them and 'did what they could, even with love'.

The history of psychiatric nursing is also a promising, yet relatively unexplored field of research. Analysing a series of Dutch textbooks for student psychiatric nurses from 1897, Cecile aan de Stegge sheds light on changing attitudes towards the use of restraint in mental institutions in the twentieth century. Although reliable data on the actual use of restraint are lacking or scarce, she shows that from the beginning, both the textbooks and the requirements of the State Inspectors reflected rejection of the use of mechanical restraint – at least of those means of restraint that had to be registered, such as straitjackets. On the whole, both textbook authors and Inspectors 'felt uneasy with mechanical measures that hampered the freedom of bodily movement'. However, as far as other techniques to restrain patients and the isolation of patients were concerned, they appeared to be more flexible and less consistent. Aan de Stegge highlights a fundamental change between the mid-1920s and the mid-1950s, when short-term 'educational seclusion' in the context of occupational therapy was considered 'appropriate'. After the introduction of psychotropic drugs, a diminishing tolerance for 'unnecessary' restriction can be detected, but should seclusion nevertheless be used, nurses were expected to be able to motivate this intervention in writing.

The other chapter on psychiatric nursing, by Gunnel Svedberg, is about Sweden and covers the period from the mid-nineteenth until the end of the twentieth century. Her focus is on professional identity, including the role of gender and class. The Swedish case is rather special in that psychiatric nursing was not established as a separate, autonomous, and asylum-based branch of training like, for instance, in the Netherlands, Britain, or Germany. As in the USA, all Swedish nurses received both general training and supplementary training in a special field, such as psychiatric nursing. Whereas in other countries men worked as psychiatric nurses, in Sweden this profession was, until the early 1950s, an exclusively female affair. In daily practice, qualified female nurses were appointed as head-nurses on both female and male asylum wards, whereas a much larger group of female and male attendants, with much less training, performed most of the nursing work. Male attendants especially were increasingly dissatisfied with this situation, which would only change when training for attendants was improved, and nursing colleges finally opened their doors to male students in 1950.

In their chapter about the 'hidden history' of psychiatric drugs, Toine Pieters and Stephen Snelders, on the basis of two case studies, examine the continuities and discontinuities with regard to the use and meaning of medication in mental institutions. The first case study concerns the European career path of the new drug hyoscine (scopolamine) in the late nineteenth century. The second, based on Dutch professional and popular publications as well as interviews with expert witnesses, focuses on the career path of chlorpromazine in the 1950s and 1960s, primarily in the Netherlands. Pieters and Snelders conclude that in both cases, continuity rather than discontinuity should be stressed. In both cases, a recurring cycle of therapeutic optimism and subsequent re-evaluation and disappointment can be discerned.

The third and final part of the volume contains two chapters with reflections on the previous contributions and has the twofold goal of comparing Dutch developments with those in other countries and presenting some new approaches and promising research topics. Frank Huisman elaborates historiographic issues and offers suggestions on how to write a (comparative) history of psychiatry, while Ido de Haan and James Kennedy, in their joint contribution, present some general and concluding reflections.

Psychiatric Cultures Compared: Results and Remaining Problems

This collection, of course, can by no means offer a final comparative history of psychiatry and mental health care. We have only made a start, and this volume illustrates some of the difficulties in attempting international comparison. An exhaustive comparison of national psychiatric cultures requires not only a certain structuring of themes that are considered worth comparing, but also thorough research on common topics. As far as the organisation and provision of mental health care and the treatments offered are concerned, we are fairly well informed – although historical research of outpatient care still leaves much to be desired. However, this is much less true, for example, of issues that are essential from the perspective of the 'history from below': the need among the population for mental health care, the way people experienced mental disorders and articulated their needs and demands, and the available options they did or did not use. These issues are covered in the three chapters on patients and their families, but they do not go beyond the first half of the twentieth century, nor do they cover the UK, France, Germany, and the USA – the major countries with which the Netherlands is compared. The patient's perspective should receive more attention, including the role of the family and patient's 'careers'. Also, the perspective of psychiatric nurses or attendants, the professional group that is most intensively involved with care for psychiatric patients, appears to be a promising topic for future research. At another level, more research into the politics and funding of mental health care may lead to new insights. In this way, this volume generates new questions, though we have certainly learned a lot from this undertaking. As far as the general trends highlighted earlier in this introduction are concerned, we are able to qualify some of them and to specify in what way Dutch mental health care in the twentieth century might be different or even unique from an international perspective.

It appears to be crucial to distinguish between ideas or ideals, rhetoric, norms, intentions and plans with respect to mental health care on the one hand, and what was actually realised on the other. It is also useful to distinguish between reporting what happened at both these levels and the extent to which the one corresponded with or diverged from the other, as well as attempting to explain why things happened as they did, or failed to happen. The reform of mental health care through de-institutionalisation and the promotion of community care in particular were frequently accompanied by high expectations and much enthusiasm, but nearly everywhere, this commitment met with financial, political, organisational or professional obstacles. The chapters in this volume contain numerous examples of outcomes that fell short of or deviated from the original intentions and expectations. To answer the question of why this happened and how we should explain the unexpected results requires a more detailed comparative analysis than can be offered here. It is beyond doubt that the growing involvement of national governments, the development of welfare states, and the impact of financial considerations were important. However, they do not in themselves account for the various policies that were implemented and the different ways in which new systems of mental health care materialised.

The shift from mental institutions to other psychiatric provisions, including 'community care', is usually seen as one of the most drastic changes in twentieth-century mental health care. The way in which and the extent to which complementary or alternative facilities were realised differed considerably, however, both in timing and cross-nationally, and even regionally within the larger nations. Moreover, the term usually used to characterise this development, 'de-institutionalisation', may be inaccurate or even misleading. What often happened was in fact 'de-mental-hospitalisation', the reduction of (long-term) hospitalisation in mental hospitals. If, in a more literal sense, de-institutionalisation is understood to mean the reduction of institutional care as such, then the care provided by, for instance, the inpatient psychiatric departments of general hospitals, institutions for the mentally handicapped, and nursing homes for demented elderly people should also be included. In such a perspective, the shift from mental hospital to alternative types of residential care should perhaps not be called de-institutionalisation, but rather, as Grob suggests, 'trans-institutionalisation'.[30] Certainly, for many patients suffering from severe and chronic mental illnesses, the range and (financial as well as geographical) accessibility of mental health services was broadened, especially in the form of outpatient or community care facilities. Although the expansion of public community care facilities was orientated towards psychiatric patients in the majority of the countries concerned, this appears to have been only partly the case in the USA and the Netherlands where, as Oosterhuis shows, a broader clientele with minor mental complaints and psycho-social problems was also included. To what extent this also happened in other countries has yet to be clarified.

To what extent can we answer the question of whether or not the Netherlands presented a special case? The contributions by Gijswijt-Hofstra and Oosterhuis as well as the concluding chapter by De Haan and Kennedy refer to this in some detail, though a relatively limited number of (large) countries has been included in our comparison. In future considerations, it would be worthwhile expanding the scope, and also including, for instance, some smaller countries like Belgium, the Scandinavian nations, Switzerland and Austria.

With respect to Dutch institutional psychiatry, it may be noted that until the last decades of the nineteenth century, most asylums were old – sometimes centuries old – and small and were situated in towns. Most remained relatively small-scale, seldom more than 800-900 beds. The Netherlands was among the first countries to introduce an insanity law emphasizing that the insane were to be treated and cured, and imposing state supervision on asylums to maintain good standards of care and treatment. The Netherlands was also among the first countries that opened asylum wards for uncertified admissions. In the context of the 'pillarisation' of Dutch society from the late nineteenth century onwards, voluntary, religiously inspired initiatives (orthodox Calvinist, Roman Catholic, Jewish, Dutch Reformed) played along with public initiatives, a prominent role in the building and administration of mental institutions. As the Netherlands is a small country, the geographical distance between the different parts of the country could be fairly easily bridged. Thus, some Roman Catholic patients from Amsterdam were sent to a relatively cheap denominational mental institution in the south of the country. It should be mentioned, however, that the Netherlands was by no means the only country where religious organisations played an important role in institutional psychiatry: this was also the case in Belgium and Germany. As in other social sectors, there has always been a delicate balance in Dutch mental health care between voluntary organisation and administration on the one hand, and public financing and government supervision on the other. If and to what extent this public/voluntary mix was specific to the Netherlands remains a question for future research.

With respect to the therapeutic regime, Dutch asylum doctors tended to follow international medical developments. However, the very prominent role of 'more active therapy' (in German: *aktivere Therapie*) in the Netherlands, from the 1920s until the 1960s, is striking. Although this form of occupational therapy

– a social and didactic rather than medical approach to mental illness – originated in Germany, it seems to have been especially popular and lasting in the Netherlands. Why this would have been the case has not become sufficiently clear. Obviously, Nazi Germany went its own way. In Britain, France and the United States this form of occupational therapy was either not introduced at all or did not become nearly as popular as in the Netherlands – and, for that matter, initially in Germany itself. Future research may shed more light on this. It seems quite probable that the overall small scale of Dutch asylums, many of them built according to the pavilion or cottage system, offered a relatively favourable environment for the introduction of active therapy, certainly if compared to the large British, French, and American mental institutions. In addition, it may well be that this therapy fitted in with a more general preference for moral, didactic and social approaches that can also be found in Dutch outpatient mental health care. Compared with their colleagues in other European countries, Germany in particular, Dutch psychiatrists were somewhat more reserved towards somatic treatments; in general, their approach was eclectic and pragmatic, and many of them had an open mind towards psychoanalysis as well as social, phenomenological and anthropological psychiatry. In contrast with pre-war Germany, the USA and some Nordic countries, eugenics never caught on in Dutch psychiatry.

Psychiatric nursing appears to have some specific Dutch features. The Netherlands is one of the few countries where this specialty developed apart from general nursing in somatic medicine and where there has been a separate training system for psychiatric nurses – both female and male – from the late nineteenth century onwards. In the Dutch training system psychological, didactic and social approaches were allotted an increasingly important place, whereas in Sweden, for instance, nursing was much more medically orientated. Other countries that, at one time or another, developed a training system for psychiatric nurses that was completely separate from general nursing were Britain, Ireland and Switzerland.[31]

With respect to Dutch extramural mental health care, public outpatient facilities were founded early (from the 1920s) and showed a stronger degree of continuity than anywhere else. This was partly caused by the influence of the Dutch pillarised social system, which facilitated more or less stable organisational structures on the basis of voluntary initiatives, and later by the generous collective funding in the Dutch welfare state. Otherwise, the role of the Dutch government remained rather passive, at least until the 1970s, when it began to formulate and implement its own policies. When from the 1980s onwards 'socialisation', being the Dutch variant of de-institutionalisation, began to be pursued – later than in the Anglo-Saxon countries and Italy – an extensive and multifaceted network of outpatient facilities was already in place. Another striking element of the Dutch outpatient mental health care sector was its wide boundaries.

From early on, it not only offered pre- and aftercare for psychiatric patients and the mentally handicapped, but also included counseling centres for problem children, for marriage- and family-related issues, for psychotherapy, and for alcohol and drug addiction. Outpatient mental health care, partly organised on a religious basis, was not just medical psychiatry or psychotherapy, to a large extent it was also (moral) education, pastoral care and social work. Moral-didactic and psycho-social approaches rather than medical treatment gained the upper hand in this respect.

The broad orientation and accessibility of Dutch extramural mental health care can also be explained by its fairly early and generally strict differentiation from institutional and clinical psychiatry. There was a strong tendency in the outpatient sector to keep patients with serious psychiatric disorders, who were difficult to treat, out of its system. In Britain, France and Germany, the public mental health sectors were more exclusively geared toward the mentally ill, while there was also a closer link with clinical psychiatry. The major role of psychotherapists – psychiatrists as well as psychologists and social workers – in Dutch outpatient mental health care, especially since the 1960s, sets the Netherlands apart from other European countries, where psychotherapy largely remained limited to the more or less elitist private practice of psychiatrists. In this respect, the developments in the Netherlands were more similar to those in the United States. In both countries, the emphasis on a multidisciplinary approach in post-war mental health care ultimately resulted in both the expansion of its domain and a strong psychological orientation.

What is perhaps most striking in Dutch psychiatry and mental health care is their openness towards various foreign examples. Before the Second World War, social psychiatry, active therapy, psychoanalysis and other forms of psychotherapy, phenomenological and anthropological approaches, and experimental and clinical psychology were adopted from Germany, Austria and, to a lesser extent, France. Whereas these innovations largely came to an end in Central Europe in the 1930s, they proved enduring in the Netherlands. The same was true of the counseling centres for alcoholism and family and marriage problems, established around 1910 and 1940, respectively. Before and after the Second World War, Dutch psychiatry also followed models from the USA and the UK: the mental hygiene movement, child guidance clinics, psychiatric social work, counseling methods and new forms of psychotherapy, and the therapeutic community. Again, some of these were longer lasting in the Netherlands than in the countries in which they originated.

Notes

*   We are indebted to our co-editor Joost Vijselaar for his comments on earlier drafts of this introduction and to Hugh Freeman for correcting the English.

1.   Pándy's study appeared in Hungarian (1905) and in German: K. Pándy, *Die Irrenfürsorge in Europa. Eine vergleichende Studie* (Berlin: Georg Reimer, 1908).

2.   See, for instance, F. de Haen (ed.), *Mental Health Care in Some European Countries. Policy, Organization and Financing of Mental Health Care in Belgium, France, England, Wales, Denmark and Switzerland* (Utrecht: National Hospital Institute of the Netherlands, 1989).

3.   For instance: H.L. Freeman, T. Fryers & J.H. Henderson, *Mental Health Services in Europe: 10 years on* (Kopenhagen: WHO, 1985).

4.   See Steen P. Mangen (ed.), *Mental Health in the European Community* (Beckenham: Croom Helm, 1985) and *Acta Psychiatrica Scandinavica*, 104 (Suppl. 410) (2001); T. Becker and J.L.Vázquez-Barquero, 'The European Perspective of Psychiatric Reform', in *Ibid.*, 8-14.

5.   Klaus Dörner, *Bürger und Irre: Zur Sozialgeschichte und Wissenschaftssoziologie der Psychiatry* (Franfurt am Main: Europäische Verlagsanstalt, 1969); English translation: *Madmen and the Bourgeoisie: A Social History of Insanity and Psychiatry* (Oxford: Basil Blackwell, 1981); J. Postel and C. Quetel (eds), *Nouvelle Histoire de la Psychiatrie* (Toulouse: Editions Privat, 1983).

6.   Roy Porter and David Wright (eds), *The Confinement of the Insane. International Perspectives, 1800-1965* (Cambridge: Cambridge University Press, 2003).

7.   By psychiatric cultures we understand 'distinct worlds of meaning' with respect to how mental illness and mental problems were/are defined, named, interpreted, and treated or prevented. See: William H. Sewell, 'The Concept(s) of Culture', in Victoria E. Bonnell and Lynn Hunt (eds), *Beyond the Cultural Turn. New Directions in the Study of Society and Culture* (Berkeley: University of California Press, 1999), 35-61: 52, 57-58. See also: Marijke Gijswijt-Hofstra, 'Introduction: Cultures of Psychiatry and Mental Health Care in Postwar Britain and the Netherlands', in *idem* and Roy Porter (eds), *Cultures of Psychiatry and Mental Health Care in Postwar Britain and the Netherlands* (Amsterdam & Atlanta: Rodopi, 1998) 1-7: 1-2.

8.   Edward Shorter, *A History of Psychiatry: From the Era of the Asylum to the Age of Prozac* (New York: John Wiley & Sons, 1997); Mark S. Micale and Roy Porter (eds), *Discovering the History of Psychiatry* (New York: Oxford University Press, 1994); Porter and Wright (eds), *op. cit.* (note 6); Gijswijt-Hofstra and Porter (eds), *op. cit.* (note 7). Joseph Melling and Bill Forsythe (eds), *Insanity, Institutions and Society, 1800-1914. A Social History of Madness in Comparative Perspective* (London & New York: Routledge, 1999); Marijke Gijswijt-Hofstra and Roy Porter (eds), *Cultures of Neurasthenia from Beard to the First World War* (Amsterdam & New York: Rodopi, 2001); Michael Neve and Harry Oosterhuis (eds), *Social Psychiatry and Psychotherapy in the Twentieth Century: Anglo-Dutch-German Perspectives*, special issue *Medical History*, 48, 4 (2004).

9.   Leonie de Goei and Joost Vijselaar (eds), *Proceedings of the 1st European Congress on the History of Psychiatry and Mental Health Care* (Rotterdam: Erasmus Publishing,

1993); F. Fuentenebro, R. Huertas, and C. Valiente (eds), *Historia de la psiquiatría en Europa: Temas y tendencias* (Madrid: Frenia, 2003).

10. See also Steen Mangen, 'Psychiatric Policies: Developments and Constraints', in: *idem* (ed.), *op. cit.* (note 4), 1-33: 4.

11. Most contributions in this collection are based on a selection of the pre-circulated papers presented at the workshop, mediated by the contributions of the invited commentators and participants.

12. Directors of the project are Marijke Gijswijt-Hofstra and Harry Oosterhuis. The other participants are in the sequence of the projects mentioned: Joost Vijselaar, Ido Weijers (assisted by Peter van Drunen), Gemma Blok, Cecile aan de Stegge, and, for the project on financing, Karin Bakker and Henk van der Velden. Up until January 2005 two individual projects have resulted in book publications: Gemma Blok, *Baas in eigen brein. 'Antipsychiatrie' in Nederland, 1965-1985* (Amsterdam: Uitgeverij Nieuwezijds, 2004); Ruud Abma and Ido Weijers, *Met gezag en deskundigheid. De historie van het beroep psychiater in Nederland* (Amsterdam: SWP, 2005).

13. See Michel Foucault, *Madness and Civilization. A History of Insanity in the Age of Reason* (London: Tavistock, 1971); Robert Castel, *The Regulation of Madness. The Origins of Incarceration in France* (Cambridge: Polity Press, 1988); Andrew Scull, *Museums of Madness. The Social Organization of Insanity in Nineteenth Century England* (London: St. Martin's Press, 1979); D.J. Rothman, *The Discovery of the Asylum. Social Order and Disorder in the New Republic* (Boston & Toronto: Little, Brown, 1971).

14. See, for instance, Robert Nye, *Crime, Madness, and Politics in Modern France. The Medical Concept of National Decline* (Princeton: Princeton University Press, 1984); Ruth Harris, *Murders and Madness. Medicine, Law, and Society in the fin de siècle* (Oxford: Oxford University Press, 1989; Edward Shorter, *From Paralysis to Fatigue. The History of Psychosomatic Illness in the Modern Era* (New York: Free Press, 1992); Joachim Radkau, *Das Zeitalter der Nervosität. Deutschland zwischen Bismarck und Hitler* (Munich & Vienna: Carl Hanser Verlag, 1998); Harry Oosterhuis, *Stepchildren of Nature. Krafft-Ebing, Psychiatry, and the Making of Sexual Identity* (Chicago: The University of Chicago Press, 2000); B. Shepherd, *A War of Nerves, Soldiers and Psychiatrists 1914-1994* (London: Jonathan Cape, 2000); Gijswijt-Hofstra and Porter (eds), *op. cit.* (note 8: *Cultures of Neurasthenia*); Eric J. Engstrom, *Clinical Psychiatry in Imperial Germany. A History of Psychiatric Practice* (Ithaca & London: Cornell University Press, 2003); Paul Lerner, *Hysterical Men. War, Psychiatry, and the Politics of Trauma in Germany, 1890-1930* (Ithaca and London: Cornell University Press, 2003); R. Castel, F. Castel and A. Lovell, *The Psychiatric Society* (New York: Columbia University Press, 1982); Andrew Scull, 'Psychiatry and Social Control in the Nineteenth and Twentieth Centuries', *History of Psychiatry*, 2 (1991), 149-69; J.C. Pols, *Managing the Mind. The Culture of American Hygiene, 1910-1950* (University of Pennsylvania, 1997); Leonie de Goei, *De psychohygiënisten. Psychiatrie, cultuurkritiek en de beweging voor geestelijke gezondheid in Nederland 1924-1970* (Nijmegen: SUN, 2001).

15. See, for instance, P. Bartlett and D. Wright (eds), *Outside the Walls of the Asylum. The History of Care in the Community 1750-2000* (London: Athlone Press, 1999).

16. Anthony Giddens, *The Consequences of Modernity* (Cambridge: Polity Press, 1990).

17.   Abraham de Swaan, R. van Gelderen and V. Kense, *Het spreekuur als opgave. Sociologie van de psychotherapie 2* (Utrecht & Antwerpen: Het Spectrum, 1979), 28-34.

18.   See C. Taylor, *Sources of the Self. The Making of Modern Identity* (Cambridge: Cambridge University Press, 1994); Mark S. Micale (ed.), *The Mind of Modernism: Medicine, Psychology, and the Cultural Arts in Europe and America, 1880-1940* (Stanford: Stanford University Press, 2004); R.H. Turner, 'The Real Self: From Institution to Impulse', *American Journal of Sociology*, 81 (1976), 989-1016; M.L. Gross, *The Psychological Society* (New York: Touchstone, 1978); R. D. Rosen, *Psychobabble. Fast Talk and Quick Cure in the Era of Feeling* (New York: Avon Books, 1979); N. Rose, *Governing the Soul. The Shaping of the Private Self* (London: Routledge, 1990); N. Rose, *Inventing our Selves: Psychology, Power, and Personhood* (Cambridge: Cambridge University Press, 1996); Anthony Giddens, *Modernity and Self-Identity. Self and Society in the Late Modern Age* (Cambridge: Polity Press, 1991); E.S. Moskowitz, *In Therapy We Trust. America's Obsession with Self-Fulfillment* (Baltimore: Johns Hopkins University Press, 2001).

19.   Dörner, *op. cit.* (note 5); Doris Kaufmann, *Aufklärung, bürgerliche Selbsterfahrung und die 'Erfindung' der Psychiatrie in Deutschland 1770-1850* (Göttingen: Vandenhoeck & Ruprecht, 1995); M. Gaudet and G. Swain, *Madness and Democracy. The Modern Psychiatric Universe* (Princeton: Princeton University Press, 1999).

20.   B. Müller-Hill, *Tödliche Wissenschaft. Die Aussonderung von Juden, Zigeunern und Geisteskranken 1933-1945* (Reinbek bei Hamburg: Rowohlt, 1985); E. Stover, E. and E.O. Nightingale (eds), *The Breaking of Bodies and Minds. Torture, Psychiatric Abuse, and the Health Professions* (New York: W.H. Freeman and Company, 1985); Paul J. Weindling, *Health, Race and German Politics between National Unification and Nazism, 1870-1945* (Cambridge: Cambridge University Press, 1989); Ian R. Dowbiggin, *Keeping America Sane. Psychiatry and Eugenics in the United States and Canada 1880-1940* (Ithaca and London: Cornell University Press, 1997).

21.   Mangen, *op. cit.* (note 4), 27-8.

22.   Matthew Thomson, 'Before Anti-Psychiatry: "Mental Health" in Wartime Britain', in Gijswijt-Hofstra and Porter (eds), *op. cit.* (note 7), 43-59; *idem*, 'Constituting Citizenship: Mental Deficiency, Mental Health and Human Rights in Inter-war Britain', in Chr. Lawrence and A.-K. Mayer (eds), *Regenerating England: Science, Medicine and Culture in Inter-war Britain* (Amsterdam, Atlanta: Rodopi, 2000), 231-50; Harry Oosterhuis, 'Self-development and Civic Virtue. Psychiatry, Mental Health, and Citizenship in the Netherlands, 1870-2005', in G. Eghigian, A. Killen and C. Leuenberger (eds), *The Self as Scientific and Political Project* (Chicago: The University of Chicago Press: forthcoming 2007).

23.   Shorter, *op. cit.* (note 9); David Healy, *The Antidepressant Era* (Cambridge MA & London: Harvard University Press, 1997). See also the contributions by Toine Pieters & Stephen Snelders, Marijke Gijswijt-Hofstra, and Hugh Freeman.

24.   See the contribution by Gemma Blok, and also by Volker Roelcke.

25.   See chapter 10 by Harry Oosterhuis, and also the contributions by Marijke Gijswijt-Hofstra, Hugh Freeman, Gerald Grob, and Franz-Werner Kersting.

26.   See the contribution by Volker Roelcke.

27.   See the concluding remarks in the contribution by Marijke Gijswijt-Hofstra.

28.   See the contribution by Ido de Haan & James Kennedy.

29.   Roy Porter, 'The patient's view: Doing medical history from below', *Theory and Society*, 14 (1985), 175-198.

30.   See the contribution by Gerald Grob, and also chapter 10 by Harry Oosterhuis.

31.   See Peter Nolan, *A History of Mental Health Nursing* (Cheltenham: Stanley Thornes Publishers Ltd, 1993); Jérôme Pedroletti, *La formation des infirmiers en psychiatrie. Histoire de l'école Cantonale vaudoise d'infirmières et d'infirmiers en psychiatrie 1961-1996 (ECVIP)* (Genève: George éditeurs, 2004). With thanks to Cecile aan de Stegge.

Overviews Psychiatry and Mental Health Care

CHAPTER I

Within and Outside the Walls of the Asylum

Caring for the Dutch Mentally Ill, 1884-2000

*Marijke Gijswijt-Hofstra**

Introduction: Law, Context, Historiography

The first Dutch insanity law of 1841 marked a break with the past. After an earlier effort to reform the asylums had largely failed, the insanity law ordained that asylums should treat and cure the insane medically rather than just provide shelter and care. Asylums which did not come up to standard had to be closed or could be assigned the status of shelter (*bewaarplaats*). A state inspectorate was instituted to monitor the standards, while the provinces were responsible from then on for providing sufficient asylum capacity for their own poor insane, if not by building their own asylums then by securing and possibly subsidising beds in other asylums. It was, moreover, the duty of local authorities to pay the asylum fees of their poor inhabitants.[1] The Poor Law of 1854 ordained that medical poor relief was the responsibility of the municipal authorities. All admissions, whether of the poor or the wealthy, had to be medically certified and subsequently authorised by the court. Authorisation for asylum admission was only considered to be justified if this was in the interest of the public order or of the sufferer himself. During the next four decades only two new asylums were built, one of them being Meerenberg, the trend-setting provincial asylum (1849) in the dunes of Noord-Holland. All others at that time were older, renovated institutions situated in towns, two of them dating from the fifteenth century. From the 1850s onwards, 'moral treatment' would be introduced into Dutch asylums.

The second insanity law of 1884 marked another turning point, in that from then on, a substantial number of new asylums were built, all situated in the countryside because this was considered to be healthy for the patients as well as cheap. It was, however, not the new legislation that prompted this building boom, but rather the overcrowding of the asylums and, where private, denominational initiatives were concerned, the mission to provide asylum care for their own people according to their own religious principles. Legal authorisation remained required.

This paper will describe briefly how Dutch institutional care of the mentally ill developed from the late nineteenth century onwards. By that time, the Netherlands had experienced the take-off of industrialisation, a substantial population increase (from three to five million between 1850 and 1900), intensified urbanisation, the emergence of labour and feminist movements, and the beginning of what came to be called 'pillarisation' (*verzuiling*): social and political compartmentalisation along denominational (orthodox Protestant, Roman Catholic) and ideological (social democratic, liberal) lines or 'pillars'.[2] Social legislation began to be introduced from around 1900 onwards, general male and female suffrage followed in 1917 and 1919, respectively. The neutral Netherlands were left relatively untouched by the First World War. The Second World War, however, brought five years of German occupation and the deportation and extermination of the majority of the Jewish population, including the patients and staff of the Jewish mental hospital, the 'Apeldoornsche Bosch'. Notwithstanding economic setbacks due to the World Wars, the economic crises of the inter-war period and the period 1973-1985, the twentieth century as a whole was a century of remarkable economic growth. It was economic prosperity that provided the foundation for the expansion of the Dutch welfare state from the 1960s onwards. In this same period, the churches began to lose their formerly firm grip on their flocks. From then on, 'de-pillarisation' could make headway. Dutch society became more egalitarian, open, and individualistic, stressing values such as tolerance, self-realization and democratisation. By 2000, the Netherlands had sixteen million inhabitants, including a substantial number of immigrants.

Dutch asylum history in many ways reflects Dutch history in general. The old town asylums bear witness to the early urbanisation of Dutch society, most stayed relatively small-scale – seldom more than 800-900 beds – and in a small country, the confessional asylums were a manifestation of and in their turn contributed to the 'pillarisation' of Dutch society. Moreover, all asylums were to a large extent publicly financed, including those in the voluntary, denominational sector. The government defined the legal requirements, public, especially local, authorities provided money, while where the voluntary sector was concerned, the 'social middle field' (*maatschappelijk middenveld*) provided the actual services to members of their own denominational group.

The government would begin to play a more active, steering role in the field of (mental) health care from the late 1960s onwards. This coincided with economic growth and the discovery of huge natural gas reserves, which provided the funds to expand collective health care provisions. It also coincided with the early stages of 'de-pillarisation' and the counter-cultural movements of the 1960s, including the rise of the anti-psychiatry movement. Regionalisation of care (mental institutions were very unevenly spread over the country), de-institutionalisation or socialisation, i.e. integrating patients in society, and the integration or co-ordination of mental health care were successively promoted as catchwords of public policy. However, the decline if not (yet) the demise of the asylum would only truly manifest itself from the 1990s onwards. De-

Within and Outside the Walls of the Asylum

institutionalisation was not hastily introduced. On the contrary: it was only after outpatient and community care had become more or less firmly organised that the capacity of psychiatric hospitals began to be seriously reduced, thereby in turn contributing to a further increase of outpatient and community care.

Starting with an overview of intramural psychiatric facilities and facilities for community care in 1900 and 2000, this article will then continue with sections on the period of the 'great building' of mental institutions (1884-1918), the promises of new therapies and social psychiatry (1918-1940), evacuation and deportation during the Second World War (1940-1945), post-war reconstruction and the psychopharmacological revolution (1945-1965), psychiatry for every-body and the turmoil of anti-psychiatry (1965-1980), and, finally, the latter days of the traditional psychiatric hospital and the role of the state (1980-2000).

Facts and Figures from 1900 and 2000

According to an inspector of the State Inspectorate for the Insane and the Asy-lums (*krankzinnigengestichten*), in 1900 the Netherlands contained: 23 asylums for the insane, including two smaller institutions with separate provisions for the insane and for nervous sufferers (*zenuwlijders*), a hospital pavilion for both insane and nervous sufferers, four asylums for idiots, three institutions for epi-leptics, four sanatoria for alcoholics, and 19 sanatoria or convalescent homes for nervous sufferers.[3]

At that time, officially recognised asylums housed some 8,000 people, while annual admissions amounted to 1,800. The capacity of the sanatoria or conva-lescent homes would have been slightly more than 500. The asylum population comprised about 0.16 per cent of the Dutch population, then just over five mil-lion. Just over 30 per cent of the people admitted to an asylum would sooner or later recover and be discharged (about 70 per cent of them within a year of admission), while some 35 per cent would die in the asylum (about 40 per cent within a year of admission). Although exact numbers are lacking, psychiatrists constantly complained about the rising numbers of chronic, incurable patients, blocking beds much needed for new admissions. *Dementia praecox* (schizophre-nia) ranked by far the highest on the list of diagnoses at 34 per cent, while *para-noia* (10 per cent), *imbecillitas* (11 per cent) and *idiotia* (9 per cent) came next. Organic disorders like *insania epileptica* and several different types of *dementia* made up 18 per cent, and mood disorders some 10 per cent of the diagnoses.[4]

A century later, the Dutch Guide for Mental Health Care 2000-2001 listed nearly twice as many psychiatric hospitals (about 45) as had existed in 1900, as well as a range of specialised mental health care institutions. Under the heading of 'intramural care' were 29 psychiatric hospitals, 56 psychiatric wards of gen-eral hospitals or psychiatric university clinics, 39 child and youth psychiatric institutions, 277 psycho-geriatric (wards of) nursing homes, 9 psychotherapeutic communities, 15 forensic clinics and 8 convalescent homes.[5] To this list should be added the integrated institutions for mental health care which had resulted from mergers – mainly from the late 1990s onwards – between psychiatric hospitals and outpatient and community mental health care organisations. If all 'psychiatric hospitals' are taken together, whether or not they are part of integrated institutions, the total comes to about 45, which just about corresponds with the number of psychiatric hospitals from before the mergers.[6]

Moreover, in addition to integrated and intramural provisions, the Dutch guide of 2000-2001 includes 269 'semi-mural' or community care facilities for mental patients such as institutions for part-time treatment, crisis intervention centres, and sheltered residences. However, it does not mention institutions for the mentally handicapped. From the mid-1950s onwards, this sector had expanded to such an extent that it had gained a more or less separate status by the early 1980s. Whereas psychiatric hospitals in the 1950s and 1960s still housed some 10,000 mentally handicapped, this number had been reduced to less than 800 by the late 1980s. In the early 1990s nearly 43,000 mentally handicapped were living in special institutions or in domestic-type homes.[7]

According to the 2000-2001 Guide, the intramural sector for mental health care – including the integrated institutions, but excluding care for the mentally handicapped – then counted about 57,000 beds. Next to this, the Guide listed nearly 5000 places in sheltered residences.[8] More than half the intramural beds (about 31,000 or 54 per cent) were situated in psycho-geriatric (wards of) nursing homes. The 'psychiatric hospitals', including the integrated institutions, were a good second with over 20,500 beds (36 per cent). Other counts come to about 23,000 psychiatric hospital beds.[9] Using these higher counts, at any moment in 2000, some 0.14 per cent of the Dutch population, then about 16 million, would be resident in 'psychiatric hospitals', which appears to be fairly similar to the percentage a century earlier.

However, much had changed in the meantime, and the psychiatric hospitals of 2000 were very different from the asylums of 1900. First of all, external differentiation has had an enormous impact on the composition of the population in mental institutions. Indeed, the development of separate forms of institutional care for the mentally handicapped and for people with psycho-geriatric problems has resulted in both a more homogeneous psychiatric clientele and a much larger capacity than before for this particular clientele. Whereas the asylums of 1900 had been populated by a broad range of patients (see above), the psychiatric hospitals of 2000 were serving a clientele that had been narrowed down to what could be called people with 'core' psychiatric problems. Moreover, this clientele consisted of short-stay cases to a much larger extent. Quite a number of them were 'revolving door' patients, admitted several times within a few years. Whereas the number of beds in mental hospitals had been gradually reduced from more than 27,000 in the 1950s to 26,000 in 1965 and 23,000 in 2000, the number of admissions had experienced a sharp rise: from over 10,000 in 1965 to over 52,000 in 2000. Although the number of short-stay admissions had been increasing, and sheltered residences had been created, a substantial number of beds – more than 10,000 of the 23,000 beds in the late 1990s – were still occupied by chronic patients, who had been there for at least two consecutive years.[10]

Even if the actual number of beds at the old sites of psychiatric hospitals may actually have been less than 23,000, the numbers nevertheless suggest that Dutch de-institutionalisation was late and also slow.[11] How this and several other developments came about will be discussed below.

The 'Great Building' of Asylums (1884-1918)

When the second insanity law came into force in 1884, the Netherlands had 14 asylums, eight of them dating from before the nineteenth century and almost all situated in towns. While the older asylums were run by local authorities or private foundations with strong links to the municipalities, the later institutions offer a more varied picture: one provincial, two in cities, and three voluntary (one Jewish, two Roman Catholic). From 1884 to the First World War, 19 more asylums were opened. Two of these were state asylums, one was the second provincial asylum in the province of Noord-Holland (the other one, Meerenberg, gaining a substantial extension), seven were city asylums or 'outlying' (*succursaal-* or *buitengestichten*) which were linked to older city asylums, and nine were built by the voluntary sector.[12] The orthodox Calvinists (*gereformeerden*) took the lead with four asylums opened between 1886 and 1907, and a combined Protestant asylum in 1909.[13] The Roman Catholic orders would follow with three asylums between 1907 and 1914, while another Jewish asylum was opened in 1909. By 1914, there were 31 asylums, some of the older ones having been closed down in the meantime.

Most of the newly built asylums were designed on the 'cottage' system, with several pavilions of varying size (20-100 beds) for different kinds of patients.[14] The total size tended to be relatively modest, the majority having between 3 and 600 beds. Only two asylums were substantially bigger: the provincial asylum Meerenberg was by far the biggest, with about 1,300 beds.

In addition to asylums for the insane, a modest number of asylums and charitable institutions for 'idiots' were built from the early 1890s onwards, as well as a few for epileptics and alcoholics.[15] This external differentiation was entirely the result of voluntary, mainly orthodox Calvinist or Roman Catholic initiatives. Moreover, in the wake of the establishment of academic psychiatry, several psychiatric-neurological university clinics were opened. The *fin de siècle* also witnessed a boom in the field of sanatoria and convalescent homes for nervous sufferers – people who suffered from neuroses (for example neurasthenia and hysteria), milder forms of psychoses, or organic nervous disorders. Since this predominantly private and only partially denominational sector fell outside the insanity law, legal authorisation was not required. Especially for people suffering from psychoses, the sanatoria and convalescent homes offered a welcome alternative to the asylum. However, with very few exceptions, only paying and therefore reasonably well-to-do patients who could afford such an alternative were admitted.[16]

Returning to the asylums for the insane and the 'great building' activities during this period, it remains to be seen if these activities produced the desired results and why they were undertaken in the first place. Even from the 1860s, it had been pointed out repeatedly, both by the inspectorate and by asylum doctors, that these institutions were becoming increasingly overcrowded and that more accommodation was needed. After 1884, both the expansion of existing asylums and the building of new ones were taken up energetically, resulting in an increase of the total capacity from about 4,800 in 1884 to 14,500 by the end of 1914, including some 800 beds in institutions for idiots.[17]

Although the public and voluntary (denominational) sectors built almost the same number of new asylums (10 and 9, respectively), the public sector contributed substantially more to the increase of capacity. Nevertheless, at least in this respect, the confessional building activities marked an important shift from the public to the voluntary sector – a shift which would gain even more impetus during the inter-war years. As mentioned above, the confessional asylums were both a manifestation of and in their turn contributed to the 'pillarisation' of Dutch society. The orthodox Calvinist asylums in particular, with Veldwijk (1886) leading, distinguished themselves by imbuing asylum life with Christian principles, attempting to organise the asylum as if it were a Christian family and to morally re-educate the insane for their eventual return to society.[18]

As mentioned above, the voluntary asylum sector was to a large extent publicly financed, e.g. through provincial loans for building and guarantees concerning the reservation of a certain number of beds for publicly financed cases and the fees to be paid. Moreover, the local authorities were liable to pay the asylum fees for their indigent insane. Around 1910, three-quarters of the asylum population was dependent on poor relief, and this percentage would rise further in later years due to rising asylum fees.[19]

Notwithstanding the building boom, the problem of overcrowding and lack of space in the asylums was still not solved. It was as if every expansion of capacity attracted a new wave of patients. This observation was substantiated by the rising numbers of the asylum population compared with the population as a whole: whereas in 1884 about 11 out of every 10,000 inhabitants were resident in an asylum, this number had risen to 23 in 1914. The number of admissions had gone up from a little more than 1,000 in 1884 to nearly 3,000 in 1914, while the average recovery rate – the percentage of recoveries (as defined by the asylum doctors) compared with admissions – was about 33 per cent in this period.[20] The inspectors and asylum doctors were very worried about the increase of the asylum population, the more so because the costs of asylum care were tending to go up as well. They asked themselves if the Dutch were becoming more insane, or whether other explanations were more plausible. Had the improved quality of asylum care, the existing accumulation of people waiting for admission, or the lessened resistance against admission on the part of the family caused the growth of the asylum population?[21]

The historian Binneveld attributed the increase before 1914 primarily to a generally lower level of tolerance on the part of society towards the insane: the more asylums there were established, the less acceptable it was found to continue looking after insane family members at home and to keep them in society.[22] Vijselaar's recent research, however, points in a rather different direction: his sample of patients' records from three Dutch asylums demonstrates that many families had been caring for an insane or mentally handicapped relative for quite some time. In these cases, it was only after the situation had become untenable, e.g. because the caring relative could not continue to provide care or the cared-for relative had become unmanageable, that admission to an asylum, as a last resort, could no longer be avoided.[23] Financial considerations may well have played a part in the wish to avoid hospitalisation of a family member, and to ask for his or her discharge as soon as possible. Even more remote relatives could be held liable for paying part of the asylum fees.[24]

Furthermore, it would go much too far to label the building activities and ensuing growth of the asylum population as a 'great confinement', at least if this refers to a systematic policy by the authorities to put away the troublesome mad forever.[25] This was certainly not the case in the Netherlands. On the contrary, admission to an asylum was surrounded with legal safeguards, and even more importantly, the asylums were explicitly meant to function as medical institutions, to make people better, and not for lifelong confinement. It cannot be denied, though, that theory and actual practice diverged. The recovery rate stuck at one-third, and the asylums were populated by a growing number of chronic patients, including many demented and mentally handicapped. It was therefore suggested that chronic patients be moved out of the asylums and placed in separate, less expensive institutions, comparable to the *bewaarplaatsen* (non-medical madhouses) that existed before 1884, to make room for acute and curable patients. This suggestion was not realised, although the establishment of several asylums for 'idiots' certainly went some way in this direction. The same goes for an amendment to the insanity law in 1904, which gave more leeway to charitable institutions to care for chronic, non-dangerous psychiatric patients.[26] The inspectorate and at least a number of asylum doctors were certainly worried about the increasing chronicity of the asylums and the negative consequences of this for their adequate functioning from a medical point of view.

They were also worried about the quality of asylum nursing care. The introduction of mental nurse training from the early 1890s and later the improvement of the terms of employment did go some way in the desired direction.[27] Although it proved difficult to attract 'civilised' female nurses – this qualification was used by asylum doctors – and the turnover remained high, the number of nurses was rising, while the average nurse-to-patient ratio improved from about one to seven around 1900 to about one to six in 1917.[28] These figures included male nurses, who made up 36 per cent of the total in 1910. The qualified nurse-to-patient ratio, on the other hand, went down as many nurses left the asylum after qualification.

With mental nurses receiving training, asylum doctors came somewhat nearer to realising what they considered to be proper treatment and care of the insane. In the 1890s bed care and, soon after 1900, prolonged baths were introduced, which required extra nursing skills and time. Medication, e.g. with bromide or opium, remained in use as part of the therapeutic repertoire. However, work was the most intensive activity for patients through the years, whether it was considered as therapy or not. Moreover, asylum doctors increasingly stressed the moral and psychological aspects of mental nursing. Some of them also advocated family care as an extension of asylum care, either as a halfway station before returning to society or as a more permanent form for quiet chronic patients. However, the actual share of family care would for the time being remain below one per cent of official asylum care.

The position of the asylum doctors themselves was far from easy. With some 150 to 300 patients for each doctor to care for, the official norm from 1884 being one to 200, little time was available for doctor-patient contacts – on average, about fifteen minutes per week. This, as well as the terms of employment, the frequently subordinate position of the senior doctor to the asylum board, and their comparatively low status in the medical world gave asylum doctors even more reason to complain. Interestingly, before the mid-1910s, few doubts about the effectiveness of the therapeutic repertoire itself were ventilated, although there had already been some discussion about the negative effects of bed care.[29]

Before 1916, when the first 'registered section' was opened (see below), all asylums were completely closed institutions. Once admitted, the door would stay shut until the doctor gave permission to leave. The quality of life in the asylums varied, depending on the types of regime, where they were situated, the size of the wards, and – not unimportant – whether it was third-class care for poor patients or first- and second-class care for more well-to-do paying patients. Third-class day- and night-rooms that housed dozens of people were no exception. According to the official norms from around 1900, the night-rooms should have 20-24 cubic metres per person, while the dayrooms could manage with only 12-15 cubic metres per person.

Some asylums, often the more expensive ones, had a better reputation than others. Notwithstanding its large size, Meerenberg was reputed to be an exemplary asylum, often the first to introduce new therapies and applying little if any mechanical restraint.[30] The orthodox Calvinist asylum Veldwijk, in many ways the opposite of Meerenberg, was likewise known as a model asylum. Its small pavilions, the friendly family-like atmosphere, and the favourable nurse-to-patient ratio all contributed to Veldwijk's positive reputation. In published writings about their asylum experiences, former patients – all of them first-class – were fairly negative about the regime and the condition of some of the older asylums (in The Hague and Zutphen), whereas Veldwijk got a considerably better press.

World War I affected the Netherlands and Dutch asylum psychiatry comparatively little. Nevertheless, food and fuel became short, which had negative health effects, costs increased, and a number of male nurses were mobilised. Yet during this same period, an initiative of Schuurmans Stekhoven, one of the inspectors of the State Inspectorate for the Insane and the Asylums, marked the first stage of the opening up of the asylums. Interpreting the 1904 amendment to the insanity law in a creative manner, he introduced in 1915 the 'registered section': an open or sanatorium section connected to an asylum. For admission to a registered section, no legal authorisation was required. By creating these sections, a number of asylums literally opened their doors for non-certified, possibly voluntary admission. For some time, this happened on a modest scale, but this situation would change once the municipalities were made liable – in 1929 – to also pay the costs of care for their indigent patients in these open sections.

Something needs to be said about the use of restraint and compulsion. In the early 1850s, the newly built provincial asylum of Meerenberg had been the first continental institution to follow British examples and abolish mechanical restraint.[31] The second insanity law of 1884 required the registration of the use of isolation and mechanical restraint (straitjacket, binding to a chair, etc.). From the early 1890s onwards, the inspectors were able to report that mechanical restraint had almost stopped and that isolation occurred less frequently. Whether this was the result of the required registration or whether bed care and later prolonged baths provided alternative ways to prevent or repress restless behaviour is difficult to say. However, it is clear that an unlisted form of restraint – the wrapping of restless patients in dry or wet sheets with a blanket and a sailcloth on top – was becoming increasingly popular. Nevertheless, it may be concluded that sensitivity to problems of restraint and freedom in and around the asylums had been growing and continued to do so.[32]

The Promises of New Therapies and Social Psychiatry (1918-1940)

Between 1918 and 1935 nine more asylums were built and one was closed, which brought the total to 39, including the 'outlying' asylums (*succursaal-* or *buitengestichten*) that were linked to older city asylums, but excluding those for the mentally deficient – the term that gradually came into use from the early twentieth century onwards. During this heyday of 'pillarisation', the confessional influence manifested itself even more strongly than in the previous period with six newly opened voluntary, denominational asylums, compared with three public asylums. Of the six voluntary asylums, three were Roman Catholic. The other three were Protestant: one orthododox Calvinist (*gereformeerd*) and two Dutch Reformed (*Nederlands Hervormd*); as such they were newcomers to the mental health market.[33] In the public sector, one more state asylum, one provincial asylum and a municipal asylum (another outlying asylum) were opened. In 1934, the government promulgated a stop to building asylums; the economic depression was then being felt deeply, and some of the more expensive asylums began to experience vacancies.[34]

The asylum population – including those for the mentally deficient – showed a further increase from 15,500 in 1918 to 25,600 in 1936.[35] This also constituted a relative increase: whereas in 1918 about 24 out of every 10,000 inhabitants were resident in an asylum, this number had risen to 29 in 1936. The annual number of admissions – excluding mutual transfers – fluctuated during this same period between 3,500 (in 1918) and 5,000 (in 1936). Between 1922 and 1928, the number of admissions went down, while they stagnated between 1932 and 1934, reflecting the combination of high asylum fees and a problematic economic situation. In those circumstances, municipalities preferred more than ever to seek cheaper solutions for their poor insane. In other words: as long as the economic situation had permitted this, the growing supply of asylum beds had more or less created its own demand. However, once there was less money available, this mechanism no longer worked. The building stop of 1934 then called a halt to a further expansion of the asylum sector.

In the meantime, much had happened both within and outside the asylums. One of the developments was the rise of a 'social-psychiatric awareness', which maintained that people with psychiatric problems should be helped to find their way back to society after a stay in an asylum and, preferably, assisted to remain in society, rather than being sent to an asylum. The rise of this ideal and its implementation had much to do with the problem of overcrowding and the rising costs of asylum care. Facilities for pre- and aftercare for the mentally ill began to be organised from around 1920 onwards, both by the asylums themselves and independently.[36]

A similar aim was at least partially served by asylum-connected family care: its share of official asylum care rose from 0.8 per cent (132 people) in 1920 to 3.4

per cent (844 people) in 1935 and 4 per cent between 1936 and 1939 (about 1,100 people in 1939 – the maximum that would be reached in the twentieth century).[37] A substantial part of this increase was realised by the newly opened asylum of the three northern provinces, Beileroord (1922), which specialised in family care. All in all, one-third of the asylums created possibilities for maintaining at least 20 of their patients in family care. Moreover, under the aegis of the Dutch inspectorate, an increasing number of Dutch patients were sent to the Belgian colony for family care at Gheel, amounting to well over 700 patients in 1935. Including these Gheel patients and others staying elsewhere in Belgium, patients in family care constituted 6.4 per cent (about 1,900 people) of the total Dutch asylum population in 1935.

During the inter-war period, a fairly large number of asylums established a 'registered section' or open section or sanatorium (see above). This was especially the case after 1929, when municipalities were made liable to pay the fees for their mentally ill poor in these new sections. By 1936, nearly two-thirds of the asylums had an open section. These were then called 'mental institutions' (*psychiatrische inrichtingen*), to distinguish them from asylums without an open section, the *gestichten*. The opening up of asylums to admission without legal authorisation meant the fulfillment of a long cherished wish on the part of both the inspectors and the asylum doctors, breaking down the barriers to a timely admission of both nervous and non-disturbed psychotic patients. Between 1928 and 1931 – the only years for which these data have been published – the number of admissions to the open sections rose from 765 to 1,374, representing an increase from 17 to 25 per cent of all admissions. In 1931, about 20 per cent of the beds in the mental institutions were in an open section, whereas the open sections received more than half the admissions to these institutions.[38] However, it remains uncertain to what extent the open sections contributed to the timely admission and 'recovery' (see above) of patients, since their average recovery rate in 1931 was only 19, compared with 30 for asylums and mental institutions altogether. Rather than encouraging timely admission and thus furthering the chances of recovery, it seems that open sections are likely to have shared the stigma of the asylum, their only real advantage being that legal authorisation was no longer needed.

The inter-war years also brought the introduction of new therapies, each at least initially holding out the promise of improving the therapeutic skills and scientific standing of psychiatry. Along with these new therapies, the older bed and prolonged bath methods continued to be used. By 1920, the malaria fever treatment was widely applied for dementia paralytica, while from around 1925, somnifen sleeping therapy became much used for schizophrenia and manic-depressive patients. From the mid- to the late 1930s, three new methods were introduced to combat schizophrenia: insulin coma therapy, cardiazol shock and electroshock. All of these were adopted from abroad – originating from Austria,

Switzerland, Germany, Hungary, and Italy, respectively – but they were further experimented with and reported on by psychiatrists working in Dutch asylums and university clinics.[39]

The therapy with perhaps the greatest impact, at least on daily life in asylums and psychiatric institutions, was the 'active' or rather '*more* active' therapy (*actievere therapie*), adopted from the German psychiatrist Hermann Simon in 1926. It was then strongly propagated by W.M. van der Scheer, the medical director of the Provincial Hospital near Santpoort, as the Meerenberg asylum had been renamed in 1918.[40] In many ways resembling the earlier moral treatment, this sought to activate patients by setting them to work and providing them with other activities, to prepare them for return to society, or at least prevent them from being restless, and socialising them within the environment of the asylum. This soon became quite popular, activating a substantial part of the Dutch asylum population, explicitly including chronic patients. It would remain a standard method in Dutch psychiatric institutions until well into the 1960s. In addition, psychotherapy, psychoanalysis in particular, had also found its way into some asylums, though still on a very modest scale. Taking stock of the therapeutic repertoire in the mid-1930s, the Deventer asylum doctor Piebenga optimistically stated that 'the time of therapeutic nihilism lies behind us'.[41]

While the new somatic therapies obviously strengthened the hospital image of mental institutions, mainly being used for recently admitted patients, Simon's 'active therapy' affected the quality of life for a majority of the patients. Especially for the nurses, these therapies implied much extra work and the need for extra psychological and social skills. How they affected the (official) recovery rates is much harder to determine. However, it took quite some time before overall recovery rates in the inter-war period equalled the level of 1914. Having gone down from 36 in 1914 to 26 in 1917 and 21 in 1918 (both years showing a much higher death rate than the previous or following years, due to under-nourishment and diseases such as tuberculosis), the recovery rates stabilised at 28-30 between 1919 and 1931. Between 1932 and 1936, the last year for which these statistics were published, the recovery rates were more or less back at the pre-war level of one-third.

Although Dutch asylum doctors were quick to adopt a number of these therapies from their German neighbours, they tended to have strong reservations with respect to the more virulent forms of eugenics. As long as social psychiatry was simply understood as pre- and aftercare, there was a fair amount of consensus. It became much more controversial, though, when 'preventive' measures were concerned, such as sterilisation to avert degeneration or, though to a lesser extent, 'therapeutic' castration in the case of sexual perversions.[42] Although not all Dutch asylum doctors were opposed to these measures, the actual number of operations appears to have remained fairly limited. That ultimately the eugenic movement remained marginal in the Netherlands should, according to Noord-

Within and Outside the Walls of the Asylum

man, be mainly attributed to resistance on the part of denominational groups – it was the heyday of 'pillarisation' – to active interference of the state in the (pro-creational) lives of families.[43]

The quality of asylum care in the inter-war period may be characterised as follows. Notwithstanding the differences between asylums, there seems to have been a general, though modest improvement of living conditions, including a more favourable nurse-to-patient ratio until the economic crisis of the 1930s. The income for these extra expenses was created by raising the asylum fees.[44] By the end of 1936, the average nurse-to-patient ratio was about one to five (compared with one to six in 1917), while on average, one doctor was available for 154 patients. The differences between the various asylums were, however, considerable.[45]

The reports from the State Inspectorate contain relatively little information about the use of isolation and mechanical restraint in the inter-war period. However, it may be assumed that the use of these measures further decreased, once the introduction of active (actievere) therapy proved to have a soothing impact on restless patients.[46] On the other hand, for the relatively few patients who were compelled to undergo shock therapies, this tended to be a fairly frightening experience.

While by no means all the promises of the new therapies and of social psychiatry came true, they did set the tone for much of what would follow after 1945. Two main trends which were often intertwined in actual asylum practice can be discerned: on the one hand, a 'socialisation' of psychiatry, manifesting itself in active therapy, institutionally linked family care, and social psychiatry in the form of pre- and aftercare; on the other hand, a 'somatisation' of psychiatry, e.g. as demonstrated by the somatic treatments. Having taken shape in the inter-war period, they would be further developed after World War II.

Evacuation and Deportation during the Second World War

The German occupation brought many kinds of both material and immaterial damage and suffering, also to the world of asylum psychiatry. Although the Germans did not implement their 'eugenic' extermination programme for the insane and mentally handicapped in the Netherlands, they did order the deportation of all Jews. Mainly in 1942 and 1943, more than 100,000 Jews (75 per cent of all Jews in the Netherlands) were deported from the Netherlands and killed in the concentration camps. This is what also happened to 869 patients and 52 nurses of the Jewish mental institution the 'Apeldoornsche Bosch' in January 1943.[47] After the deportation of these patients and staff, the Sicher-heitspolizei removed another 175 Jewish patients from other mental institutions.[48]

The other effects of the war were of a different order, but nonetheless serious for those concerned. Because of the building of the *Atlantikwall*, nearly all mental institutions that were situated in the coastal provinces were forced to evacuate in the course of 1942 and 1943. Most patients and staff were moved to other mental institutions. In addition to the obvious problems of overcrowding, the situation became very serious during the 'hunger winter' of 1944-1945. Food and fuel shortages were dramatic, resulting in a high number of deaths. Furthermore, some other mental institutions had to be evacuated because of the threat of war damage. The orthodox Calvinist mental institution Wolfheze suffered heavy casualties when it found itself in the firing lines during the battle of Arnhem in 1944: 81 patients and staff were killed, and most of the buildings were severely damaged.[49]

When the war ended, the asylum population had substantially declined from about 25,000 in December 1941 to about 21,000 in December 1945.[50] Nearly one quarter of this reduction was due to the deportation of the 'Apeldoornsche Bosch'. How many of the others were killed or died of starvation and deficiency diseases remains unknown. A substantial group of patients returned home because of the evacuations or war damage, or to make room for others. Moreover, the number of admissions inevitably dropped during the course of the war. As for people in hiding: an unknown number of Jews and members of the resistance found shelter in mental institutions, while young men applied to be student nurses in order to avoid *Arbeitseinsatz* (compulsory labour) in Germany.[51]

Post-war Reconstruction and the Psychopharmacological Revolution (1945-1965)

It would take many years before the material damage to mental institutions was restored, not to speak of the irreparable and long-lasting human misery. Except for the Dutch Reformed mental institution Hulp en Heil (1949) and the Jewish Sinai Clinic at Amersfoort (1960) which replaced the 'Apeldoornsche Bosch', no new institutions would be opened until 1965. At the end of 1949, inspector Pameyer listed 34 mental institutions with a total capacity of just over 24,000 beds, and 8 institutions for the mentally handicapped with a total of nearly 3,000 beds.[52] By 1958, according to the Central Bureau of Statistics, there were 38 mental institutions – institutions for mentally handicapped not included – with more than 27,000 beds. Six of these mental institutions housed more than 1,000 patients.[53] In the 1960s, there was a slight increase to 39 mental institutions, and a reduction of the number of beds to about 26,000. The number of admissions, including re-admissions, rose from a little more than 8,000 in 1955 to well over 10,000 in 1965. During this same period, the number of institutions for the

Within and Outside the Walls of the Asylum

mentally handicapped increased from 19 to 56, while their capacity went up from well over 8,000 to just over 13,000.[54]

The reconstruction period was also characterised by a serious shortage of staff. Female nurses especially were hard to recruit, due to the tight labour market, comparatively low salaries, and poor working conditions – the 45-hour working week was only introduced in 1961 – as well as the negative reputation of mental institutions. The shortage of nurses increased to such an extent – from 9 per cent in 1953 to 20 per cent in 1957 – that waiting lists for admission were introduced by the mid-1950s, and a number of institutions even closed wards.[55] It would take until well into the 1960s before the situation improved.

The problems were aggravated by the growing numbers of long-stay patients, many of them elderly, resulting from improved hygiene and medical care.[56] From the mid-1950s onwards, a solution to this problem would be sought in external differentiation by building special institutions for mentally handicapped and psycho-geriatric patients, together with an intensification of pre- and aftercare. This process of course created more room for 'psychiatric' patients. Special institutions were also established for other, less numerous groups of patients, including forensic clinics and a first child psychiatric clinic.

While economic growth since the 1950s – the Marshall Plan was of great help to the Netherlands – and the discovery of natural gas reserves in the early 1960s provided the necessary financial scope for these developments,[57] it was the psychopharmacological revolution of the 1950s that significantly, but by no means exclusively, contributed to reducing the period of hospitalisation, if not the number of admissions. The introduction of anti-psychotic drugs, beginning with chlorpromazine in 1953, actually had a double effect, for they also reduced the amount of unrest and aggression in the institutions themselves.[58] Antidepressants like imipramine were soon to follow.[59] With the exception of electroconvulsive therapy and prolonged narcosis, the introduction of the new psychopharmacological drugs marked the end of the older somatic therapies in the years to come.[60]

It would, however, give a fairly one-sided impression of what went on in the 1950s and early 1960s, and indeed of what had been happening before, if all changes in the mental hospital regime would be attributed to or even identified with the introduction of the psychopharmacological drugs. Already in the late 1940s, inspector Pameyer was able to report that the percentage of discharges had become higher than ever before, thanks to active therapy and to the intensification of aftercare services.[61] Once the new drugs had been introduced, this social regime could be intensified and expanded. Socio- or community therapy was developed, creative therapy and psychomotor or movement therapy received much more attention, while both individual and group psychotherapy gradually became part of the therapeutic repertoire, thereby changing the atmosphere in mental hospitals.[62] This was also the time that 'ABC-therapists' – for work (arbeid), movement (*beweging*), and creative activities (*creativiteit*) – and clinical psychologists entered mental institutions, although at first with the specific task to test rather than treat patients. Physicians and social workers were also added to the staff.

Dutch post-war psychiatry, in fact, very much resembled its pre-war self in being eclectic and favouring mixed approaches, using both social and somatic therapies and to an increasing extent also psychological therapies. Whereas shock therapies and the new psychopharmaceuticals were mainly used to suppress symptoms, the social and psychological therapies were thought to at least have the potential to make people function and communicate in a more satisfactory way. It hardly needs saying that post-war inspiration no longer came from the eastern neighbours, but primarily from the UK, the USA, and to some extent France. Indeed, as in these countries, Dutch public concerns in the post-war period were to a large extent directed towards problems of mental hygiene or mental health. Solving these problems seemed to hold the promise of a better and sounder society.[63] The intramural psychiatric sector, being primarily associated with the seemingly insoluble problem of chronic patients, attracted much less public attention at the time, although a substantially larger part of the public budget was spent on this than on the ambulant sector.[64]

Whereas it would take until 1994 before the old insanity law of 1884 would be replaced by new legislation, the years after the war did bring a number of organisational changes at the national level. In 1947, the State Inspectorate for the Insane and the Asylums was moved from the Ministry of the Interior to the Ministry of Social Affairs. In 1957, the inspectorate was renamed the Medical Inspectorate for Mental Health (*Geestelijke Volksgezondheid*). Four years later, it became integrated into the State Inspectorate for Public Health. Looking back, the inspectors reported that the moment had finally come in which the inspectorate no longer had to work within the sphere of the Poor Law and could consider the broader field of mental health care as its undisputed sphere of activity.[65]

This was by no means an isolated development. It formed part of the post-war expansion of government and the construction of the welfare state under successive coalitions of the Roman Catholic People's Party and the Labour Party (up to 1958 and again in 1965). This process gained momentum from about 1960, when Dutch government spending began to take the lead compared with other European countries.[66] The establishment of the Ministry of Social Work in 1952 was an early and in many ways trend-setting example of changing conceptions about the responsibilities of the government vis-à-vis the governed. In the 1960s, when Dutch society became increasingly secularised, and 'de-pillarisation' was in its early stages, this ministry would in fact become an important moral entrepreneur, attempting to implement the values of well-being, happiness, self-development, health, responsibility and freedom.[67]

Meanwhile, the mental institutions were clearly in the process of developing their hospital function – and also their rehabilitation function – as measured by

Within and Outside the Walls of the Asylum

the rising admission and discharge rates. However, they by no means lost their asylum or care function.[68] Notwithstanding the creation of separate facilities for the mentally handicapped and, on a still modest scale, nursing homes for the demented elderly, the majority of the beds was still taken up by chronic patients.[69] The opening up of the mental institutions to admissions without legal authorisation made good progress. By 1951, all but three had an open section, while in the period to come, ever more wards would be assigned for patients without legal authorisation.[70] In 1953, the Rotterdam mental institution Maasoord was the first to establish its own polyclinic for outpatient care. It would, however, take ten more years before a second polyclinic would follow. In 1961, the first psychiatric day hospital was opened by one of the orthodox Calvinist mental institutions, Wolfheze.

How did these post-war developments affect the patients? Initially, the quality of care in mental institutions was quite problematic because of the overcrowding and shortage of staff. Yet, many initiatives were still undertaken, especially in the spheres of therapies and regime. If chlorpromazine could not do more than suppress symptoms, it at any rate helped to reduce restless and aggressive behaviour and thus contributed indirectly to a more homelike atmosphere, less restraint, and a greater receptivity to therapy.[71] Much attention was paid to activating and socialising patients, both through the old formula of active therapy and through socio-therapy, psychotherapy and several other forms of therapy (see above). In addition to admitting an increasing number of patients without legal authorisation, the mental institutions also became more open in other ways: visits by the family were encouraged, and patients were increasingly given leave of absence.[72] Their chances of being discharged, sooner or later, improved in the course of this period. Moreover, from the 1950s, patients began to be taken on short holidays, and around 1960, television made its entrance within the institutions.[73]

The post-war period was clearly one of renewal and also of reflection on the position and future of mental institutions. Once the asylums (*gestichten*) had been transformed into and renamed mental institutions (*psychiatrische inrichtingen*), meaning that they had open sections for voluntary admission without legal authorisation, the next transformation – from mental institutions into mental hospitals (*psychiatrische ziekenhuizen*) – occurred from around 1960, by renaming if not in actual practice.[74] This last development more or less coincided with the establishment of psychiatric wards in general hospitals (later called PAAZ).[75]

Psychiatry for Everybody and the Turmoil of Anti-psychiatry (1965-1980)

By the second half of the 1960s, the Netherlands had become both affluent and culturally exciting. Counter-cultural movements like Provo gave Dutch society a thorough shake-up, the introduction of the contraceptive pill secured sexual liberation, the emancipation of both homosexuals and women gathered momentum, while in the wake of '1968', the call for democratisation at all levels of society became very strong.[76] Self-development, individual freedom and equality ranked high on the list of slogan-like ideals. Traditional taboos were criticized, including the ban on drugs, abortion and euthanasia.[77] Secularisation and the ensuing breakdown of the traditional 'pillars' were very much part of this process.

The year 1968 also brought the end of the connection between institutional mental health care and poor relief. While short-term psychiatric hospitalisation had already become eligible for coverage by the Sickness Fund Act in the early 1950s, the new Exceptional Medical Expenses Act (AWBZ) now covered the expenses after the first year of stay. In the course of the 1970s and 1980s, outpatient services and consultations with private practitioners also became eligible for reimbursement from AWBZ funds.[78] The AWBZ was in fact the final piece of the Dutch social security system, which received a strong impulse from the old-age pension act of 1956.[79]

Financially speaking, mental health care thus became equally accessible to everybody, beginning with the intramural sector. Notwithstanding the shift from local to national funding of mental health care, the traditional mix of public funding and voluntary providers remained intact. The shift would, however, have a considerable impact in terms of policymaking, for AWBZ funding provided the state with more control and steering instruments than before. During the 1970s, policy concepts were developed that would mainly be implemented in the next decades. Both for general health care and for mental health care, regionalisation (*regionalisatie*) – the organisation of health care provisions by region – and *echelonnering* – the organisation of health care provision according to the level of specialisation – became leading concepts.[80]

The implementation of regionalisation especially was to have far-reaching effects on the organisation of intramural mental health care. To mention but one aspect, it would tackle the long-standing problem of distance between mental institution and home.[81] The mental institutions were very unevenly spread over the country, many of them being remotely situated in the countryside and having a specific denominational status. Patients were often sent to far-off institutions, thereby isolating them from family and friends. The Sint Franciscushof at Raalte, opened in 1965, would be the last traditional, denominational mental institution to be built, although it did have a regional function for Roman Catholics. The four mental hospitals, or 'centres', that were opened between 1973 and 1982 had an explicitly regional, all-round function as well as a neutral, non-denominational status.[82] This implied a clear break with the past.

As the mental health care budget increased and mental hospitals got rid of their 'poor' image, more and better trained nursing and other staff could be attracted.[83] The 1970s would in fact bring quite a few changes for both patients – or clients as they were now called – and for nurses and other members of staff. As more professions entered the mental hospital, therapies became more differentiated. Moreover, as budgets increased, the renovation of old mental hospitals and even more the substitution of old by new, small-scale buildings would finally be embarked on.[84] This was no luxury, for in 1977, an investigation initiated by the government showed that more than half the 'psychiatric beds' were below acceptable standards. A governmental committee was then set up with the task to improve the situation quickly. In the first phase, the Action Housing Psychiatry (*Actie Huisvesting Psychiatrie*) resulted in the renewal of more than 6,000 beds (half of those below standard) around 1982. In the second phase, the renewal would be linked to a better spread of capacity throughout the country.[85]

Although the capacity of the mental hospitals was reduced slightly from about 26,000 beds in 1965 to about 25,000 beds in 1980, and the number of beds per 1,000 inhabitants also decreased during this same period from 2.2 to 1.7, the actual number of beds available for psychiatric patients became higher instead of lower as a result of the exodus of the mentally handicapped and demented elderly.[86] Notwithstanding this, a considerable number of beds would remain occupied by long-stay patients. In 1989, it was reported that 40 per cent of the beds in mental hospitals were still occupied by people who had been there for more than five years.[87] The actual increase consisted rather of more beds becoming available for short-stay patients. The number of admissions or re-admissions rose from 10,000 in 1965 to more than 27,000 in 1980. Between 1965 and 1983, legally certified admissions would go down from 25 per cent to about 15 per cent.[88] Moreover, most mental hospitals had by that time established outpatient clinics.[89]

The older, institutionally linked family care was clearly on the wane. Whereas between 1955 and 1965 some 700 patients were maintained in family care, this number would show a continuously downward trend from then on. By 1989, the number of patients in family care had gone down to 188, which was about 1 per cent of the total mental hospital capacity.[90]

The ideas of foreign critics of psychiatry such as Laing and Cooper fell on fertile soil, and the Dutch also had their own idol of 'anti-psychiatry', the psychiatrist Jan Foudraine.[91] They also had their own conflict in the early 1970s – the Dennendal experiment and its aftermath, the forceful eviction of staff by police and the closing down of Dennendal after conflicts had escalated.[92] In this institution for mentally retarded people, the director, psychologist Carel Muller, and his personnel had introduced 'an alternative caring culture of extremely informal manners, a relaxed but inspired attitude to work, and above all, an attitude of "being yourself"'.[93]

Although the Dennendal experiment became a symbol for the Dutch counter-movement in mental health care, it was by no means the only or earliest example of attempts at renewal in this field. Therapeutic communities had already been introduced in a number of mental hospitals by the late 1960s.[94] Concepts of the sick-making family, personal growth through crisis, and the 'schizophrenogenic mother' were promoted as guiding principles. As Gemma Blok has shown, this was not only the case in therapeutic communities, like Amstelland, belonging to the mental hospital 'Santpoort', but also in other situations, e.g. observation wards of mental hospitals or the newly opened psychiatric centre Welterhof in the province of Limburg.[95] By no means all mental hospitals were as quick to embrace renewal. Delta mental hospital near Rotterdam and Endegeest near Leiden, for example, would only join in these changes from the mid-1970s onwards.[96]

The 'medical model' was fiercely criticized as being inhumane and needing to be replaced by the 'social model'.[97] This was thought to guarantee a more humane, less hierarchical form of care, as in Dennendal. In the case of psychiatric patients, however, their own responsibility for their state of well-being was emphasized much more, including the importance of social relationships and communication. 'Hospitalisation', in the sense of getting used to and becoming dependent on hospital care, was to be avoided at all costs. The social model also implied that the staff would 'humanize' and democratise their treatment of both short-stay and long-stay patients. All members of staff alike, whether doctors, psychologists or nurses, were to be involved in the therapeutic process. Attempting to diminish the outward distinction between the patients and themselves, they exchanged their uniforms for civilian clothes. Even more revolutionary was the pulling down of the traditionally strict barriers between male and female patients in the course of the 1970s.

The psychiatric reform movement, and mental hospitals in particular, received much public attention. In addition to Foudraine's bestseller *Who is made of wood...*, the *Gekkenkrant* (the Fools' Paper) provided an important forum for criticism, while several former patients wrote books in which they reported critically on what they had experienced during their stay in a mental hospital. The interests of 'clients' were moreover promoted by the *Cliëntenbond*, a patients' association established in 1971.[98] Patients' rights would become an increasingly important topic for the government from the mid-1970s onwards. The Van Dijk Committee, established in 1975, published its final report on the legal position of patients in 1980, and a few months later, the Minister of Justice issued directives to meet the requirements of the European Court of Human Rights. Indeed, one of the most concrete results from the 1970s may well prove to be the establishing of patients' rights, as they materialised in the ensuing decades in, e.g., the ombudsman, the mediator for mental patients, patients' councils, and new legislation (see below).[99]

Although pleas for the closing down of mental hospitals had already been made in the early 1970s, including by Foudraine himself, they did not have a

Within and Outside the Walls of the Asylum

serious impact for the time being. It was only in the early 1980s, after attempts at renewal had in their turn come to a stop or were being criticized and the medical or biological model was slowly regaining ground, that adherents of critical psychiatry, inspired by American, English and Italian reforms, felt urged to demand further changes. These included a 'moratorium', a temporary building stop for psychiatric hospitals, arguing that the money that the Action Housing Psychiatry (see above) was planning to invest in building small-scale, regionally focused hospitals would be better spent on community and outpatient mental health care. Their actions were successful in that. Parliament decided in 1983 to reconsider the building plans for psychiatric hospitals.[100]

If the 1970s are assessed in terms of what they brought patients, then it has to be stated that the differences between mental hospitals and also between institutions for the mentally handicapped were considerable. Even between different wards of the same mental hospital, the situation could diverge considerably. However, the general trend of scaling down, both with respect to the size of mental hospitals – 500 beds becoming the maximum norm – and with respect to the size of the buildings and rooms, will have made a difference.[101] This trend, of course, reflected changes in the norms for housing and privacy in society at large.

While material conditions in the mental hospitals clearly improved, it remains to be considered how the new therapeutic regimes and treatment affected patients and their relatives. As Blok's research in the psychiatric admission ward Conolly at Deventer demonstrates, patients were put under great pressure to show initiative and work on their own recovery.[102] Family therapy may have been popular among members of staff, but it tended to be harsh on those who had to undergo it. After several years, the initial, well-meant enthusiasm on the part of staff tended to wear off or develop into conflicts. Although this did have consequences for the therapeutic regime and internal hierarchy, it did not seriously affect achievements in the way of more egalitarian relationships between patients and staff, and between staffmembers themselves.

While short-stay patients were the main targets of therapeutic renewal, long-stay patients generally had to wait somewhat longer before renewal, at least in the sphere of sheltered residences and other forms of 'socialisation' (vermaatschappelijking), would gain momentum. For the time being, these patients primarily profited from the more general changes in the climate of care.

The Latter Days of the Traditional Psychiatric Hospital and the Role of the State (1980-2000)

The 1980s and 1990s brought important reorganisations in the by then 'de-pillarised' (see above) but still highly fragmented field of mental health care.

It began in the outpatient mental health care sector with the establishment of the Regional Institutes for Ambulatory Mental Health Care (RIAGGS) in the early 1980s.[103] The mergers of the 1990s (and after) between mental hospitals and RIAGGS, to mention the most important bodies, brought a further integration of the field. To an important extent, these new developments were initiated (in the case of mergers) or at least promoted and supported (the RIAGGS) by the state by means of legislation and funding. They were also a manifestation of a process that may best be described as 'pragmatisation', in the sense that pragmatic and managerial considerations became ever more important. Already before the mergers took place, the appointment of managing directors in mental hospitals was a clear example of pragmatisation.

The Dutch economy developed from a state of 'Dutch disease' around 1982 to what came to be called 'the Dutch miracle' during the last decade of the twentieth century.[104] As elsewhere the ideology, or at least the rhetoric of the market came to reign supreme, and the privatisation of public services and organisations was taken up energetically. As most of the mental hospitals were voluntary institutions anyway, this development left the intramural sector relatively untouched. The mental hospitals were much more affected by progressive government intervention in the field of health care, including economy measures. As mentioned above, the Exceptional Medical Expenses Act (AWBZ) provided the government with an important instrument of control with respect to mental health care, although health care in general had become very much the concern of the state from the 1970s onwards.

Except for regionalisation and the organisation of health care provisions according to the level of specialisation (*echelonnering*), legislation on hospital provision, dating from the 1970s and after, also had an important impact on the intramural mental health sector, the policy being to build small-scale and regionally dispersed mental hospitals.[105] The previously mentioned action in the early 1980s for a *moratorium* on the building and renovation of mental hospitals was initiated by adherents of critical psychiatry, including the clients' organisation; it was Parliament that supported this initiative, after which the Ministry of Health shifted priorities, not by proclaiming a building stop but by explicitly stimulating the substitution of mental hospital beds by places in sheltered residences, day treatment facilities, outpatient clinics, etc.[106] It was not downright de-institutionalisation, but 'socialisation' (*vermaatschappelijking*) that was launched as government policy in 1984, representing the wish to prevent hospitalisation and to integrate chronic patients in society by means of sheltered residences and other forms of non-institutional care.[107] It had been hoped that the gap between intramural and outpatient care would finally disappear.[108] This was no easy task.[109]

What came to be called the Amsterdam model offers an interesting, though at the time exceptional example. Urged on by adherents of critical psychiatry and the responsible Communist alderwoman in 1984, the Amsterdam city council

Within and Outside the Walls of the Asylum

unanimously approved the plans to reform mental health care into a de-institutionalised, decentralised, and integrated system of care, in which the functions of treatment, care, living, and shelter would be separated from each other as much as possible. Next to sheltered residences, day activities centres (DACS), and other facilities, Social Psychiatric Service Centres (SPDCS) would be established with some 20-40 beds for short-term treatment in various parts of the city. Within the framework of regionalisation, it was decided to transfer capacity (and patients) from the provincial mental hospital Santpoort to Amsterdam. In late 1986 and 1987, the first chronic patients were moved from Santpoort to sheltered housing facilities in Amsterdam, thereby also implementing the policy of 'socialisation'. In 1988, the first SPDC opened its doors to Santpoort patients, to be followed by two more in 1994. Although initially not planned as such, the transfer of Santpoort patients to Amsterdam and the subsequent closing down of wards would ultimately lead to Santpoort's final closure, in March 2002.[110]

However, both in Amsterdam and elsewhere, the need for coherence, co-ordination and co-operation between the various types of mental health care provision – essential for implementing the policy of 'socialisation' – made itself increasingly felt. The establishment of the RIAGGS from 1982 onwards had indeed decreased fragmentation in the field of outpatient mental health care, and thereby strengthened the field as a whole. In the early 1990s, the organisational integration of outpatient and intramural mental health care provisions in the different regions – about 40 – became a primary policy target, to be realised by the establishment of 'Multi-Functional Units' (see below).[111] A special government fund for care renewal (*Zorgvernieuwingsfonds*) was instrumental in triggering such new initiatives.[112] The appointment of case managers who assisted individual clients to find their way in the complicated field of mental health care and ensured that their clients received appropriate care was one such step towards implementing the target of organisational integration. The mergers between mental hospitals and RIAGGS, that gained momentum from the mid-1990s onwards, represented another, more structural step in this direction.[113]

What difference did all this make?[114] Looking at simple numbers, the capacity of mental hospitals went down from about 25,000 beds in 1980 to about 23,000 in 2000. Facilities in sheltered residences went up from about 3,000 places in 1984, when substitution was promoted to be official policy, to about 5,000 in 2000 – the number that had been targeted for 1990.[115] Although this type of care had become eligible for funding by the Exceptional Medical Expenses Act (AWBZ) in 1985, it was fairly slow to develop. The community care sector furthermore expanded thanks to an increase of facilities for part-time treatment and crisis intervention centres. As already indicated, external differentiation made further headway during this period, especially with respect to psycho-geriatric wards of nursing homes, totalling about 31,000 beds in 2000.

While at the end of 1980 0.15 per cent of the Dutch population was resident in a mental hospital, this percentage was down to 0.13 at the end of 1996.[116] The number of admissions or re-admissions in mental hospitals continued rising, from over 27,000 in 1980 to over 52,000 in 2000. Re-admissions rose from 23 per cent of all admissions in 1980 to 32 per cent in 1996. The number of short-stay patients, remaining less than three months in a mental hospital, increased from 59 per cent in 1980 to 72 per cent in 1996.[117]

As mentioned above, in the late 1990s, the mental hospitals still housed some 10,000 chronic patients, hospitalised for at least two years, half of whom had been resident for at least ten years. Another count, using the criterion of a stay of at least one year, identified more than 12,000 chronic patients in mental hospitals in 1996, and just over 5,000 patients in sheltered residences. According to this definition, nearly two-thirds (62 per cent) of the mental hospital population in 1996 consisted at any time of chronic patients.[118] These numbers clearly demonstrate that 'extra-muralisation' or de-institutionalisation was only slowly making headway. Integrating hospitalised chronic mental patients into society proved to be a complicated and difficult task, that in actual practice may have enjoyed less priority than government policy had indicated.[119]

Yet it cannot be denied that the directives of the government with respect to the formation of Multi-Functional Units (MFES), mentioned earlier, were indeed followed-up. In the course of the 1990s, most psychiatric hospitals entered into co-operation with a regional institution for ambulatory mental health care (RIAGG) or a psychiatric ward of a general hospital (PAAZ). Altogether, some 80 Multi-Functional Units were formed, offering a broad range of decentralised, small-scale forms of psychiatric care for part of the region, near to where people were living, or even at home. Psychiatric intensive home care, case-management, day treatment, day activities centres – all of these were directed towards helping patients to remain or become self-sufficient, and to live at home as much as possible. Patients in need of more help could be placed in sheltered residences. The idea was that transfers between intramural, community, and outpatient care would become easier as the barriers were lifted and 'care circuits' were formed. Stimulated by special funding, many small-scale care projects of this kind were started.

The plan was that about 50 per cent – some 10,000 beds – of the original capacity of the mental hospitals would be transferred to these MFES. Moreover, the number of general psychiatric hospitals fell from 41 in 1993 to 37 in 1998, due to mergers between eight of these hospitals. By that time, 16 mental hospitals had merged with at least one RIAGG, thereby forming a 'transmural' regional mental health organisation. By 2000, about 80 per cent of the original 41 general psychiatric hospitals had merged or were about to merge.[120]

Whether the integration of chronic patients into society will be substantially furthered by the Multi-Functional Units and the mergers is by no means certain.

Within and Outside the Walls of the Asylum

It has been pointed out that there is no clarity about the desired character and size of the 'asylum' function, and that strategic, solidly based choices for long-term policy are lacking.[121] However, a study on the need for 'asylum' provision stated that for half the chronic patients in mental hospitals, the care or asylum function is most important. It recommends a varied and flexible array of facilities for chronic patients, and stresses the need for adequate and humane care.[122]

So far, nothing has yet been said about the development of the therapeutic regime in the 1980s and 1990s and about the treatment of psychiatric patients in general, including matters of restraint. With respect to aetiology, the most striking feature was the increasing dominance of biological psychiatry, especially in the course of the 1990s. Mental disorders came to be primarily interpreted as disorders of the brain and diagnosed by means of DSM III or IV. The therapeutic regime, on the other hand, consisted of a mixed bio-psycho-social approach. Although medication was most frequently used, and electroshock functioned as an *ultimum remedium*, other types of therapy, including individual psychotherapy, group therapy and cognitive behavioural therapy, also remained in use or were added to the repertoire. With rehabilitation a primary goal, brief, problem-directed treatment and domestic training have come to be part of the standard repertoire. Therapies directed at acquiring social and practical skills, self-reliance, and the ability to cope with one's illness are considered to be more effective than those directed at personal discovery and change. This may well count as another instance of growing pragmatism. It should be added that whereas in the 1970s the patient's family had all too often functioned as scapegoat, it was allocated a much more constructive and supporting role in the decades to follow.

As mentioned above, the old insanity law of 1884 was finally replaced by new legislation, the law on hospitalisation in psychiatric hospitals (BOPZ: *Wet Bijzondere Opnemingen in Psychiatrische Ziekenhuizen*). After years of discussion in Parliament, the final version was passed in 1992, coming into force two years later. Whereas the old law had covered all admissions to mental institutions except for those to the 'registered sections' after 1916, the new one was only concerned with compulsory admission to mental hospitals. Compulsory, legally certified admission now became the exceptional route to a mental hospital and 'voluntary', legally non-certified admission the normal route, as had in fact been the actual practice in the post-war period.[123] In accordance with modern ideas about individual autonomy, integrity and personal responsibility of patients, the law formulated strict criteria for compulsory hospitalisation – when someone poses a threat to himself and/or others. Moreover, since the 1970s, patients' rights, including their own view with respect to treatment, had become one of the central issues. Treatment plans and agreements had already become part of the standard procedures for voluntarily admitted patients in the 1970s, and patients' rights had become anchored in general laws. The new law BOPZ explicitly granted the right to refuse psychiatric treatment to compulsorily admitted patients.[124] In practice, this has given rise to serious problems. Its emphasis on the protection of patients' rights has had the unintended effect that growing numbers of people with serious psychiatric problems no longer receive the treatment and care they need.

Concluding Remarks

Between 1884, when the second Dutch insanity law came into force, and 2000, nearly one decade after the bopz law had been passed, Dutch institutional care of the mentally ill has experienced numerous changes. Many of these also occurred in other Western countries, and in some cases at a somewhat earlier stage, thus potentially serving as an example. From a historical point of view, the interesting thing is to determine which examples were followed by whom and which not. Until World War ii, Dutch asylum psychiatry got its inspiration mainly from Germany and to a somewhat lesser extent from other Central European countries. This included asylum architecture (e.g. pavilions), therapies (bed-rest and prolonged baths, somatic therapies of the inter-war period, active therapy), and social psychiatry in the form of pre- and aftercare. Dutch psychiatrists were, however, by no means inclined to copy the German 'eugenics' programme. After World War ii, apart from the rapid international spread of psychopharmacology, the examples followed were mainly British and American (therapeutic communities, ideas connected with 'anti-psychiatry', Community Mental Health Centres), as well as French (socio-therapy) and Italian (de-institutionalisation).

Although American and British de-institutionalisation had started earlier, it was rather the Italian example that stirred the imagination of adherents of the Dutch psychiatric counter-movement. However, its immediate impact remained limited. It was not the closing down of mental hospitals, but the substitution of part of hospital provision by community and outpatient care that was promoted to official policy in 1984, with the aim of integrating patients into society as much as possible ('socialisation'). The implementation of substitution and 'socialisation' has been slow, except in the case of Amsterdam. This 'soft' variant of de-institutionalisation has stayed free of the excesses that did occur in countries that proceeded more drastically.

Apart from focusing on the reception of innovative examples from other countries or regions, it may be useful to examine similarities and differences between and within countries or regions, and between different time periods. Leaving more specific international comparisons to other parts of this volume, some comment will be made here on the central themes that have been discussed in this contribution.

Within and Outside the Walls of the Asylum

The development from closed asylums to open mental institutions or hospitals and from mainly or exclusively legally certified admissions to mainly 'voluntary', uncertified admissions has been a fairly general trend in the history of Western institutional psychiatry. Paradoxically, one of the aims – along with therapeutic and custodial ones – of the Dutch insanity law of 1884 (like that of 1841) was to guard the civil rights of both the insane and the sane, and to ensure that admission to an asylum took place in an orderly, lawful way. However, once admitted, the insane could be subjected to an almost prison-like lack of freedom and a high degree of dependence, although actual practice could be different.[125] It may well have been the unintended effect of this law, requiring legal authorisation for all admissions without exception, that Dutch doctors attempted to get around these rules at a comparatively early stage (1916). They wished to transform the asylum into a more hospital-like setting where patients could be admitted more expeditiously and on a more voluntary basis. An earlier amendment to the insanity law (1904) provided the loophole to do so.

The mix of public funding and, to an increasing extent, voluntary provision of care may have originated and developed as an integral part of Dutch pillarisation, but it also outlived pillarisation, having become more firmly established than ever. The Exceptional Medical Expenses Act (AWBZ) of 1968 provided the state with an important instrument to control and steer, while the actual provision of care has been even more delegated to the voluntary sector. The question remains to be answered if and to what extent this public/voluntary mix was specific to the Netherlands.

The processes of internal and external differentiation that Dutch mental institutions have been passing through are part of a wider international pattern. External differentiation eventually resulted in narrowing down the population of mental hospitals to patients with psychiatric problems. The reduction of the number of beds in mental hospitals since the 1960s stands primarily for specialisation rather than the reduction of hospitalisation. Whether counted separately or together, intramural care for psychiatric patients, mentally handicapped and geriatric patients has increased instead of getting less. Although dispersal of chronic psychiatric patients to sheltered residences or other facilities outside the mental hospital has been official policy since 1984, the actual results have been fairly modest up till now.

It may nevertheless be concluded that the hospital or therapeutic function, compared with the asylum function of mental institutions, has been strengthened. Short-stay patients have become much more numerous, especially from the 1960s, both relatively and absolutely speaking. This is not to say that substantially more patients become 'cured'.[126] Medical aspirations for treating and curing the insane have been frustrated repeatedly. Moreover, most therapeutic innovations were directed at relatively small groups of patients who were thought to be curable. Only 'active therapy' (*actievere therapie*) was more widely used. It is equally clear from Vijselaar's contribution on the first half of the twentieth century that a considerable number of patients who were discharged with the qualification 'recovered' or 'improved' may not have received any form of specific treatment. The difference between the first and second half of the twentieth century was rather that an increasing number of patients could be helped, through medication and otherwise, to cope with their problems, both inside and outside the mental institution. Pre- and aftercare and other forms of services to patients outside the hospital have reinforced this process.

It is, finally, not a simple matter to assess the quality of institutional or other types of care of the mentally ill as it developed in the course of the twentieth century. It makes a significant difference whether the quality of care is judged by past or present standards. Using present standards implies a serious risk of anachronism, if not presentism. Even if past standards are being used, it can make a difference depending on which standards are taken into account: those of doctors, nurses, patients and their families, whether poor or well-to-do, etc. Although the voices of doctors, including the inspectors, tend to be much more strongly represented in the available historical sources than those of nurses and patients, they at least provide us with relevant information. It is clear that standards for sufficient or good quality of care have been subject to enormous change in the course of the twentieth century. Time and again, this has resulted in pointing out shortcomings that were formerly not recognised as such.[127]

Notes

*   With thanks to Catharina Th. Bakker, Leonie de Goei, Harry Oosterhuis and Joost Vijselaar for their comments on earlier versions of this paper, and to Hugh Freeman who both corrected the English and offered some more comments.
1.   The Poor Law of 1854 ordained that medical poor relief was the responsibility of the municipal authorities.
2.   The standard account on pillarisation in English is A. Lijphart, *The Politics of Accommodation: Pluralism and Democracy in the Netherlands* (Berkeley: University of California Press, 1968).
3.   A.H. van Andel, *Les établissements pour le traitement des maladies mentales et des affections nerveuses des Pays-Bas, des colonies Néerlandaises et de la Belgique en 1900* (Leiden & Antwerp: Van Doesburgh, De Nederlandsche Boekhandel, 1901).
4.   J.H. Schuurmans Stekhoven, *Ontwikkeling van het krankzinnigenwezen in Nederland 1813-1914* ('s-Gravenhage: Algemeene Landsdrukkerij, 1922), table VIII: 174-5. The overview of diagnoses concerns the asylum population on 31 December 1909.
5.   *Gids geestelijke gezondheidszorg 2000-2001* (Utrecht & Houten: Trimbos Instituut & Bohn Stafleu Van Loghum, 2000). The guides distinguish between intra-, semi-, and extramural care. Intramural care refers to institutional care. Semi-mural

care refers to particular forms of care in the community (institutions for part-time treatment, crisis intervention centres, sheltered residences) and has been translated as community care. Extramural care refers to ambulatory care and has been translated as outpatient care.

6.   See, for example, the *Gids geestelijke gezondheidszorg 1996-97* (Utrecht & Houten: NvGv & Bohn Stafleu Van Loghum, 1996). This guide mentions 47 general psychiatric hospitals with 23,532 beds.

7.   G.H.M.M. ten Horn, 'Care for People with a Mental Handicap', in A.J.P. Schrijvers (ed.), *Health and Health Care in the Netherlands. A Critical Self-Assessment by Dutch Experts in the Medical and Health Sciences* (Utrecht: De Tijdstroom, 1997), 132-40: 136. Of a total of 42,770 places, 17,000 were in family-replacing homes. Cf. the *Statistisch Jaarboek* of the Centraal Bureau voor de Statistiek ('s-Gravenhage: SDU-uitgeverij, 1990 etc.). This statistical yearbook mentions for 1990 31,454 places for the mentally handicapped, for 1995 33,723 places, and for 2000 35,309 places.

8.   The *Gids geestelijke gezondheidszorg 2000-2001* mentions under the heading of semi-mural care nearly 4,600 places in sheltered housing facilities, and under the heading of integrated institutions nearly 300.

9.   There are several different censuses of psychiatric hospital beds, using different criteria. See for example: H. Rigter et al., *Brancherapport GGZ-MZ '98-'01* (s.l.: Ministerie van Volksgezondheid, Welzijn en Sport/Trimbos-instituut, s.a.), 25-6. Rigter mentions for the year 2000 over 23,500 'permitted' beds, including other categorial institutions. The number of permitted beds appears to be higher than the actual number in use. The *Statistisch Jaarboek* mentions for this same year nearly 23,000 beds in integrated institutions and psychiatric hospitals, not counting psychiatric wards of general and academic hospitals.

10.   See Paul Schnabel, 'Dutch Psychiatry after World War II', in Marijke Gijswijt-Hofstra and Roy Porter (eds), *Cultures of Psychiatry and Mental Health Care in Postwar Britain and the Netherlands* (Amsterdam & Atlanta: Rodopi, 1998), 29-42: 32. Over 5,000 of these 10,000 patients had been hospitalised for at least ten years.

11.   See note 9. Some of the beds that have been listed as in psychiatric hospitals, will no longer be situated in or at the old sites of these hospitals, having been moved to small-scale intramural or sheltered housing facilities elsewhere, e.g. in the city.

12.   Only three of the four outlying asylums have been counted here, because the fourth one, near Delft, was officially merged with the city asylum within ten years after its opening.

13.   The Dutch religious map is quite complicated, especially in relation to the Calvinist Protestants. The *Gereformeerde Kerken*, established in 1892, combined two different groups of dissenters that had separated from the official Dutch Reformed Church, the *Nederlands Hervormde Kerk*. The one group consisted of the majority of the so-called Secession Communities (*Afscheidingsgemeenten*) of 1834, the other was the secession movement (*Doleantie*) of 1886, which was headed by the leader of the so-called Anti-Revolutionary Party, Abraham Kuyper. It was primarily these *gereformeerden*, hereafter called orthodox Calvinists, that were to constitute the Protestant 'pillar' in Dutch society.

14.   The orthodox Calvinistic asylum Veldwijk, opened in 1886, was the first Dutch asylum to be built according to the cottage system. German asylums served as an example.

15.   It concerns five asylums for 'idiots' which were under the aegis of the State Inspectorate for the Insane and the Asylums. Next to these, a small number of charitable institutions and about ten boarding schools for mentally handicapped were established at the time. In the Netherlands, the establishment of special institutions for the mentally handicapped began relatively late compared with countries like the USA, Germany and the UK. See Inge Mans, *Zin der zotheid. Vijf eeuwen cultuurgeschiedenis van zotten, onnozelen en zwakzinnigen* (Amsterdam: Prometheus, 1998), 164.

16.   A. Kerkhoven and J. Vijselaar, 'De zorg voor zenuwlijders rond 1900', in Giel Hutschemaekers and Christoph Hrackovec (eds), *Heer en heelmeesters. Negentig jaar zorg voor zenuwlijders in het christelijk sanatorium te Zeist* (Nijmegen: SUN, 1993), 27-59; Marijke Gijswijt-Hofstra and Roy Porter (eds), *Cultures of Neurasthenia from Beard to the First World War* (Amsterdam & New York: Rodopi, 2001).

17.   In other Western countries a similar building boom had already started earlier.

18.   G.A. Lindeboom and M.J. van Lieburg, *Gedenkboek van de Vereniging tot christelijke verzorging van geestes- en zenuwzieken, 1884-1984* (Kampen: Kok, 1984); J.A. van Belzen, *Psychopathologie en religie. Ideeën, behandeling en verzorging in de gereformeerde psychiatrie, 1880-1940* (Kampen: Kok, 1989).

19.   Catharina Th. Bakker and Henk van der Velden, *Geld en gekte. Verkenningen in de financiering van de GGZ in de twintigste eeuw* (Amsterdam: Universiteit van Amsterdam, 2004), 16-9: 17.

20.   Schuurmans Stekhoven, *op. cit.* (note 4).

21.   See for example: J.H. Schuurmans Stekhoven, 'Voorloopig algemeen overzicht der beweging in de Nederlandsche krankzinnigengestichten over het jaar 1909', *Psychiatrische en Neurologische Bladen*, 14 (1910), 444-54. See also Gerard Kraus, *Krankzinnigheid in Nederland. Een sociaal-psychiatrische studie* (Groningen: Wolters, 1933), 156-60.

22.   J.M.W. Binneveld, *Filantropie, repressie en medische zorg. Geschiedenis van de inrichtingspsychiatrie* (Deventer: Van Loghum Slaterus, 1985), 195.

23.   See the contribution by Joost Vijselaar.

24.   With thanks to Catharina Th. Bakker for this information.

25.   See Michel Foucault, *Histoire de la folie* (Paris: Librairie Plon, 1961). And also Andrew Scull, *Museums of Madness. The Social Organization of Insanity in Nineteenth Century England* (London: Allen Lane, 1979); Dirk Blasius, 'Einfache Seelenstörung'. *Geschichte der deutschen Psychiatrie 1800-1945* (Frankfurt am Main: Fischer, 1994).

26.   This amendment allowed institutions under public administration (e.g. psychiatric university clinics) and institutions which were governed by charitable organisations to apply for the status of a 'registered institution'. This status made it possible to care for more than two insane people without having to comply with the rules of the insanity law, including magisterial certification.

27.   See Geertje Boschma, *The Rise of Mental Health Nursing. A History of Psychiatric Care in Dutch Asylums 1890-1920* (Amsterdam: Amsterdam University Press, 2003).

28. Nurse-to-patient ratios considerably differed between the asylums, but also between different classes within asylums.

29. Cox stressed that psychotherapeutic treatment was largely lacking in the asylums. W.H. Cox, 'Psychiatrie contra wet', *Psychiatrische en Neurologische Bladen*, 19 (1915), 467-83: 470.

30. Joost Vijselaar (ed.), *Gesticht in de duinen. De geschiedenis van de provinciale psychiatrische ziekenhuizen van Noord-Holland van 1849-1994* (Hilversum: Verloren, 1997).

31. Joost Vijselaar, 'Zeden, zelfbeheersing en genezing. De zedenkundige behandeling en het 'non-restraint' in Meerenberg, 1849-1884', in Vijselaar (ed.), *op. cit.* (note 30), 41-73.

32. See also the contribution by Cecile aan de Stegge.

33. See note 13.

34. P.J. Piebenga, 'Voordracht', in Conferentieverslag Antonia Wilhelmina Fonds, *De verhouding tusschen Psychiatrische Inrichting, Gezinsverpleging en Voor- en Nazorg* 10 ([Utrecht]: Antonia Wilhelmina Fonds, 1936), 20-39: 23-6.

35. After 1936 no more reports from the State Inspectorate for the Insane and the Asylums would be published until 1969.

36. See the contribution by Harry Oosterhuis (ch. 2). See also *idem*, 'Between Institutional Psychiatry and Mental Health Care: Social Psychiatry in The Netherlands, 1916-2000', *Medical History* 4 (2004), 413-28; Leonie de Goei, *De psychohygiënisten. Psychiatrie, cultuurkritiek en de beweging voor geestelijke volksgezondheid in Nederland, 1924-1970* (Nijmegen: SUN, 2001).

37. Antonia Wilhelmina Fonds, *Gezinsverpleging van geestelijk gestoorden.* 17e Conferentie, 5 oktober 1957 ([Utrecht]: Antonia Wilhelmina Fonds, 1957), 16. World War 11 brought a serious decrease with 350 patients in family care in 1945, after which the numbers rose to 850 patients in family care in 1954.

38. *Verslag van het Staatstoezicht op krankzinnigen en krankzinnigengestichten over het jaar 1931* ('s-Gravenhage: Algemeene Landsdrukkerij, 1933), 124-5: Bijlage 11: Algemeen overzicht der beweging in de psychiatrische inrichtingen.

39. The recently opened Roman Catholic mental institution St. Willibrord, for example, was the first to introduce the insulin coma therapy, and to further develop and experiment with this therapy. Catharina Th. Bakker and Leonie de Goei, *Een bron van zorg en goede werken. Geschiedenis van de geestelijke gezondheidszorg in Noord-Holland-Noord* (Amsterdam: SUN, 2002), chapter 111. It remains to be seen to what extent Dutch academic psychiatry – university clinics, handbooks, medical training, etc. – has had an effect on (changes in) the institutional treatment and care of the mentally ill in the course of the twentieth century. This influence may well have been fairly modest. With thanks to Harry Rooijmans for raising this point.

40. W.M. van der Scheer, *Nieuwere inzichten in de behandeling van geesteszieken* (Groningen: Wolters, 1933); W.M. van der Scheer and W. Hemmes, 'Les tendances actuelles de la psychiatrie en Hollande', *Annales médico-psychologiques : revue psychiatrique*, 94 (April 1936), 554-80. See also Gemma Blok, 'Proefmaatschappij in de duinen. De invoering van de actievere therapie, 1918-1940', in Vijselaar (ed.), *op. cit.* (note 30), 122-50.

41.   P.J. Piebenga, 'De medische staf in onze psychiatrische inrichtingen', *Psychiatrische en Neurologische Bladen*, 40 (1936), 270-79: 272.

42.   J. Noordman, *Om de kwaliteit van het nageslacht. Eugenetica in Nederland 1900-1950* (Nijmegen: SUN, 1989), chapter 6; Harry Oosterhuis, *Homoseksualiteit in katholiek Nederland. Een sociale geschiedenis 1900-1970* (Amsterdam: SUA, 1992), chapter 3. See also: A.L.C. Palies and J.J. Wuite, 'Therapeutische castratie bij zedendelinquenten', *Psychiatrische en Neurologische Bladen*, 45 (1941), 511-36.

43.   Noordman, *op. cit.* (note 42), 260-6.

44.   Rising costs of personnel and inflation also necessitated a rise of asylum fees.

45.   *Verslag van het Staatstoezicht op krankzinnigen en krankzinnigengestichten over de jaren 1932-1936* ('s-Gravenhage: Algemeene Landsdrukkerij, 1938), 33-4.

46.   See, however, also the contribution by Cecile aan de Stegge.

47.   R.G. Fuks-Mansfeld and A. Sunier (eds), *Wie in tranen zaait... Geschiedenis van de Joodse geestelijke gezondheidszorg in Nederland* (Assen: Van Gorcum, 1997), 104-10.

48.   Gemma Blok, 'Opname in het Derde Rijk 1940-1945', in Gemma Blok and Joost Vijselaar, *Terug naar Endegeest. Patiënten en hun behandeling in het psychiatrisch ziekenhuis Endegeest 1897-1997* (Nijmegen: SUN, 1998), 131-8: 134.

49.   Noor Mens, *De architectuur van het psychiatrisch ziekenhuis* (Wormer: Inmerc bv, 2003), 179. Also: A. Kerkhoven et al., *Beeld van de psychiatrie 1800-1970. Historisch bezit van de psychiatrische ziekenhuizen in Nederland* (Zwolle: Waanders, 1996), 205-6; Leonie de Goei, 'Psychiatrie en de Tweede Wereldoorlog: een verkenning te Zeist', in Hutschemaekers and Hrachovec (eds), *op. cit.* (note 16), 197-216.

50.   P.J. Piebenga, 'De toekomst van de psychiatrische inrichting', *Folia psychiatrica, neurologica et neurochirurgica neerlandica*, 54 (1951), 356-64: 356. These numbers do not include the institutions for the mentally handicapped.

51.   See on the Provinciaal Ziekenhuis nabij Santpoort and Endegeest: Gemma Blok, '"Situaties welker primitiviteit iedere beschrijving tart..." De provinciale ziekenhuizen tijdens de tweede wereldoorlog', in Vijselaar (ed.), *op. cit.* (note 30), 151-65. Blok, *op. cit.* (note 48).

52.   J.H. Pameyer, 'De wettelijke bepalingen betreffende de zorg voor geesteszieken in Nederland', *Maandblad voor de Geestelijke Volksgezondheid*, 6 (1951), 173-80: 179. With a total population of ten million and a total asylum population of just over 28,000 on 31 December 1949 (including the institutions for the mentally handicapped and institutional family care), 28 out of every 10,000 Dutch inhabitants were staying in a mental institution or an institution for the mentally handicapped.

53.   Kerkhoven, *op. cit.* (note 49), 231.

54.   Centraal Bureau voor de Statistiek, *Statistisch zakboek '68* ('s-Gravenhage: Staatsuitgeverij, 1968), 32.

55.   Zr. F. Meyboom, 'De taak van de verplegenden in een psychiatrische inrichting', *Maandblad voor de Geestelijke Volksgezondheid*, 7 (1952), 25-9; Kerkhoven, *op. cit.* (note 49), 235-6.

56.   It has been estimated that in 1960, 90 per cent of the patients in mental hospitals were 'long-stay' patients, i.e. patients who were not resident in the clinical wards. In 1962 68 per cent of the patients in the mental hospitals in the province of Noord-Holland had been staying there for more than five years. J.A. Valk, 'Proble-

men rondom de huidige en toekomstige structuur van het psychiatrisch centrum', *Het Ziekenhuiswezen*, 37 (1964), 395-400: 397.

57.   See for the important impact of money on the development of mental health care: Schnabel, *op. cit.* (note 10).

58.   P.A.F. van der Spek, 'Largactil en geestelijke gezondheid', *Maandblad voor de Geestelijke Volksgezondheid*, 15 (1960), 361-5. Also: H. van Andel, 'Wijzigingen en verschuivingen in structuur en werkmethoden in de psychiatrische inrichting', *Maandblad voor de Geestelijke Volksgezondheid*, 15 (1960), 5-14.

59.   See Healey's studies on the history of psychopharmacology. David Healy, *The Anti-depressant Era* (Cambridge MA & London: Harvard University Press, 1997); *Idem, The Creation of Psychopharmacology* (Cambridge, MA: Harvard University Press, 2002).

60.   Leucotomy was introduced soon after the war and was used on a relatively modest scale, amounting to some 200 operations before 1972. See: Gemma Blok, 'Wetenschap en wederopbouw 1945-1965', in Blok and Vijselaar, *op. cit.* (note 48), 147-86: 165.

61.   As cited in Piebenga, *op. cit.* (note 50), 357. See also Bakker and De Goei, *op. cit.* (note 39), 133-71.

62.   P.A.F. van der Spek, 'Verpleging in psychiatrische inrichtingen', *Maandblad voor de Geestelijke Volksgezondheid*, 14 (1959), 145-51.

63.   T. van der Grinten, *De vorming van de ambulante geestelijke gezondheidszorg. Een historisch beleidsonderzoek* (Baarn: Ambo, 1987); De Goei, *op. cit.* (note 36); *Idem*, 'Psychiatry and Society: The Dutch Mental Hygiene Movement 1924-1960', in Gijswijt-Hofstra and Porter (eds), *op. cit.* (note 10), 61-78. See also the contribution by Harry Oosterhuis (ch. 2).

64.   In 1970, the ambulant sector received 9 per cent of the national mental health budget; in the 1980s this would rise to about 20 per cent. With thanks to Catharina Th. Bakker and Henk van der Velden for this information.

65.   Staatstoezicht op de Volksgezondheid, *Verslag over de jaren 1969-1974 van de Geneeskundige (hoofd-)inspectie voor de geestelijke volksgezondheid* ('s-Gravenhage: Staatsuitgeverij, 1976), 1-2.

66.   Piet de Rooy, *Republiek van rivaliteiten. Nederland sinds 1913* (Amsterdam: Mets & Schilt, 2002), 235-6.

67.   Ido de Haan and Jan Willem Duyvendak (eds), *In het hart van de verzorgingsstaat. Het Ministerie van Maatschappelijk Werk en zijn opvolgers (CRM, WVC, VWS), 1952-2002* (Zutphen: Walburg Pers, 2002), 13-4.

68.   Cf. N. Speijer, 'De toekomst der psychiatrische inrichtingen', *Tijdschrift voor Psychiatrie*, 25 (1983), 19-25. This is a reprint from the original publication in 1962. See also J.P. de Smet, 'De plaats van de psychiatrische inrichting in het totaal van de geestelijke gezondheidszorg', *Het ziekenhuiswezen*, 40 (1967), 322-5.

69.   See note 56. Precise data are hard to come by for lack of published reports from the State Inspectorate.

70.   Pameyer, *op. cit.* (note 52), 177. In 1951 the capacity of the open sections is likely to have been less than half of the total capacity of the mental institutions.

71.　Mens, *op. cit.* (note 49), 166. Van der Spek, *op. cit.* (note 58). Again, no data on restraint and isolation have been published for this period.

72.　Van der Spek, *op. cit.* (note 62), 148.

73.　Blok, *op. cit.* (note 60), 176.

74.　Although Meerenberg had already been renamed Provinciaal Ziekenhuis nabij Santpoort (*ziekenhuis* meaning hospital) in 1918, this example was not followed at the time. The Rotterdam mental institution Maasoord was renamed Delta ziekenhuis in 1958. The *Statistisch zakboek* made the switch from mental institution (*psychiatrische inrichting*) to mental hospital (*psychiatrisch ziekenhuis*) in or just before 1975. See also J.P. de Smet, 'Enkele beschouwingen over het geneeskundig werk in de psychiatrische inrichting', *Folia psychiatrica, neurologica et neurochirurgica neerlandica*, 55 (1952), 411-9: 411.

75.　L. Neijmeijer and G. Hutschemaekers, *GGZ in het algemeen ziekenhuis. Een verkenning van de GGZ-praktijk in algemene en academische ziekenhuizen* (Utrecht: NcGv, 1995), 9-23. See also the Guides for Mental Health Care from 1958 onwards.

76.　James C. Kennedy, *Nieuw Babylon in aanbouw. Nederland in de jaren zestig* (Amsterdam & Meppel: Boom, 1995); Hans Righart, *De eindeloze jaren zestig. Geschiedenis van een generatieconflict* (Amsterdam: De Arbeiderspers, 1995); Jan Willem Duyvendak, *De planning van ontplooiing. Wetenschap, politiek en de maakbare samenleving* (Den Haag: Sdu Uitgevers, 1999). See for an international overview: Arthur Marwick, *The Sixties. Cultural Revolution in Britain, France, Italy, and the United States, c.1958-c.1974* (Oxford & New York: Oxford University Press, 1998).

77.　James Kennedy, *Een weloverwogen dood. Euthanasie in Nederland* (Amsterdam: Bert Bakker, 2002).

78.　Schnabel, *op. cit.* (note 10), 33-4.

79.　Kees Schuyt and Ed Taverne, *1950. Welvaart in zwart-wit* (Den Haag: Sdu Uitgevers, 2000), 287-96.

80.　See, for example, the *Structuurnota Gezondheidszorg* of 1974.

81.　From the early twentieth century onwards, asylum doctors expressed their concern about the remoteness of asylums and/or patients being sent to far-off asylums for the sake of cost-reduction and/or denominational considerations. See also De Goei, *op. cit.* (note 36), 249-53.

82.　See on the concept of mental centre: De Smet, *op. cit.* (note 68), 325.

83.　Staatstoezicht op de Volksgezondheid, *Verslag over de jaren 1969-1974 van de Geneeskundige (Hoofd-)Inspectie voor de geestelijke Volksgezondheid* ('s-Gravenhage: Staatsuitgeverij, 1976), chapter 5; Joost Vijselaar, '"Vrijheid, gelijkheid en broederschap". Een revolutie in de psychiatrie 1965-1985', in *idem* (ed.), *op. cit.* (note 30), 192-237: 194.

84.　Mens, *op. cit.* (note 49), 221-31.

85.　Jos de Wit, *Hoe provinciaal is de GGZ? Formele en informele betrokkenheid van de provinciale overheden bij de GGZ, 1884-1991* (Utrecht: NcGv, 1991), 56-8.

86.　Centraal Bureau voor de Statistiek, *Statistisch zakboek 1980* ('s-Gravenhage: Staatsuitgeverij, 1980), 60. Idem, *Statistisch zakboek 1983* ('s-Gravenhage: Staatsuitgeverij, 1983), 59.

　　　　　　　　　　　　　　　Within and Outside the Walls of the Asylum

87. H.H. Hoekstra en I.M. Mur-Veeman, 'De langdurig opgenomen psychiatrische patiënt: afgeschreven voor beschermd wonen?', *Maandblad voor de Geestelijke
Volksgezondheid*, 44 (1989), 1300-8: 1300. In 1970 this percentage was still nearly 60
per cent. See: W.J. Schudel, *Opgenomen..., opgegeven? Een exploratief onderzoek naar
het gebruik van de bedden in psychiatrische ziekenhuizen* (Deventer: VanLoghum Slaterus, 1976), 23.
88. J. Veerman, 'Ontwikkeling en structurele opbouw der voorzieningen', in Antonia Wilhelmina Fonds (ed.), *Psychisch gestoorden tussen gezin en inrichting*. 22e Conferentie 18 oktober 1969 ('s-Gravenhage: Stichting Antonia Wilhelmina Fonds, 1970),
10-25: 11; Tom van der Grinten, 'Mental Health Care in the Netherlands', in Steen P.
Mangen (ed.), *Mental Health Care in the European Community* (London: Croom
Helm, 1985), 208-27: 209.
89. Joost Mastboom, *Poliklinieken van psychiatrische centra. Een beschrijvend onderzoek naar ontstaan, werkwijze, personele opbouw, taken en funkties van de psychiatrische
poliklinieken van psychiatrische centra (ppc's) en een nadere positiebepaling binnen de
geestelijke gezondheidszorg in Nederland in 1978* (Utrecht: NcGv, 1981). As mentioned
above, the Rotterdam mental institution Maasoord was in 1953 the first mental institution to establish its own polyclinic.
90. Meindert-Jan Haveman and Marian Maaskant, 'De patiënten van de psychiatrische gezinsverpleging', *Maandblad voor de Geestelijke Volksgezondheid*, 45 (1990),
635-50: 635-7.
91. Foudraine published an 'anti-psychiatric' bestseller in 1971. See Gemma Blok,
Baas in eigen brein. 'Antipsychiatrie' in Nederland, 1965-1985 (Amsterdam: Uitgeverij
Nieuwezijds, 2004); *Idem*, '"Messiah of the Schizophrenics": Jan Foudraine and
Anti-Psychiatry in Holland', in Gijswijt-Hofstra and Porter (eds), *op. cit.* (note 10),
151-67.
92. Evelien Tonkens, *Het zelfontplooiingsregime. De actualiteit van Dennendal en de
jaren zestig* (Amsterdam: Prometheus, 1999).
93. Ido Weijers, 'The Dennendal Experiment, 1969-1974. The Legacy of a Tolerant
Educative Culture', in Gijswijt-Hofstra and Porter (eds), *op. cit.* (note 10), 169-83:
172.
94. P. Bierenbroodspot, *De therapeutische gemeenschap en het traditionele ziekenhuis*
(Meppel: Boom 1969). See also Vijselaar, *op. cit.* (note 83), 197-9; Bakker and De
Goei, *op. cit.* (note 37), chapters VIII and IX on the 'Oosthoek'.
95. Blok, *op. cit.* (note 91: 2004); *Idem*, '"Tall, Spanking People": The Idealisation
of Adolescents in a Dutch Therapeutic Community', in Marijke Gijswijt-Hofstra and
Hilary Marland (eds), *Cultures of Child Health in Britain and the Netherlands in the
Twentieth Century* (Amsterdam & New York: Rodopi, 2003), 265-85; Gemma Blok,
'Een droominstituut', in *idem* and Joost Vijselaar (eds), *De weg van Welterhof. 25 jaar
psychiatrie in Oostelijk Zuid-Limburg* (Utrecht: Matrijs, 1999), 11-42.
96. Joost Vijselaar, 'De woelige jaren van het Deltaziekenhuis (1975-1985), in
Catharina Th. Bakker, Gemma Blok and Joost Vijselaar (eds), *Delta. Negentig jaar
psychiatrie aan de Oude Maas* (Utrecht: Matrijs, 1999), 121-66.
97. See for example: Cornelis J. Trimbos, 'In Search of New Models in Psychiatry',
Folia psychiatrica, neurologica et neurochirurgica neerlandica, 75 (1972), 251-9;

P. Bierenbroodspot, 'De reorganisatie in het psychiatrisch ziekenhuis', *Maandblad Geestelijke volksgezondheid* 29 (1974), 85-92.

98. The sector of outpatient mental health care took the lead in this respect.

99. Hanneke van de Klippe, *Dwangtoepassing na onvrijwillige psychiatrische opname. Een juridische beschouwing* (Nijmegen: Ars Aequi Libri, 1997); J. Legemaate, *De rechtspositie van vrijwillig opgenomen psychiatrische patiënten* (Arnhem: Gouda Quint, 1991).

100. Flip Schrameijer, 'Het Amsterdamse model; van droom naar daad en terug', *Maandblad Geestelijke volksgezondheid*, 46 (1991), 603-22.

101. De Wit, *op. cit.* (note 85), 60-1.

102. See the contribution by Gemma Blok. And also: *idem, op. cit.* (note 91: 2004).

103. See the contribution by Harry Oosterhuis (ch. 2).

104. De Rooy, *op. cit.* (note 66), 267-72.

105. H.G. Bijker, *De doelmatigheid en effectiviteit van het spreidingsbeleid inzake de klinisch psychiatrische voorzieningen met behulp van de Wet Ziekenhuisvoorzieningen* (Assen: Van Gorcum, 1994).

106. E. van der Poel et al., *Het psychiatrisch ziekenhuis in diskussie. Verslag van de actie Moratorium Nieuwbouw APZ'en* (Amsterdam: Initiatiefgroep 'Moratorium Bouw Psychiatrische Ziekenhuizen', 1985). Schrameijer, *op. cit.* (note 100); Ministerie van WVC. Staatssecretaris Van der Reijden, *Nieuwe Nota Geestelijke Volksgezondheid* (Rijswijk: SDU, 1984).

107. M.H. Kwekkeboom, 'Sociaal draagvlak voor de vermaatschappelijking in de geestelijke gezondheidszorg. Ontwikkelingen tussen 1976 en 1997', *Tijdschrift voor gezondheidswetenschappen*, 78 (2000), 165-71; *Idem, Zo gewoon mogelijk. Een onderzoek naar draagvlak en draagkracht voor de vermaatschappelijking in de geestelijke gezondheidszorg* (Den Haag: Sociaal en Cultureel Planbureau, 2001); H.J. Wennink, *De ongelukkige relatie tussen maatschappij en geestelijke gezondheidszorg. Een bezinning op 25 jaar rumoer in de (sociale) psychiatrie* (Maarssen: Elsevier/De Tijdstroom, 1998); H.J. Wennink et al., 'De metamorfose van de GGZ. Kanttekeningen bij vermaatschappelijking', *Maandblad Geestelijke volksgezondheid*, 56 (2001), 917-36.

108. See on the traditionally problematic relationship between intramural and outpatient care, in particular 'mental hygiene' and 'mental health': De Goei, *op. cit.* (note 36). Bakker and De Goei, *op. cit.* (note 39). See also the contribution by Harry Oosterhuis (ch. 2).

109. Kwekkeboom, *op. cit.* (note 107: 2001), chapter 2.

110. Gemma Blok, 'Enkele reis op z'n retour. Santpoort en het Amsterdamse model', in Vijselaar (ed.), *op. cit.* (note 30), 238-67; Schrameijer, *op. cit.* (note 100); Mens, *op. cit.* (note 49), chapter 8.

111. Ministerie van WVC. Staatssecretaris Simons, *Onder Anderen. Geestelijke gezondheid en geestelijke gezondheidszorg in maatschappelijk perspectief* (Rijswijk: SDU, 1993).

112. Els Borgesius and Wim Brunenberg, 'Nieuwe zorg van het psychiatrisch ziekenhuis. Een inventarisatie van zorgvernieuwingsprojecten', *Maandblad Geestelijke volksgezondheid*, 51 (1996), 1267-81.

113. See for a detailed description of the process of regional integration in the northern part of the province of Noord-Holland: Bakker and De Goei, *op. cit.* (note 39), chapter x by Joost Vijselaar.

114. For brevity's sake no attention will be paid to the development of staff in psychiatric hospitals, including psychiatric nursing, or the demand for psychiatric care on the part of immigrants (by 2000 some 10 per cent of the Dutch population) or problems related to, e.g., homeless persons with psychiatric problems.

115. D. Kal, *Werken aan ruimte voor mensen met een psychiatrische achtergrond* (Amsterdam: Boom, 2001), 7.

116. E. Borgesius and W. Brunenberg, *Behoefte aan asiel? Woon- en zorgbehoeften van 'achterblijvers' in de psychiatrie* (Utrecht: Trimbos-instituut, 1999), 10. The numbers presented earlier in this paper for 2000 are based on the capacity of mental hospitals and therefore concern the percentage of the Dutch population that *could* be resident in a mental hospital, which was some 0.14 per cent.

117. *Ibid.*

118. It has, moreover, been estimated that in this same year, the total number of chronic patients in the Netherlands – this time defined as patients who receive formal or informal care and suffer from serious and protracted mental disorders and restrictions – may well have been between 50,000 and 75,000. This means that only a minority of all 'chronic patients' were staying in mental hospitals or sheltered residences. *Ibid.*, 11.

119. *Ibid.*, chapter 5. See also: Ministerie van wvc. Staatssecretaris Simons, *op. cit.* (note 111), 14.

120. D.P. Ravelli and A.J.P. Schrijvers, 'Eindtijd van de Nederlandse apz-en. Omvang, aard, aanleiding, doelen en gevolgen van de transmurale integratiegolf in de geestelijke gezondheidszorg sinds 1993', *Maandblad Geestelijke volksgezondheid*, 54 (1999), 490-504: 491-4.

121. *Ibid.*, 500-2.

122. Borgesius and Brunenberg, *op. cit.* (note 116).

123. Certified admissions would remain at the level of about 15 per cent.

124. Van de Klippe, *op. cit.* (note 99); Legemaate, *op. cit.* (note 99); J. Legemaate, 'Normen en grenzen in de psychiatrische behandeling: beschouwingen over juridisering', *Tijdschrift voor Psychiatrie*, 38 (1996), 251-62.

125. Vijselaar's contribution on the first half of the twentieth century provides examples of certified patients who were sent on probationary release – something provided for by the insanity law of 1884. He also shows that families could exert a clear influence upon the discharge of their relatives.

126. Words like 'recovery' and 'cure' are problematic. It is hard to establish what degree of improvement these terms represent in different time periods and for different actors.

127. In the 1990s, several reports have been published in which shortcomings in treatment and care have been stressed, especially with respect to chronic patients, one of the dilemmas being the matter of care versus autonomy or rights of the patient. See, for example: Jeanette Pols, 'Enforcing patient rights or improving care? The interference of two modes of doing good in mental health care', *Sociology of*

Health & Illness, 25 (2003), 320-47; Ido Weijers and Evelien Tonkens, 'Autonomy, Solidarity, and Self-Realization: Policy Views of Dutch Service Providers', *Mental Retardation*, 37 (1999), 468-76; Borgesius and Brunenberg, *op. cit.* (note 116); B. van Wijngaarden, M.E.M. Bransen and H.J. Wennink, *Een keten van lege zondagen. Tekorten in de zorg voor langdurig zorgafhankelijke patiënten in het APZ, vergeleken met een standaard* (Utrecht: GGZ Nederland, 2001).

Within and Outside the Walls of the Asylum

CHAPTER 2

Insanity and Other Discomforts

A Century of Outpatient Psychiatry and Mental Health Care in the Netherlands 1900-2000

*Harry Oosterhuis**

Throughout the nineteenth century, psychiatry in the Netherlands, as in other countries, primarily developed in relation to the care of the insane in asylums. Around 1900, however, it also gained ground in clinics tied to universities, in sanatoria and other facilities for mental and neurotic patients as well as alcohol addicts, and in private practice. After the First World War, psychiatrists began to treat more and more individuals who were not institutionalised. The 1920s and 1930s saw the emergence of the mental health movement and the establishment of Pre- and Aftercare Services for the mentally ill and the mentally retarded as well as counselling centres for problem children. In the Second World War the first public facility for psychotherapy was established, followed by Centres for Family and Marriage Problems.

In the nineteenth century psychiatry centred on the notion that the mentally ill could be cured by temporarily removing them from society, but in the twentieth century, the opposite view gradually won ground. It was now thought better to treat those with either serious disorders or minor psychic and behavioural problems in ways that enhanced their social functioning and allowed them to remain in their everyday environments as much as possible. In the last decades of the twentieth century, this approach gained prominence in Dutch mental health care.

In this general overview, I will map all the various extramural organisations, facilities, and practices in the Netherlands in which psychiatrists and other professional groups have played a role during the twentieth century. My discussion is chronologically divided into four periods: (1) before the Second World War, when the first outpatient facilities and the first mental health organisations were established, with specific contradictions coming to the fore from the beginning; (2) the years of the German occupation and post-war reconstruction (1940-1965), when the fairly small-scale mental health care system rapidly expanded and professional expertise was increasingly emphasized; (3) the years between the mid-1960s and early 1980s, marked by a substantial increase in scale of the mental health system as a whole, a growing involvement and funding by the government, and a striving for greater uniformity in the fragmented outpatient care sector; and (4) finally, the 1980s and 1990s, a period in which the limitations of the sector's unbridled growth became visible and the emphasis shifted from building an independent outpatient sector towards closer collaboration with institutional psychiatry. Moreover, my discussion is organised around four themes: (1) the formal and institutional development of outpatient mental health care, including its funding; (2) the professional groups that shaped it and its various groups of patients and clients; (3) the kinds of approaches and treatments adopted by the mental health facilities; and (4) finally, the larger socio-cultural context.

Germination and Fragmentation (1900-1940)

The first form of outpatient psychiatry in the Netherlands developed in private practice. At the end of the nineteenth century, 'nerve doctors' were active in this field. The growing medical attention paid to nervous disorders, neurasthenia in particular, and a larger social sensitivity for these complaints caused doctors, and some nurses also, to focus on this new group of patients, who were not insane and therefore not eligible for certification and institutionalisation.[1] This emerging clientele allowed Dutch psychiatrists to expand their practice beyond the confines of the mental asylums and enlarge their professional standing. It was in the psychiatric setting of private practice and sanatoria for nervous sufferers that the first forms of psychotherapy were developed. Initially, these were largely didactic in nature: the doctor's personality exerted a strong moral influence on patients in order to strengthen their will-power and self-control. In 1887, the Dutch pioneers in this field, A.W. van Renterghem and F. van Eeden, established an institute for psychotherapy in Amsterdam that was geared towards the treatment of psychosomatic and nervous as well as psychological disorders. They practised hypnosis and suggestion and, later on, influenced by psychoanalysis, also applied talking-cure.

After the First World War, when psychoanalysis began to make headway, more psychiatrists began to focus on offering psychotherapeutic treatment in private practice. Their number must have been slight, though, given that the market for private psychotherapy was extremely small: only a few individuals could pay for a lengthy and expensive analysis, assuming they already saw its usefulness and possessed the proper verbal and introspective skills. As a result, psychoanalytic therapy was necessarily elitist and exclusive.[2] As a theory, psychoanalysis received favourable attention from leading Dutch psychiatrists even before the First World War, but its institutionalisation was delayed by the various internal conflicts and rivalries that plagued the Dutch Association for Psychoanalysis, established in 1917. Disagreements on the proper interpretation of

Insanity and Other Discomforts

theoretical aspects and questions as to whether laypersons should be allowed to practise psychoanalysis, whether future psychoanalysts had to undergo analysis as part of their training, and who was qualified to train new analysts caused divisions within the Association. In the 1930s and 1940s, these conflicts even led to secessions. The arrival of foreign psychoanalysts, most of them refugees from Nazi Germany, also stirred up disputes, pitting nationally and internationally orientated analysts against each other. These antagonisms were resolved only in the post-war period. The Psychoanalytic Institute, established in Amsterdam in 1946, became the leading national centre for training and professional practice.

A second extramural domain in which Dutch psychiatrists were active during the first decades of the twentieth century was the fight against alcohol addiction.[3] In the wake of the emergence of a social movement against (excessive) alcohol consumption, which emphasized the social and moral aspects, the development of a medical-psychiatric approach and the foundation of some sanatoria signalled the beginning of individualised care for alcohol addicts. In 1909, the first counselling centre for alcohol abuse was established in Amsterdam, with psychiatrist K.H. Bouman as one of its initiators. By emphasising the centre's medical character, he sought to define this new health facility in contrast to the excessively moral effort of the temperance movement. Nevertheless, the centre's regime basically consisted of a form of moral re-education, aimed at building self-discipline and promoting social re-integration, with special attention for the surveillance and rehabilitation of convicted alcoholics. Soon, other Dutch cities would establish similar provisions.

In the 1910s, some psychiatrists began to advocate the necessity of social and psychiatric support for and supervision of the insane and mentally disturbed who were not yet or no longer hospitalised. This awareness of the significance of aftercare followed in the footsteps of various Dutch philanthropic associations which were established – some as early as the mid-nineteenth century – to offer both material and social support for discharged patients. Yet the call by psychiatrists for pre- and aftercare facilities was also closely tied to the overcrowding of asylums and the growing costs of hospitalisation. Between 1884 and 1915, the number of institutionalised patients almost tripled, from about 4,800 to over 14,000.[4] The rising costs to local governments, who were financially responsible for the institutional care of the indigent, as stipulated by the Poor Relief Law, and increasing doubts about the effectiveness of hospitalisation caused both psychiatrists and government officials to look for alternative care options. The Amsterdam psychiatrist F.S. Meijers was instrumental in the birth of psychiatric pre- and aftercare in the Netherlands when he established the city's outpatient service in 1916. It provided help to discharged mental patients, as well as to mentally ill, mentally retarded and other disabled individuals who had not (yet) been institutionalised. He also set up an association aimed at serving their social interests and promoting his social-psychiatric approach in other parts of the nation. By the 1920s and 1930s, psychiatrists, assisted by nurses, did consultations in some 20 Dutch towns and cities.[5]

In the 1920s, mental asylums also began to organise outpatient facilities to support discharged patients and prevent (re-)admission by giving consultations, paying home visits, and providing social support. Some leading psychiatrists in this field argued that mental illness in itself constituted no sufficient cause for institutionalisation and that only patients whose behaviour was intolerable or dangerous needed to be certified as insane, and indeed be hospitalised.[6] The introduction in asylums of the new approach called 'active therapy', adopted from Germany, also reflected growing confidence in the possibility of making patients more responsible for their own behaviour. This didactic approach, geared towards the social rehabilitation of the mentally ill through work, opened up new opportunities to look after patients extramurally, for example in sheltered workshops. Some psychiatrists viewed its beneficial effects as evidence of the major influence of the social environment on the behaviour of the mentally ill.

To a large extent, the growth of pre- and aftercare in the Netherlands during the 1930s, when about half of the country's 39 mental institutions established such services, was advanced by the endeavour of local and provincial governments to cut down on their expenses for psychiatric patients.[7] In a decade marked by economic depression, they were faced with tighter budgets, and taking care of psychiatric patients in society was seen as a less expensive solution than institutionalisation. The small-scale outpatient facilities were supervised by psychiatrists, who held office hours, but most of the work was carried out by nurses. They mobilised social support and paid home visits. However, given the uneven geographical spread of asylums and the religion-based identities of half of them, their outpatient facilities did not always operate effectively. In contrast to institutions that only admitted patients on a regional basis, many catered to patients from their own religious constituency (Catholic, orthodox Protestant, Dutch Reformed or Jewish), and these generally came from all over the country. Because of this spread and the distances involved, it was difficult to realise effective pre- and aftercare. For this reason, some cities and provinces began to establish facilities that operated on a local or regional basis, more or less independently of the mental institutions.[8]

In Amsterdam, A. Querido, the director of Amsterdam's public outpatient service, developed a comprehensive social-psychiatric approach: psychiatrists and nurses held office hours, offered crisis intervention, visited patients at home, provided medication, looked for alternatives to hospitalisation, and served as intermediary in case of a person's institutionalisation. Querido, who (not quite correctly) advertised himself as the pioneer of social psychiatry in the Netherlands, claimed that his approach was successful, at least in the sense that the number of admissions stabilised.[9] Some other Dutch cities followed the example of Amsterdam, but most new pre- and aftercare facilities that operated autono-mously were established on the basis of private and religious initiatives, as well as longer standing home nursing services. These received subsidies from provincial and local governments, who thus tried to justify a lowering of their subsidies to mental institutions. The two largest Social-Psychiatric Services, those of Amster-dam and Rotterdam, had a clientele of some 1,500 to 2,000 each year. But all the other services were fairly small, employing just one psychiatrist and a few nurses and serving not more than a few hundred patients at most.[10]

In the 1930s, pre- and aftercare was also designated as 'social psychiatry'. However, this term had a broader meaning, referring in a general way to a psy-chiatric approach to mental illness that focused on its social origins and back-grounds. In this interpretation, social psychiatry was closely linked with the psycho-hygienic goal of preventing mental disorders. In 1924, K.H. Bouman, Professor of Psychiatry in Amsterdam, took the initiative towards laying the groundwork for the Dutch mental hygiene movement.[11] Those involved in-cluded doctors, but also teachers, educational experts, sociologists, psycholo-gists, criminologists, lawyers and social workers. Concerned about the perceived increase in mental and nervous disorders in modern society, they argued for a containment of it by preventive measures, an approach that had proven effective in the fight against epidemics and contagious diseases. The professional domain they claimed stretched from the care for socially disabled, mentally retarded, psychopathic and insane individuals to the treatment of minor psycho-logical flaws and behavioural problems of basically healthy people. It covered family life, procreation, sexuality, education, alcoholism, crime and leisure activ-ities. For inspiration, this movement looked in particular to eugenics and educa-tion. The theory of heredity and the interventions in the field of procreation that were based on it supposedly offered opportunities for preventing mental defects. A new branch of medical pedagogy targeted 'abnormal' and 'retarded' children and sought to provide for early treatment and special educational pro-grammes, so as to limit the occurrence of mental disorders among them at a later age.

The underlying reasoning of psycho-hygienists was rooted in a more broadly shared cultural pessimism about the assumed harmful effects of the modernisa-tion process, as well as in an optimistic belief in the potential of science to solve them. In addition to heredity, they viewed society's rapid changes and mounting complexity as a major cause of the presumed increase in mental and nervous disorders. An increasing number of people would have trouble keeping up with the rapid technological advances and high-paced lifestyle of urbanised and industrialised society. From the late nineteenth century, a wide array of prob-lems, including illness, poverty, poor housing, unemployment, bad labour con-ditions, neglected children, crime, immoral conduct and educational disadvan-tages, had given rise to a broadly shared social activism, aimed at improving the living conditions of the lower classes and 'civilising' them. These efforts had been initiated by the liberal bourgeoisie, but since the turn of the century, they became entangled with both religious and socialist politics, aimed at furthering the social emancipation of their constituencies. As political and social democratisation progressed, it seemed all the more essential to improve the overall population morally. Responsible citizenship required self-control, a sense of duty and a sense of community.[12] With their particular understanding of 'public mental health', the leading psycho-hygienists closely aligned themselves with the paradigm of an orderly mass society that was based on the adaptation of the individual to nationally shared civil norms and values.

In addition to moral-didactic activism, professional interests equally played a role in the emergence of the mental hygiene movement. Psychiatrists, educators and eugenicists turned to psycho-hygiene to forge a professional alliance and legitimise or enlarge their professional domains.[13] Confronted with overpopulation, financial shortages and the low improvement rates of mental asylums, psychiatrists tried to extend their professional competence by focusing on society. Experts in special education, teachers and school medical officers concerned with abnormal children used mental hygiene to promote the medical status of their new area of expertise. While advocates of eugenics considered mental hygiene a potentially helpful notion for spreading their doctrine, psychiatrists and remedial education experts referred to the significance of genetics so as to give their concern for mental hygiene a scientific outlook.

Despite their ambitions, the psycho-hygienists did not establish a strong or broad movement. It is possible to single out three major reasons for this failure.[14] First, psychiatrists who were interested in psychological approaches to mental disorders, influenced by psychoanalysis and phenomenology, mainly kept apart, because mental hygiene was defined either as a form of social psychiatry or as a branch of biomedical psychiatry, with an emphasis on heredity. Second, mental hygiene and eugenics proved hard to combine into one approach. Some eugenicists rejected the social-psychiatric objective of keeping the mentally ill as much as possible in society, because they believed the mentally ill should not procreate, and apart from sterilisation, social isolation by means of institutionalisation provided the best guarantee for this. When it came to implementing concrete measures like sterilisation and forced isolation, however, many social psychiatrists proved rather sceptical of eugenics. In both social psychiatry and in the mental hygiene movement as a whole, confidence in the possibility of reforming human beings, which in the Netherlands was strongly rooted in the tradition of moral education and social work, won out over biological determinism. Furthermore, Catholics and orthodox Protestants, whose views could not be ignored given the prominent social and political role of religious denominations in the Netherlands, also believed eugenics to be at odds with Christian principles.[15] Third, in a more general way Christian groups were hesitant about a neutral mental health movement based only on scientific principles. Its domain comprised education, marriage, family and sexuality and, as such, was closely intertwined with core religious values. Therefore, in the early 1930s, they established their own organisations in these areas based on Cathoiic, Dutch Reformed and orthodox Protestant views respectively.[16] This fully fitted the increasingly 'pillarised' structure of Dutch society, its segmentation along religious-ideological lines.

The first initiative of the neutral mental hygiene movement failed, then, mainly because of professional and religious rivalries, but it received a new impulse from outside the psychiatric world. In 1928, on the initiative of E.C. Lekkerkerker, a lawyer, the first Dutch Child Guidance Clinic, geared towards troubled children and young delinquents, was established in Amsterdam, followed by five more clinics in the 1930s. This new type of facility, although staffed by psychiatrists and psychiatric social workers, was rooted not so much in medical psychiatry but in the judicial domain, child welfare organisations and the educational system. Stressing the hygienic aim of prevention, Lekkerkerker and her associates claimed that the effort should focus in particular on maladjusted behaviour of children and that therefore, ordinary families were the main targets of intervention. They distanced themselves from the institutional care of the insane, so as to avoid scaring off parents and educators, as well as from the moralistic and repressive approach that was the prevailing pedagogical response at the time. Applying insights and methods from psychology, social work and psychiatry, the staff of the Child Guidance Clinics defined problems in psychological and especially psychoanalytic terms. Much emphasis was put on 'becoming aware' of problems and making them into a topic of discussion. Treatment applied not only to the child's mental condition, but also to the parents' attitudes.

If the first Dutch initiative in the area of psycho-hygiene was tied directly to the problems of mental asylums and largely based on eugenics and German social-psychiatric models, the Child Guidance Clinic model was adopted from the United States. The American mental hygiene movement had changed its focus from the reform of institutional psychiatry and the prevention of mental disorders with adults to the treatment of children and their families on the basis of psychological insights. Because of Lekkerkerker's input and the participation of several leading Dutch psycho-hygienists in the First International Congress on Mental hygiene in Washington in 1930, the Dutch movement increasingly tended towards the American model. This caused a much more autonomous development of mental health care, disconnected from the institutional care of the insane and, to a lesser extent, also from pre- and aftercare.[17] Psychiatrists who wanted to open up the closed asylum system by integrating institutional and social-psychiatric care into the broader field of mental health failed to realise their goal, also because of financial policies. Whereas the mental asylums, which were not funded and administered as health care but on the basis of the poor relief system and the judicial requirements of institutionalisation, were co-ordinated by the Ministry of Domestic Affairs, mental hygiene facilities fell under the aegis of the health section of the Ministry of Social Affairs. A new umbrella organisation, the National Federation for Mental Health, was established in 1934 to maintain contacts with the health section of the Ministry of Social Affairs and distribute public health funds aimed at prevention. In part because of Lekkerkerker's influence, most of the funding went to the Child Guidance Clinics, while most pre- and aftercare facilities were excluded because they were the responsibility of the Ministry of Domestic Affairs as part of its monitoring task regarding the care of the insane. Many psychiatrists felt that Lekkerkerker's concept of prevention was an overly one-sided interpretation of mental hygiene and basically left the insane out in the cold. On the eve of the Second World War, the competing views on what belonged to psycho-hygiene and what did not caused a split between institutional psychiatry and extramural mental health care, while pre- and aftercare hovered uneasily in between.

Growth and Professionalisation (1940-1965)

During and after the war, the National Federation for Mental Health undertook several major efforts aimed at reorganising the fragmented Dutch mental health care system. In addition to proposing more governmental supervision and funding, some psychiatrists favoured a closer link between institutional and outpatient care as well as more collaboration among the various extramural facilities. Apart from the existing Pre- and Aftercare Services and Child Guidance Clinics, two separate Institutes for Psychotherapy and a growing number of Centres for Marriage and Family Problems was set up in the 1940s.[18] Some psychiatrists strongly advocated an integrated mental health care system, in which social psychiatry would play a pivotal role as an intermediate between the mental asylums and psycho-hygienic provisions. Others, however, rejected such proposals: they favoured a strict separation between intramural psychiatry and extramural mental health care, not just because of the stigma associated with the mentally ill but also because in their opinion, psycho-hygiene comprised much more than just medical psychiatry.

The 1948 international meeting of the World Federation of Mental Health in London, much like the 1930 Washington conference, provided a major incentive for the Dutch psycho-hygienic movement. The notion 'mental health' replaced 'mental hygiene', underscoring that not only the prevention and treatment of mental problems mattered, but also that it was important to ensure maximal health and general well-being for all citizens. The National Federation for Mental Health focused on developments in Great-Britain and America, where various psycho-social approaches were providing alternatives to the medical-psychiatric view. In extramural mental health care, the biomedical perspec-

Insanity and Other Discomforts

tive was now superseded by the view that education and environment (especially family life) constituted the main factors in the aetiology of psychological disorders. Even more strongly than before, emphasis was put on the need for a multidisciplinary approach by teams of various professional groups: psychiatrists, psychologists, educators, psychiatric social workers and social-psychiatric nurses. In particular, the psychoanalytic model, which was already central in Child Guidance Clinics, became more prominent, even though the most common form of treatment in outpatient services was more akin to social casework and counselling. Although many of the post-war reform proposals proved unproductive, from the late 1940s on, mental health care provisions expanded, received more government funding and saw increased professionalisation. Worries about social disruption and moral decay in the wake of the German occupation, followed by concern about the harmful psychological effects of economic and social modernisation, gave psycho-hygienists a strong argument in support of their cause. They argued that many people were unable to cope with social pressure and change, mainly because of individual shortcomings, behavioural defects, and difficulties with personal relationships; these were treatable and could thus be prevented from degenerating into more serious mental disorders.

In 1940, just after the beginning of the German occupation, the first public facility for psychotherapy was established in Amsterdam: the Institute for Medical Psychotherapy. It was geared towards those who were suffering mentally from exposure to the war's violence. After the war, the psychiatrists who staffed this institute described the common occurrence of neuroses and the loss of a sense of security in a rapidly changing society as reasons for legitimising psychotherapy. Among the Institute's staff, a split developed between those who favoured classical psychoanalysis, aimed at providing insight, and those who favoured shorter, didactic forms of treatment, geared towards solving concrete problems. The latter group won out, in part because of the institute's public funding, but also because the Psychoanalytic Institute, established in 1946, specialised in psychoanalytic therapy. Until the 1960s, these two Amsterdam-based facilities, together with one that was set up in Utrecht in 1954, were the only psychotherapeutic institutes in the Netherlands. Their annual number of clients rarely exceeded a few hundred.[19] The total clientele of psychotherapy did not increase until the second half of the 1960s and in the 1970s, when more institutes were established in other Dutch cities. In addition to the limited funding opportunities, the public's lack of familiarity with psychotherapy curbed its growth. Initially, it was unclear to many what kind of problems these institutes actually addressed and who was eligible for treatment. Few people were familiar with the therapists' specific expectations and mode of interpretation. What is more, psychotherapy itself invited selection on the basis of rather specific personal aptitudes, such as being introspective, the ability to verbalise, and a willingness to reveal one's inner life in front of a stranger.[20]

In addition to the public's limited familiarity with psychotherapy, several concrete forms of resistance in Christian circles obstructed its spread. Catholics in particular viewed therapy as a threat to Roman ethics. Around 1950, psychotherapy and psychoanalysis were the main issue in conflicts between clergy and conservative doctors on the one hand and some psychiatrists and psychologists on the other. These antagonisms reflected a struggle about expertise between the established moral and medical authorities and the psycho-hygienic newcomers, who began to challenge Catholicism's rigid sexual morality. The latter claimed that people's sexual health and emotional balance were better protected by psychological guidance than by the Church's moral preaching and sanctions. Despite religious resistance against psychotherapy, some priests and ministers began to be interested in psychotherapeutic insights and techniques, and they used these new views to improve their own spiritual care practice. In both Protestant and Catholic circles, study groups were established in which clergy and mental health professionals reflected together on how to bridge the gap between the Christian faith and the insights of psychology and psychiatry. The gist of these discussions was that clergymen ought to have more concern for people's individual circumstances, their psychological barriers, and their personal conscience, so that religious morality became easier to live with. In this sense, psychotherapeutic insights were considered to be helpful in their work. From the late 1950s, both Protestant and Catholic clergymen began to be concerned with acquiring psychological knowledge and skills. Especially, Rogers' non-directive counselling method was seen as useful for renewing pastoral care by shifting the balance from dictating and moralising toward understanding and empathy. In this way, around 1960, some leading Catholic and Protestant psychiatrists and clergymen openly advocated a new approach to marriage, birth control, sexuality and homosexuality, stressing acceptance, tolerance and individual responsibility. Genuine moral conduct could not be imposed from outside or above, they argued, but was a product of inner reflection and conviction.[21]

Whereas the specialised psychotherapeutic institutes remained small and limited in number until the 1970s, the Child Guidance Clinics and Centres for Family and Marriage Problems, which focused on psycho-social (especially relational and family) problems, saw a substantial growth.[22] They employed psychiatrists with psychotherapeutic expertise as well as other doctors, psychologists, educators and social workers, their approach being largely based on social work and simple psychological methods such as counselling. The psychiatric social worker gradually turned into the key figure of both organisations. Frequently, she was not only responsible for managing daily affairs, but also took charge of the intake of new clients and also began to play a role in their treatment. Psychiatric social workers – all female – were social workers trained in both social casework and mental health care. The rise of this specialisation was closely linked with the professionalisation of social work, whereby new methods designed in

Insanity and Other Discomforts

the United States replaced older approaches that were mainly tied to the traditions of philanthropy, poor relief and moral edification. Social casework was meant to improve not only the clients' social adaptation, but also their sense of autonomy and self-reliance. The reasoning was that their proper social functioning was obstructed by their psychological shortcomings rather than by their immorality. The social worker had to approach them with an open mind and avoid a moralising stance. It was crucial to observe and listen to clients carefully, build a relationship of trust with them and encourage them to face up to the motives underlying their behaviour. The casework method relied on conversational techniques and psychological interpretation and aimed at solving clients' problems by talking about them, improving their self-knowledge and self-awareness, and bringing about changes in the way they related to their partners, children and others.

As with the application of psychotherapy, mental health workers in Catholic Centres for Family and Marriage Problems met with resistance from clergy members and general practitioners, who saw this innovation as a threat to their own authority in family matters. In particular, the plea of psychiatrists and psychologists for a more flexible way of dealing with birth control caused fierce polemics. The pivotal element of the new conjugal and sexual ethics they propagated in the 1950s and 1960s was the forming of healthy personal relationships. The mistrust in religious circles regarding their approach disappeared in the 1960s, mainly because many doctors and clergy members liberalised their views on marriage and sexuality. The differences between the Catholic centres and the neutral, humanist and Protestant equivalents, where the psychological mode of treatment was accepted earlier, had basically faded. The care providers looked for the causes of marital and family problems in relational difficulties, which on the basis of psychoanalytic notions were traced back to the personality structure of those involved. To solve the problems of clients, it was necessary for them to express their emotions and become aware of their behaviour, attitudes, motivations and feelings.

A psychological perspective and the use of psychotherapeutic techniques set the tone in Child Guidance Clinics, Centres for Marriage and Family Problems, and Institutes for Psychotherapy. To be eligible for treatment, clients were expected to have some capacity for introspection, verbal talent, initiative and willingness to change, which automatically excluded the mentally ill and other 'troublesome' clients – such as alcohol addicts and, later, drug addicts. The Pre- and Aftercare Services, which barely survived the war but were restored in the late 1940s, failed to win a solid footing in this new extramural mental health care network, although they employed more psychiatrists and served more patients than the other facilities, and almost all of them had broken away from the mental institutions. Whereas other outpatient facilities were financed by the national health care Prevention Fund, social psychiatry was dependent on support from local and provincial governments, which only provided money obtained after cutbacks in their financial contributions to the mental institutions. Not until 1961, when the pre- and aftercare facilities were officially renamed the Social-Psychiatric Services, was their funding formally regulated on a national basis.

On the other side, neither was there a close relationship between social and institutional psychiatry. Because of the uneven regional spread of mental hospitals, many of which admitted patients from their own religious constituency from all over the country, the psychiatric hospitals gradually gave up organising outpatient services themselves, although many institutional psychiatrists worked part-time for them. Nearly all Social-Psychiatric Services operated largely autonomously, and their size and quality varied substantially. The public facilities in some large cities were best equipped, whereas the provincial services, found in less densely populated regions, tended to be small. Usually, the latter employed just one part-time psychiatrist, not specially trained for the job, and a few full-time social-psychiatric nurses.

Social psychiatry held little prestige among psychiatrists, mainly because of the high pressure of work and the irregular shifts, and also because often they were not allowed to give patients medical treatment to avoid competition with other doctors. In many ways, in fact, social psychiatry was social work rather than medicine. Because universities devoted little attention to this branch of psychiatry, it hardly attained any academic status. In actual practice, much of the work required mainly pragmatism and a talent for improvisation.[23] Psychiatrists held office hours, and the social-psychiatric nurses, as the key players, either paid home visits or provided help to clients in collaboration with other care-providing facilities and social institutions. The Social-Psychiatric Services not only catered to people with serious psychiatric symptoms but also the mentally retarded, demented elderly, epileptics, alcoholics and 'psychopathic' delinquents on probation. For some patients who had been discharged from the hospital but could not live on their own, half-way houses were set up. From the 1950s, the introduction of new psychopharmacological drugs, which allowed more patients to be treated at home, contributed to the growth of these services.[24] Also, in the 1960s, when psychologists began to work in this field, family and group therapy was introduced.

The Counselling Centres for Alcohol Addiction, which expanded their activities in the late 1960s to include drug addiction, played a rather marginal role in the mental health care system. Previously, medical-psychiatric views had replaced socially and morally inspired approaches to alcohol addiction, at least in theory, but few services were able to put the new views into practice. Because of a shortage of psychiatrists, their lack of interest in this problem, and the centres' major role in the rehabilitation of delinquents, social workers gained the upper hand, which meant that the social aspects of addiction continued to receive the most attention. The medical orientation mainly served strategic goals, associated with the facilities' recognition and acquisition of public health funds. In the 1960s, however, the medical model lost ground to psycho-social approaches.

Heyday and Integration (1965-1980)

In the view of many mental health experts, the structural changes in post-war everyday life in the Netherlands caused by industrialisation and urbanisation threatened both the mental stability of individuals and the overall social cohesiveness, which is why countermeasures were called for. Initially, they stressed the significance of collective morality, discipline and regenerating people's spiritual life. But in the course of the 1950s their attitude towards social-economic modernisation changed. Accepting it as inevitable, they began to underline the urgency of enhancing the resilience and psychological attitudes that people needed to function properly in a changing society. Their task was, so psycho-hygienists believed, to prepare people for the dynamics of modern life. They advocated an individualising and psychologising perspective, in which people's inner orientation became centre-stage. It was the individual's task to develop into a 'personality' and to achieve a certain measure of inner autonomy regarding the outside world. Individuals were expected to follow their own convictions, but also to do this in line with social expectations involving a morally responsible mode of life. The internalisation of social norms and values in an autonomous self was crucial. The mentally healthy were not those who uncritically subjected themselves to rules and regulations, but those who were independent, conscientious and responsible – who knew how to take decisions on their own, strove for optimal self-development and thoughtfully adapted to social change. Therefore, constant reflection on individual conduct and motivation was called for, to find the right balance between guidance and supervision on the one hand, and autonomy and individual freedom on the other.[25]

Although mental health experts pointed to the significance of social factors in the emergence of individual problems, they did not go so far as to claim that these were caused by society. Mental health care in the 1950s and early 1960s was geared towards individual shortcomings, and it looked for a solution to them in changes in personality and psychological functioning. However, during the 1960s, mental health workers increasingly voiced self-criticism. The number of those among them with training in the behavioural sciences and sociology grew, and their attention was increasingly geared towards the social wrongs that supposedly led to psychological difficulties. Fuelled by the protest movement of the 1960s and anti-psychiatry, both of which rejected people's adaptation to the existing social order, the very foundation of mental health care, individual treatment, became subject to debate. It was argued that the causes of problems should not be looked for in the psyche of the individual or their defective social integration, but in the 'social structures' that caused intolerable situations.[26] People needed to be liberated from the unnecessary restrictions imposed by society, and the realization of this objective seemed more dependent on social welfare work and political activism than on mental health care. Also, clients began to protest about what they saw as undemocratic relationships and a structural absence of their own voice in the care-providing system.

The fierce debates in the 1960s about the unfavourable effects of society on individuals, which became fused with the anti-psychiatry movement's critique of the medical institutionalisation and treatment of the mentally ill, once more accentuated the contrast between intramural psychiatry and extramural mental health care. Despite the new therapeutic energy in mental hospitals after the introduction of psycho-tropic drugs and socio-therapy and the significantly enhanced quality of care as a result of more funding, institutional psychiatry's reputation hardly improved. On the contrary, the anti-psychiatry movement caused its public image actually to deteriorate, not so much because of the absence of sufficient medical forms of treatment, which had hampered psychiatric hospitals before the 1950s, but precisely because of the dominance of the medical regime. Anti-psychiatry aimed its shots at clinical psychiatry rather than mental health care as such. It argued for its improvement, that is a demedicalised psychiatry in the community, much in the way as in the outpatient sector, which since the 1930s had repeatedly distanced itself from medical psychiatry and since the 1950s had largely a psycho-social orientation. Mental health workers, many of whom did not have a medical background but a psychological or sociological one, embraced some of anti-psychiatry's basic principles. Ultimately, the 1960s movement and anti-psychiatry led to more mental health services: supported by the expanding and generous welfare state, psycho-social and psychotherapeutic facilities increased in both size and number throughout the 1970s.[27] Furthermore, psychiatric hospitals and the psychiatric departments of general hospitals also began to offer extramural treatment in a growing number of outpatient clinics. In the early 1970s, the number of clients in extramural facilities surpassed the number of admissions to psychiatric hospitals. Essentially, though, this eventful era constituted no break in the basic development of twentieth-century mental health care in the Netherlands. Dissatisfaction with psychiatry as practised in mental institutions as well as the unacknowledged impotence to treat serious and chronic mental illness prompted the expansion of extramural mental health care, which attracted new groups of clients.

While engaging in heated debates on the political implications of their work, mental health professionals widened their domain to include the welfare sector that experienced enormous growth in the 1970s. Now that the welfare state guaranteed material security, the solution to immaterial needs came into focus; consequently, mental health experts and social workers began to count on the government's approval as well as its financial support. In the course of the 1970s, a

Insanity and Other Discomforts

comparatively generous system of collective funding was put in place, which allowed the expansion of mental health care and promoted its accessibility. As the scale of its services grew, the number of care providers and their professional diversity increased correspondingly. In the 1940s and 1950s, psychiatrists, psychiatric social workers, and social-psychiatric nurses dominated the field. From the 1960s, they began to be confronted with a growing number of social and clinical psychologists, specialised psychotherapists, social workers, sociologists and educational experts. Both psychiatrists and other mental health experts appeared as inspired advocates of personal liberation in the areas of religion, morality, relationships, sexuality, education, work and drugs. They advocated the emancipation of women, the young, the lower classes, traumatised war victims and other disadvantaged groups such as homosexuals and ethnic minorities. Influenced by the welfare ideology, the objective of prevention received a boost and also a broader interpretation. Many mental health workers were not so much involved in the treatment of the mentally ill, but they rather focused on the improvement of people's psycho-social welfare, their self-development opportunities, social participation, and assertiveness. Their clients had to 'liberate' themselves from fixed traditions and conventions and become autonomous and emancipated.

The 1970s constituted the heyday of psychotherapy in the Netherlands. It was practised by psychiatrists, psychologists and social workers alike, and in the public mind, constituted the *pars pro toto* of mental health care. The Dutch Association for Psychotherapy and the psychotherapeutic institutes played a crucial role in its development into a separate, interdisciplinary profession that achieved formal governmental recognition in the middle of the 1980s. Not only did the number and size of the psychotherapeutic institutes grow, but various psychotherapeutic approaches were also applied in other outpatient facilities and private practice. More and more people began to consider it appropriate to seek psychotherapeutic help for all sorts of discomforts. Simply by virtue of their engaging in therapy, both clients and therapists viewed themselves as members of a cultural avant-garde: psychotherapy would liberate individuals from unnecessary inhibitions and provide them with opportunities for self-discovery, self-confidence and personal growth. The humanist ego-psychology, which began to replace psychoanalysis, constituted a major source of inspiration. Most clients had a middle-class background and tended to be young, well-educated, non-churchgoing and either studying or professionally active in service sectors such as health care, social work and education.[28] What drove many of them to knock on the psychotherapist's door were concerns situated on the intersection of individual experience and changing social conditions: problems with social contacts, personal relationships, and sexuality, but also complaints associated with nervousness, obsessions, feelings of fear or aggression and psychosomatic disorders. Confronted with the new and much more liberal social and personal ideals of the 1960s and 1970s, not everyone succeeded in bringing these into line with their own views, attitudes and feelings. At the individual level, more opportunities for being autonomous and independent and having more options could cause confusion and uncertainty. Problems arose especially for those who had trouble bridging the gap between the new liberties and their old ways of thinking, feeling and behaving.[29]

The strong growth of psycho-social care during the 1970s – psychotherapy in particular – reflected a 'psychologisation of everyday life' that influenced the personal lives of ever more people: a change of mentality prompted by a combination of growing individualisation, internalisation and recognition of emotions.[30] From the 1960s, individual character traits and one's self-chosen lifestyle began to replace more traditional identity-providing structures like family background, class, property, profession and religion. Fixed conventions and rules of conduct that were linked with formalised and hierarchical social relations gradually began to lose their significance. People's conduct was increasingly a reflection of personal wishes, inner motives and feelings. Yet at the same time, increased equality also forced people to reckon more with others and, paradoxically perhaps, show more restraint in social interactions. As the authority of explicit rules and formal conventions eroded and individual social conduct became less predictable, the significance of self-regulation, subtle negotiation and mutual consent grew accordingly. To find the proper balance between assertiveness and compliance, people needed social skills, empathy, self-knowledge and an inner, self-directed regulation of emotions and actions. Thus, the interactions between people and the ways in which they evaluated each other became determined more and more by psychological insight. The less coercion and interference from outside, the more they were expected to know how to guide themselves and find their own way, and the more troubled they were in the event of failing to do so. The higher the expectations regarding the individual's pursuit of self-development, the larger the disillusion if this pursuit turned out to generate few rewards or even failure. People were given more space than before to fashion their life according to their own views and fulfil their personal wishes, without having to bother with sanctions or moral restrictions. But if they failed, they could only blame it on themselves.

Although the Social-Psychiatric Services and Counselling Centres for Alcohol and Drugs also expanded as a result of more lavish funding and a growing number and variety of professional workers, they were more or less forced on the defensive vis-à-vis other mental health care facilities. This could be seen in the prolonged debates about their merging into Regional Institutes for Ambulatory Mental Health Care (RIAGG), modelled after the American Community Mental Health Centers.[31] The serious overhaul of the Dutch extramural sector initiated in the 1970s partly by the national government, was aimed at forging a more coherent ensemble of all the various therapies, approaches, target groups and ideologically divided facilities. However, mental health workers were deeply divided as to

Insanity and Other Discomforts

what course the planned system should embark on. The Institutes for Psycho-therapy, the Centres for Family and Marriage Problems and the Child Guidance Clinics all distanced themselves (again) from care provision for psychiatric patients as well as alcohol and drug addicts, and emphasized their identity as wel-fare facilities with a psychotherapeutic orientation.[32] Workers in social psychiatry and outpatient clinics for addicts, on the other hand, feared that their patients would receive less attention in a new organisation that mainly focused on ap-proachable and treatable clients and that kept the chronic, serious mentally ill and unmanageable addicts at bay. In their view, the new system would allow – if not cause – 'difficult' cases to slip through the net. The city-run Social-Psychiatric Services in large urban areas resisted their integration into the new system until the very end, fearing that the accessibility or public character of social and emer-gency psychiatry, which was their main function, would suffer. They mainly pro-vided care to groups that were hard to approach, such as the homeless, who had physical and social problems in addition to psychiatric ones, who generally did not ask for help on their own initiative and were shut out from other forms of care, but did cause trouble and social inconvenience. Eventually, the social-psy-chiatric facilities, in contrast to the outpatient clinics for alcohol and drug addicts, merged into the RIAGG system, which was fully operative by 1983.[33]

The two key factors that triggered the emergence of the RIAGG were pressure from the government, which wanted to reinforce the extramural sector as a counterbalance against institutional psychiatry, and the growing need to control rising costs: the economic crisis in the second half of the 1970s put an end to the unbridled growth of the preceding years. The new system, which comprised divergent forms of care provision and mental health professions, aimed at a broad spectrum of problems, from personal existential problems to mental suf-fering and serious psychiatric disorders, and engaged in a range of activities – including social-psychiatric care, psychotherapeutic treatment, counselling, prevention, advice and emergency psychiatry. With almost 60 facilities the RIAGG system had a regional basis, well spread throughout the country, and each covering a catchment area of between 150,000 and 300,000 residents.

Consolidation and Reorientation (1980-2000)

In spite of the crisis of the welfare state and the downsizing of social work from the late 1970s, outpatient mental health care saw further expansion in subse-quent years. Three reasons account for the fact that mental health workers kept their professional field intact, while welfare workers failed to do so. First, the mental health sector was now paid for by collective medical insurance, and thus it had grown entirely independent of funding that was tied to collective social services. Second, further growth of the extramural sector was stimulated by the ongoing effort to push back institutional psychiatry and develop community care; in the 1980s and 1990s, this was a governmental priority. Third, the mental health sector managed to adapt better to changing social circumstances, notably the de-politicisation of social issues, coupled with ongoing individualisation. New cultural values like professionalism, efficiency and rationalization took the place of the lofty ideals of the 1960s movement that had defined politicised social work. Increased attention to free market forces and people's own sense of responsibility went hand in hand with the development of a more formal, legally based relationship between client and care provider, while specific rights and responsibilities were fixed into laws, rules and procedures.

In part because of cutbacks in government spending and the larger role of the market, the issue of costs and benefits began to weigh heavily in the 1980s, as well as the issue of who was eligible for care and who was not. Immediately after the RIAGG was created, in fact, several critics already argued that it was geared towards the wrong clientele, that is individuals with minor psycho-social problems and psychological disorders, a group that constituted the target group of psychotherapists. But mental health care, some claimed, had to concentrate on marginal groups that were not so pleasant to deal with, but that really were in need of care: those who suffered from serious and chronic mental disorders that were hard to treat and those with serious behavioural problems, who were troublesome and potentially aggressive. In the previous decades, these patient categories had been rather neglected by the leading outpatient facilities because they did not fit their therapeutic optimism. Now, social psychiatry, which in the Dutch extramural sector had always been sizeable but never prominent, would have to become a priority.

In the 1980s and 1990s, the government repeatedly argued the need to shift attention away from those with minor afflictions to those with serious disorders, not only to control the increasing demand for mental health care, but also in order to reduce admissions to psychiatric hospitals. From the 1970s on, the isolation of these hospitals was broken down and their size reduced while outpatient and half-way facilities, such as sheltered housing, expanded. Increasingly, psychiatric patients were living outside treatment facilities, so as to advance their social integration, while the number of long-term admissions significantly dropped. Only people with serious psychiatric problems who were unable to get by in society on their own without hurting others or themselves would be eligible for (temporary) hospital care. All other psychiatric patients, including those with chronic disorders, should receive the help they needed from extramural provisions, which included – apart from the RIAGG system – domiciliary care, day care, crisis intervention, mobile psychiatric task forces, outpatient psychiatric clinics and special shelter and housing projects.[34]

This policy, which prioritised social psychiatry, was (again) partly motivated by financial concerns, as outpatient care was supposed to be cheaper than hospi-

Insanity and Other Discomforts

talisation, but it also echoed some of the ideals of the anti-psychiatry movement: the need to counter the social isolation of psychiatric patients, improve their autonomy, and respect their civil rights. The government's mental health policies of the 1980s and 1990s, described as 'socialisation', moved away from the historically developed constellation of Dutch mental health care, which ever since the 1930s had been marked by a division between institutional psychiatry and the outpatient facilities. The socialisation of mental health care required collaboration between extra- and intramural facilities, as well as between the mental health sector and adjacent ones such as social welfare, care of drug and alcohol addicts, special housing and the justice system. In the late 1990s, to improve cooperation between psychiatric hospitals and the RIAGGS in particular, the government pressured these organisations to merge at a regional level. Both the outpatient facilities and the psychiatric hospitals were increasingly replaced as separate organisations by so-called 'care circuits' and 'multifunctional units' for specific categories of patients and 'case-management' for individuals. These would represent a coherent system of intra- and extramural as well as half-way services tuned to specific care demands. This signified the emergence of a new organisational principle in mental health care. Its basic tenet was no longer the supply of care by a number of separate institutions, but meeting the constantly changing tasks and functions that have to be performed for various client groups.

This recent change in the government's dominant mental health policy, however, should not obscure the high level of continuity in the development of the Dutch mental health care sector. First, contrary to the United States, Great Britain and Italy, large-scale, radical de-institutionalisation did not happen. Despite protests, new psychiatric hospitals were built, aimed at downscaling and a more even regional spread. After a small reduction in the number of beds in psychiatric hospitals in the years 1975-1985, this number slightly grew in the ensuing decade.[35] Polarisation and a radical break were averted by gradually integrating new practices in existing institutional frameworks. Second, in light of the government's persistent effort to shift attention away from psycho-social problems and towards psychiatric disorders, it is questionable to what degree this shift was in fact realised. The prevailing approach of the RIAGG network basically followed the one established earlier by the Child Guidance Clinics, Centres for Family and Marriage Problems, and Institutes for Psychotherapy. They focused on psycho-social problems and psychotherapeutic treatment, which their staff seemed to value more highly than medical and social-psychiatric activities. Although the 1970s euphoria about psychotherapy diminished while the biomedical approach gained ground, the number of people who received psychotherapeutic treatment doubled in the 1980s and 1990s, funding continued to facilitate broad accessibility, and the number of psychotherapists also increased. The RIAGGS, like the psychiatric outpatient clinics, continued to treat many individuals with more or less serious psycho-social problems.[36] Only as the 1990s evolved did they begin to give priority to more serious psychiatric disorders and to their social-psychiatric responsibilities.

By the 1990s psychotherapy had basically lost its special appeal in the Netherlands. Its discourse had become an integral part of mainstream life where – in its popularised form as 'psycho talk' – it influenced the actions and thinking of ever more individuals. If in the 1960s and 1970s the preoccupation with personal feelings and inner emotions was mainly found among young, urban and well-educated groups, while the articulation of these concerns was largely restricted to the therapeutic setting, by the end of the century psychotherapy's popular status was obvious. It was more common for people to talk about others or themselves in psychological terms and to refer to their mood or feeling as a way to legitimate their behaviour. Although medication and behavioural therapy have meanwhile become more prominent in mental health care at the expense of psychological approaches, the psychotherapeutic frame of mind has permeated both the private and public spheres. Promoted in mass media and self-help books and by all sorts of therapists, trainers, advisors and consultants, psychotherapeutic jargon has fully become part of everyday language – albeit in a watered-down version.

In the context of the dichotomy between minor psycho-social complaints and serious psychiatric illness, the coverage and accessibility of the mental health sector continued to be an issue of debate. In response to the pleas of politicians and some psychiatrists to discourage the growing demand for mental health care, others argued that this sector, in contrast to somatic medicine, still hardly received its due share, so a further expansion could well be justified. Either way, between 1980 and 2000 the growth of the mental health sector was explosive. The total number of individual registrations – which is not the same as the number of individual clients as some of them may register several times or at different facilities – increased from 2.66 per cent of the population in 1980 to 6.92 per cent in 1997, or from an annual total of some 380,000 to over a million. In the mid-1990s, about 5 per cent of the Dutch population, or between 700,000 and 750,000 people, who suffered from a wide range of serious and mild psychological disorders and complaints, came into contact with the mental health care system, while 4 per cent was actually accepted for treatment. The large majority of them, around 80 per cent, were treated in outpatient facilities, the RIAGGS in particular.[37]

Under the influence of the ongoing expansion of care use and prognostic data that even suggested a further acceleration, in the 1990s the concern with the social dimension of psychic disorders and their possible prevention grew, whereby a familiar cultural pessimism resurfaced. The supposed increase of mental problems was seen as effected by the high pace and intensity of social change, social atomisation, the loss of cohesive and normative frameworks, and the excessively high demands made on people in terms of their flexibility, social

Insanity and Other Discomforts

skills and mental resilience. The optimistic view espoused by many mental health workers in the 1970s, in which emancipated and motivated individuals would be able to solve their own problems, was replaced with concern about the loss of public morals and a sense of community. Furthermore, the positive evaluation of self-determination began to be questioned, since it allowed deranged individuals to refuse psychiatric treatment, even if they could not take care of themselves or caused social trouble. Pleas for more pressure and coercion in social-psychiatric care and for new experiments in special outreaching services for those in particular problem groups who were unwilling to co-operate or hard to reach, put earlier ideals of individual liberation and self-development into perspective.[38]

Dutch Outpatient Psychiatry and Mental Health Care: Basic Characteristics and Trends

The first forms of outpatient psychiatry in the Netherlands took shape around 1900, when nerve doctors catered to private patients who wanted to avoid any association with insanity or the asylum. By contrast, the initiatives of the 1920s in the area of pre- and aftercare were closely bound up with the mental institutions and shared their problems. This new form of care was an effort to break away from the closed-off tradition of institutional psychiatry and renew it. In the 1930s, the psycho-hygienic movement embarked on a different course, which in time would become the dominant one. First, the Child Guidance Clinic began to distance itself from institutional psychiatry by stressing that its clients had little to do with the mentally ill. After World War Two, the Child Guidance Clinics, the Centres for Family and Marriage Problems and, from the 1960s on, the Institutes for Medical or Multidisciplinary Psychotherapy set the tone in outpatient mental health care, while social psychiatry and the Counselling Centres for Alcohol Addiction were pushed into the background. In the 1980s social psychiatry was formally integrated into the new network of RIAGGS, but the persistent critique that this system neglected psychiatric patients with serious disorders indicates that the split between hospitals and outpatient care was still a major factor. The latest developments, pressured by government policies, suggest that, finally, the public mental health sector will become fully integrated, as a result of a planned merger between the various intramural, extramural and half-way facilities.

The development of extramural mental health care in the twentieth century was motivated by professional and organisational concerns rather than by public demand. The establishment and spread of the various facilities were mainly triggered by a dynamic on the supply side: the initiatives of socially concerned individuals, the aspirations of various professional groups, the rivalry among the religious-ideological pillars and, finally, funding opportunities. It is hard to ignore the impression that there has been a strong tendency in most outpatient services to keep patients with serious psychiatric disorders out of its system, especially those who might be annoying, dangerous, or frightening to others and difficult to treat. In this respect, this effort followed in a long tradition within psychiatry: the recurrent alternation and juxtaposition of therapeutic optimism and pessimism. Time and again, experts argued that the existing facilities fell short in providing adequate treatment for patients, let alone cure them. Alternative ways of organising care and establishing new facilities, they believed, would lead to successes where prior efforts had failed. Repeatedly, newly established provisions caused an expansion of psychiatry and mental health care, as well as the emergence of new groups of patients, whereby a distinction was made between those who were treatable and those who were not. This frequently implied that attention for the former led to the neglect of the latter.

Around 1900, increasing doubts were raised about the beneficial effects of a patient's stay in a closed asylum. As a result, the therapeutic optimism began to be orientated towards other institutions: the specialised sanatoria and clinics for patients with nervous disorders and alcohol addicts, private practice, and mental wards and hospitals where acute and 'neurotic' patients were admitted and treated on strictly medical grounds, without certification. From a therapeutic perspective, however, the partly open and partly closed institutions for the mentally ill continued to be a source of concern, especially given their overcrowding with chronic cases. In the 1920s, this therapeutic pessimism led to new outpatient facilities for psychiatric patients, the Pre- and Aftercare Services, and to the psycho-hygienic effort to prevent mental disorders. This second objective caused a substantial expansion of psychiatry's domain: children and youngsters with learning, educational and developmental problems were now potentially included, as were adults with problems in the sphere of marriage, family, relationships, procreation, sexuality and work. From the 1960s, mental health expanded to comprise welfare and individual well-being as well: to a large extent psychotherapy catered to people who were basically healthy but who nevertheless were troubled by personality flaws, relational problems, existential uncertainties and their potential for self-development. Only since the mid-1980s, partly because of financial considerations, did the continuing expansion of the mental health sector begin to be questioned more often, and attention focused again on the seriously and chronically mentally ill.

From the 1930s onward, the psycho-hygienic movement and most outpatient facilities tried to hook up with the overall health care sector, and they indeed managed to do so, which meant that they kept their distance from institutional psychiatry, closely associated as it was with poor relief and the judicial system. On the other hand, extramural services also displayed a clear affinity with the traditions of charitable aid and social work. In the Netherlands these sectors were strongly developed, both emphasising a close link between the alleviation of material want

Insanity and Other Discomforts

and moral or spiritual elevation. In their moral-didactic approach, they focused on the social environment and efforts to reform individuals, while the principle of social integration gained the upper hand, rather than the principle of isolating or excluding problem groups. The eugenicist perspectives of the first psycho-hygienists lost ground, while the influence of medical psychiatry remained limited, at least until the 1990s. In the 1970s, when the number of social workers in mental health care rose sharply, it even seemed that it would soon merge into welfare work. However, in the 1980s and 1990s, mental health workers retreated into the more limited professional domain of health care and thus avoided falling prey to the government's cutbacks on welfare services.

Until the 1970s, most mental health facilities were tied to Dutch society's 'pillarised' system, which meant that religious motivations played a major role. Many services were rooted in Catholic and, albeit to a lesser degree, orthodox Protestant and Dutch Reformed doctrine; they basically served the aim of maintaining the central role of religion. But from 1950, leading psychiatrists and psychologists, as well as several reform-minded clergymen, began to question the subordination of issues associated with mental well-being to the church's norms and values. Based on psycho-hygienist views, they tried to bridge the gap between religious doctrine and modern life. That the confessional groups of the population had their own mental health facilities raised the chances of religious people coming into contact with a more psychological approach to normative issues. Religion-based mental health induced individualisation at a moral level and provided a basis for the more radical liberation of individuals from the second half of the 1960s, when a massive secularisation process took off.

The prominence of the confessional groups in the area of mental health and the wide variation in facilities were made possible in part by the Dutch government's low profile in the health care sector until the mid-1960s. Its role was restricted to control and supervision, leaving the actual provision and organisation of care to local and private initiatives. Although the national government raised its subsidies in the 1950s and 1960s, its role in non-institutional mental health basically remained restricted to regulation and inspection. Only from the mid-1960s did collective funding enable the welfare state to grow and implement large-scale policies. As the money for mental health care increasingly came out of national funds, the need for a large variety of more or less autonomous facilities began to be debated increasingly, while the government issued more and more regulations concerning the implementation and organisation of care provision. It played an active role in the realization of the RIAGG-network and the increasing integration of intra- and extramural care. The policies that in the 1990s promoted deregulation and the free market diminished the input of government once again, although collective funding was maintained.

The modernisation of Dutch society and the evolving views of democratic citizenship provided the socio-political context for the pursuit of mental health;

either a cultural pessimism or an optimistic belief in society's progress prevailed. In this respect, it is possible to identify a radical break around 1950. At that point, defensive responses to the modernisation process and strict adherence to Christian bourgeois morality were exchanged for a much more accommodating stance, while in the reflection on citizenship there was a shift from an unconditional adaptation to collective values and norms to individual self-development. People's inner motivations came to be centre-stage. Between 1950 and 1965, the mental health sector accommodated to rapid social change: individuals had to shape their personality, develop their autonomy and flexibility, be open for renewal and achieve self-realization in a responsible way. In the 1960s and 1970s, mental health workers embraced personal liberation, democratisation and assertiveness as core values. Subsequently, in the last two decades of the twentieth century, they approached their clients as mature, autonomous and self-responsible citizens, whose freedom to make choices as members of a pluralist market society was perceived as self-evident. At the close of the twentieth century, worries about social cohesion resurfaced, and as attention focused on groups suffering from serious mental and behavioural disorder, the emphasis on individual autonomy was brought up for discussion.[39]

Throughout the twentieth century the size of the Dutch mental health care system increased, in both absolute and relative terms. In 1900, the number of people who received psychiatric care and treatment did not exceed 0.2 per cent of the general population. At least 80 per cent of those who received any care and treatment were hospitalised. Around 2000, the number of clients and patients in mental health care was about 750,000, or a little under 5 per cent of the population; outpatient facilities catered for 80 per cent of those who received mental care. The Netherlands, together with the United States, Canada and Australia, belonged to the countries with the highest number of psychiatrists and psychotherapists in proportion to the size of the population.[40] The strong growth of the extramural sector, especially after 1970, might give the impression that ever larger numbers of Dutch people suffered from mental afflictions. This, however, is hard to substantiate. There are indications that no correlation exists between the incidence of mental disorders in a population and the degree to which its members make use of care-providing facilities. Studies from the 1980s and 1990s reveal that about one quarter of the adult population between the age of 18 and 64 suffered from a DSM-listed psychiatric disorder or serious psychosocial problem every year. Although this number was significantly higher than that of patients who ended up in the mental health system (which increased from over 2 per cent to almost 5 per cent of all adults), it remained steady over the years and was similar to that of many other countries.[41] These data cast doubt on the view that the population's increasing demand for care also reflected the occurrence of a growing number of disorders and mental problems. It suggests that many people with mental problems did not look for professional help and that general practitioners only considered a portion of the complaints they identified as serious enough for referral to mental health services. It cannot be denied, however, that between 1980 and 2000, more and more individuals found their way to the mental health facilities, especially in the outpatient sector: there was, in fact, more than a doubling of the number of registrations.[42]

Apart from political decisions on funding, social and cultural factors have probably had a greater influence on the consumption of care than any measure of mental disorders. In the case of psycho-social problems, to which many of the outpatient facilities were geared, the definitions of disorders tend to change and expand. The way in which individuals experienced them and looked for ways of dealing with them was subject to change during the twentieth century. Individual problems are of all times, but their specific interpretation as mental health complaints has been strongly determined by the availability of specialised services, their specific treatment options and the psychological discourse used by experts. They rendered a host of tacitly experienced problems visible and identifiable and, most importantly, offered a concrete context for talking about them. Social factors influenced what counted as a problem, which complaints were identified and discussed, and who was asked to treat them. In the psycho-social and psychotherapeutic mental health sector, the growing supply of professional care created the increasing demand for care, rather than the other way around. In contrast, institutional and social (pre- and aftercare) psychiatry focused on the core group of severely mentally ill individuals. This group remains the heart of the psychiatric domain, and its relative size has remained fairly stable over time in the population at large.[43]

An extensive network of extramural mental health facilities came into being in the Netherlands over the course of the twentieth century, and especially from the 1960s, it acquired a large clientele. In this country, which in social and cultural terms used to be quite bourgeois, conservative and Christian, the cultural revolution of the 1960s was more sweeping than in others, because it coincided with rapid secularisation and de-pillarisation.[44] Once the solid, familiar moral frame began to be discussed publicly, it soon lost its relevance for many. The ensuing spiritual vacuum was partially filled by the new psychotherapeutic ethos.[45] Since the 1960s, Dutch society experienced an accelerated democratisation of public and everyday life, which replaced hierarchy, group coercion and formal power relations with self-development, emancipation and informal manners. This subsequently required self-control, subtle social regulation and psychological insight from individuals. The focus on discussion, accommodation and consensus, which has long been characteristic of Dutch political elites, became a characteristic of society as a whole. With their emphasis on self-reflection and raising sensitive issues, mental health workers articulated new values and offered a clear alternative for the outdated morality of dos and don'ts. They not only adapted their views to the continuously changing social circumstances but also functioned as major agents of social-cultural renewal, especially in the 1950s, 1960s, and 1970s. Talking was their preferred strategy for solving problems, which not only linked them with the Dutch culture of negotiation and consensus, but also with the practice of everyday life of many Dutch people.

Since the 1930s, the largest segment of the working population has been active in the services sector, in which communications grew increasingly central.[46] In the densely populated and highly urbanised Netherlands, therefore, proper social functioning depended greatly on personality traits associated with verbal and communicative skills, flexibility and the subtle regulation of emotion. Finally, the strong inclination toward psychologisation dovetailed with how the Dutch culture of consensus addresses social and ethical issues. It is a culture in which experts figure prominently because of their supposedly objective professional stance, thus neutralising social conflicts over sensitive issues. In the articulation of policies on sexuality, birth control, abortion, euthanasia, drugs and disability, for example, experts such as doctors, psychiatrists, psychologists, and others had a large say. They generally contributed to formulating solutions that are both pragmatic and well-considered, while also taking individual conditions, attitudes and motivations into account as much as possible.

Notes

* I am indebted to Marijke Gijswijt-Hofstra and Joost Vijselaar for their comments on earlier drafts of this article, and to Ton Brouwers and Hugh Freeman for correcting the English.
1. See the articles of J. Vijselaar, J. Slijkhuis and M. Gijswijt-Hofstra, in M. Gijswijt-Hofstra and R. Porter (eds), *Cultures of Neurasthenia. From Beard to the First World War* (Amsterdam, New York: Rodopi, 2001). See also the article by Gijswijt-Hofstra in this volume.
2. On the history of psychotherapy and psychoanalysis in the Netherlands, see W.J. de Waal, *De geschiedenis van de psychotherapie in Nederland* ('s-Hertogenbosch: De Nijvere Haas, 1992); I.N. Bulhof, *Freud en Nederland. De interpretatie en invloed van zijn ideeën* (Baarn: Ambo, 1983); C. Brinkgreve, *Psychoanalyse in Nederland. Een vestigingsstrijd* (Amsterdam: Uitgeverij De Arbeiderspers, 1984).
3. On the history of alcoholism and its treatment, see J.C. van der Stel, *Drinken, drank en dronkenschap. Vijf eeuwen drankbestrijding en alcoholhulpverlening in Nederland. Een historisch-sociologische studie* (Hilversum: Verloren, 1995).
4. P. van der Esch, *Geschiedenis van het staatstoezicht op krankzinnigen* 1 (Leidschendam: Ministerie van WVC, 1975), 81-2; J.H. Schuurmans Stekhoven, *XXVste Verslag van het Staatstoezicht op krankzinnigen en krankzinnigengestichten over de jaren 1915-1929* ('s-Gravenhage: Algemeene Landsdrukkerij, 1932), 172.
5. Nederlandsche Vereeniging voor Geestelijke Volksgezondheid, *Gids betreffende de geestelijke volksgezondheid (psychische hygiëne) in Nederland* (Amsterdam: F. van Rossen, 1936), 74-6.

Insanity and Other Discomforts

6.   R. de Schepper, *De Pameijer Stichting (1926-1991): Een geschiedenis van de sociale psychiatrie en verstandelijk gehandicaptenzorg te Rotterdam* (Rotterdam: Pameijer Stichting, 1991); G. Blok and J. Vijselaar, *Terug naar Endegeest: Patiënten en hun behandeling in het psychiatrisch ziekenhuis Endegeest 1897-1997* (Nijmegen: SUN, 1998), 94-9.

7.   Nederlandsche Vereeniging voor Geestelijke Volksgezondheid, *op. cit.* (note 5), 67-74.

8.   T. van der Grinten, *De vorming van de ambulante geestelijke gezondheidszorg: Een historisch beleidsonderzoek* (Baarn: Ambo, 1987), 36-56.

9.   On Querido see: A.J. Heerma van Voss, 'Querido, een levensverhaal', *Maandblad Geestelijke volksgezondheid*, 46 (1991), 722-811; J. van Limbeek and V. van Alem (eds), *Querido's legacy: Social psychiatry in Amsterdam from 1932-1991* (Amsterdam: GG & GD, 1991); A. Dercksen and S. van 't Hof, *Uitgereden: Bladzijden uit de geschiedenis van de Amsterdamse Centrale Riagg Dienst* (Utrecht, Amsterdam: Nederlands Centrum Geestelijke Volksgezondheid, 1994).

10.   Inspectie van het staatstoezicht op krankzinnigen en krankzinnigengestichten, *Verslag van het staatstoezicht op krankzinnigen en krankzinnigengestichten over de jaren 1932-1936* (Den Haag: Algemeene Landsdrukkerij, 1938), 84-6.

11.   On the history of the Dutch mental hygiene movement, see L. de Goei, *De psychohygiënisten: Psychiatrie, cultuurkritiek en de beweging voor geestelijke volksgezondheid in Nederland, 1924-1970* (Nijmegen: SUN, 2001). On the relation between mental hygiene, social psychiatry, and pre- and aftercare see also H. Oosterhuis, 'Between institutional psychiatry and mental health care: social psychiatry in The Netherlands, 1916-2000', *Medical History*, 4 (2004), 413-28.

12.   H. te Velde, 'How high did the Dutch fly? Remarks on stereotypes of burger mentality', in A. Galema, B. Henkes and H. te Velde (eds), *Images of the Nation. Different Meanings of Dutchness 1870-1940* (Amsterdam, Atlanta: Rodopi, 1993), 59-79; R. van Ginkel, *Op zoek naar eigenheid. Denkbeelden en discussies over cultuur en identiteit in Nederland* (Den Haag: Sdu Uitgevers, 1999).

13.   De Goei, *op. cit.* (note 11), 28-32.

14.   *Ibid.*, 52-68.

15.   On the history of eugenics in the Netherlands, see J. Noordman, *Om de kwaliteit van het nageslacht: Eugenetica in Nederland 1900-1950* (Nijmegen: SUN, 1989).

16.   On the Catholic mental hygiene movement, see H. Westhoff, *Geestelijke bevrijders: Nederlandse katholieken en hun beweging voor geestelijke volksgezondheid in de twintigste eeuw* (Nijmegen: Valkhof Pers, 1996).

17.   De Goei, *op. cit.* (note 11), 69-102.

18.   Nationale Federatie voor de Geestelijke Volksgezondheid, *Gids voor de Geestelijke volksgezondheid in Nederland* (Amsterdam: NFGV, 1949), 54-75.

19.   C. Brinkgreve, J.H. Onland and A. de Swaan, *Sociologie van de psychotherapie 1: De opkomst van het psychotherapeutisch bedrijf* (Utrecht, Antwerp: Het Spectrum, 1979), 36-41, 48, 65.

20.   A. de Swaan, R. van Gelderen and V. Kense, *Sociologie van de psychotherapie 2: Het spreekuur als opgave* (Utrecht, Antwerpen: Het Spectrum, 1979), 29-32; Brinkgreve et al., *op. cit.* (note 19), 149-58.

21.   On mental health care, religion and sexuality, see D.A.M. van Berkel, *Moeder-schap tussen zielzorg en psychohygiëne: Katholieke deskundigen over voortplanting en op-voeding 1945-1970* (Assen, Maastricht: Van Gorcum, 1990); H. Oosterhuis, *Homosek-sualiteit in katholiek Nederland: Een sociale geschiedenis 1900-1970* (Amsterdam: Sua, 1992); C.N. de Groot, *Naar een nieuwe clerus: Psychotherapie en religie in het Maand-blad voor de Geestelijke Volksgezondheid* (Kampen: Kok Agora, 1995); H. Oosterhuis, 'The Netherlands: neither prudish nor hedonistic', in F.X. Eder, L.A. Hall and G. Hekma (eds), *Sexual cultures in Europe: National histories* (Manchester, New York: Manchester University Press, 1999), 71-90; Westhoff, *op. cit.* (note 16).

22.   Nationale Federatie, *op. cit.* (note 18), 54-65; Nationale Federatie voor de Geestelijke Volksgezondheid, *Gids voor de Geestelijke Gezondheidszorg in Nederland* (Amsterdam: NFGV, 1962), 240-6, 303-13.

23.   See H. Bakker, L. de Goei and J. Vijselaar, *Thuis opgenomen: Uit de geschiedenis van de sociale psychiatrie in Nederland* (Utrecht: Nederlands Centrum Geestelijke Volksgezondheid, 1994).

24.   Nationale Federatie, *op. cit.* (note 18), 17-31; Nationale Federatie, *op. cit.* (1962) (note 22), 199-218.

25.   J.W. Duyvendak, *De planning van ontplooiing: Wetenschap, politiek en de maak-bare samenleving* (Den Haag: Sdu Uitgevers, 1999); E. Tonkens, *Het zelfontplooiings-regime: De actualiteit van Dennendal en de jaren zestig* (Amsterdam: Bert Bakker, 1999).

26.   De Goei, *op. cit.* (note 11), 194-7, 218-24, 267-77.

27.   Nationale Federatie voor de Geestelijke Volksgezondheid, *Gids voor de Geeste-lijke Gezondheidszorg in Nederland* (Amsterdam: NFGV, 1965), 20-40, 59-64, 68-75, 241-52; Nationaal Centrum voor Geestelijke Volksgezondheid, *Gids Geestelijke Ge-zondheidszorg 1981* (Utrecht: Nederlands Centrum Geestelijke Volksgezondheid, 1981), 43-241; D. Ingleby, 'The View from the North Sea', in M. Gijswijt-Hofstra and R. Porter (eds), *Cultures of Psychiatry and Mental Health Care in Postwar Britain and the Netherlands* (Amsterdam, Atlanta: Rodopi, 1998), 295-314; C.Th. Bakker and H. van der Velden, *Geld en gekte. Verkenningen in de financiering van de GGZ in de twin-tigste eeuw* (Amsterdam: Universiteit van Amsterdam, 2004), 65.

28.   Brinkgreve et al., *op. cit.* (note 19), 97, 104, 124.

29.   P. van Lieshout and D. de Ridder (eds), *Symptomen van de tijd: De dossiers van het Amsterdamse Instituut voor Medische Psychotherapie (IMP), 1968-1977* (Nijmegen: SUN, 1991).

30.   See C. Brinkgreve and M. Korzec, *'Margriet weet raad': Gevoel, gedrag, moraal in Nederland 1938-1978* (Utrecht, Antwerpen: Het Spectrum, 1978); A. de Swaan, 'Uit-gaansbeperking en uitgaansangst: Over de verschuiving van bevelshuishouding naar onderhandelingshuishouding', *De Gids*, 142/8 (1979), 483-509; W. Zeegers, *Andere tijden, andere mensen: De sociale representatie van identiteit* (Amsterdam: Bert Bakker, 1988); C. Wouters, *Van minnen en sterven. Informalisering van omgangsvor-men rond seks en dood* (Amsterdam: Bert Bakker, 1990); R. Abma et al. (eds), *Het ver-langen naar openheid. Over de psychologisering van het alledaagse* (Amsterdam: De Balie, 1995).

31.   'Ambulant' is the Dutch term for outpatient or extramural.

32.   Nationale Federatie (1965), *op. cit.* (note 27), 241; A. A. Fischer, 'De ontwikkeling van de psychotherapie in de instituten voor psychotherapie', *Nederlands Tijdschrift voor Psychiatrie*, 12/2-3 (1970), 44; M.A.J. Romme (ed.), *Voorzieningen in de Geestelijke Gezondheidszorg: Een gids voor consument en hulpverlener* (Alphen aan den Rijn, Brussel: Samson Uitgeverij, 1978) 32, 120; Nationaal Centrum (1981), *op. cit.* (note 27), 17; Van der Stel, *op. cit.* (note 3), 406, 427; C. Willemsen, *De belofte van het hiernumaals: Zeventig jaar ambulante geestelijke gezondheidszorg in het gewest Breda 1929-1999* (Nijmegen: SUN, 2001), 228-9.

33.   On the development of the RIAGG: Van der Grinten, *op. cit.* (note 8); T. Festen et al., *Van dichtbij en veraf: 15 jaar RIAGG / 25 jaar NVAGG* (Utrecht: NVAGG, 1997).

34.   H.J. Wennink, *De ongelukkige relatie tussen maatschappij en geestelijke gezondheidszorg: Een bezinning op 25 jaar rumoer in de (sociale) psychiatrie* (Maarssen: Elsevier/De Tijdstroom, 1998); M.H. Kwekkeboom, *Naar draagkracht: Een verkennend onderzoek naar draagvlak en draagkracht voor de vermaatschappelijking in de geestelijke gezondheidszorg* (Den Haag: Sociaal-Cultureel Planbureau, 1999).

35.   M.A.J. Romme, 'Deïnstitutionalisering in de psychiatrie; een emancipatieproces', in B.P.R. Gersons et al. (eds), *In het spoor van Kees Trimbos: Denkbeelden over preventieve en sociale psychiatrie* (Deventer: Van Loghum Slaterus, 1990), 44. See also the article by Marijke Gijswijt-Hofstra in this volume.

36.   F. Lemmens et al., 'Psychotherapie in de RIAGG: een balans', *Maandblad Geestelijke volksgezondheid*, 45 (1990), 356-72; G. Hutschemaekers and H. Oosterhuis, 'Psychotherapy in the Netherlands after World War II', *Medical History*, 4 (2004), 429-48.

37.   G. Hutschemaekers, 'Wordt Nederland steeds zieker? Kerngetallen en achtergrondanalyses', *Maandblad Geestelijke volksgezondheid*, 55 (2000), 316-7; P. Schnabel, *De Geestelijke gezondheidszorg: goed voor verbetering – voortgaan met het vernieuwingsbeleid* (Utrecht: Nationaal Fonds Geestelijke Volksgezondheid, s.a.), 9.

38.   P. Schnabel, R. Bijl and G. Hutschemaekers, *Geestelijke volksgezondheid in de jaren '90: Van ideaal tot concrete opgave* (Utrecht: Nederlands Centrum Geestelijke Volksgezondheid, 1992), 38.

39.   Duyvendak, *op. cit.* (note 25).

40.   Van der Esch, *op. cit.* (note 4), 81; P. Schnabel, 'The Mental Health Services: more than psychiatry alone', in A.J.P. Schrijvers (ed.), *Health and Health Care in the Netherlands* (Utrecht: De Tijdstroom, 1997), 121; G. Hutschemaekers, 'Hoe meer psychiaters, des te groter het tekort? De psychiater en de arbeidsmarkt', *Maandblad Geestelijke volksgezondheid*, 48 (1993), 1178-9.

41.   R.V. Bijl, G. van Zessen and A. Ravelli, 'Psychiatrische morbiditeit onder volwassenen in Nederland: het NEMESIS-onderzoek II, prevalentie van psychiatrische stoornissen', *Nederlands Tijdschrift voor Geneeskunde*, 141 (1997), 2453-60; Wennink, *op. cit.* (note 34), 77; Schnabel, *op. cit.* (note 37), 10, 13.

42.   Hutschemaekers, *op. cit.* (note 37), 317.

43.   P. Schnabel, *Het recht om niet gestoord te worden: Naar een nieuwe sociologie van de psychiatrie* (Utrecht: Nederlands Centrum Geestelijke Volksgezondheid, 1992).

44.   J. Kennedy, *Nieuw Babylon in aanbouw: Nederland in de jaren zestig* (Amsterdam, Meppel: Boom, 1995); H. Righart, *De eindeloze jaren zestig: Geschiedenis van een generatieconflict* (Amsterdam, Antwerpen: De Arbeiderspers, 1995).

45.   See G. Blok, *Baas in eigen brein: 'Antipsychiatrie' in Nederland, 1965-1985* (Amsterdam: Uitgeverij Nieuwezijds, 2004).

46.   H. Knippenberg and B. de Pater, *De eenwording van Nederland: Schaalvergroting en integratie sinds 1800* (Nijmegen: SUN, 1990), 128-130.

Insanity and Other Discomforts

CHAPTER 3

Madness and Autonomy

The Moral Agenda of Anti-psychiatry in the Netherlands

Gemma Blok

Introduction

In 1974, a young man called Piet was admitted to Conolly – a closed ward for acute admissions of the psychiatric hospital Brinkgreven in the Dutch town of Deventer. Piet was admitted because of restlessness and derailed behaviour, and was diagnosed as suffering from 'problems in breaking away from his parents'. Family therapy (the preferred method of treatment at Conolly) was tried, but Piet's parents did not want to participate. Next, the Conolly staff tried to provoke Piet into making personal 'change'. 'Piet's way of dealing with people', one of them wrote in his patient file, 'is such that they all get mad at him. Are we not allowed to like you, Piet?' After returning from an unnerving trip into town with Piet, a nurse commented: 'Perhaps one could go on a nice outing with him, if only he would learn to control himself a little. But maybe you just like to continue playing this part, don't you, Piet? It's so nice to act out like that, and if anyone objects, well, then you're crazy, aren't you, Piet?"[1]

Labelling Piet's behaviour as a part he played is typical of the way in which the Conolly personnel of the 1970s regarded mental illness. They believed psychiatric patients were not ill at all, in a physical or neurological sense. 'Crazy behaviour', they argued, was a strategy people (subconsciously) chose to escape from stressful circumstances, to bring to light problems within the family or to avoid responsibility. Either way, 'madness' was fundamentally functional and an expression of individual autonomy. As the British psychiatrist R.D. Laing (1927-1989) – who was a big influence on the people working at Conolly – put it: 'The schizophrenic is playing at being mad.'[2]

Laing is commonly referred to as an 'anti-psychiatrist', together with – amongst others – Thomas Szasz, David Cooper, Franco Basaglia and Michel Foucault. During the 1960s and 1970s, they all argued that psychiatry was not really a medical science but rather an instrument of social control. Psychiatric hospitals were filled with the pariahs of Western society. Szasz even compared psychiatry with the Inquisition. Laing especially became immensely popular, selling millions of books world-wide in which he expressed a general cultural criticism as well as a critique of his own profession. Laing argued that Western society was pathogenic, since creativity, spirituality, sexuality and emotional openness were all stifled while materialism, competition and outward conformism were stimulated. Psychiatrists, together with parents and school teachers, were part of this massive oppression of individual freedom. They declared insane all those who couldn't or wouldn't conform while, in fact, Western culture itself was crazy.

This was not the first time clinical psychiatry had fallen under attack. Roughly between 1875 and 1900, psychiatric patients, journalists, artists and some psychiatrists in Western countries attacked the alleged abuse and neglect of patients in psychiatric hospitals and the lack of control surrounding psychiatric incarceration.[3] However, the criticism of the 1960s and 1970s was different. First of all, it was expressed for a large part by psychiatrists themselves. Secondly, the criticism now became more widespread than ever before, as a result of the new mass media and the higher level of education in the West. Finally, the anti-psychiatric critique of the 1960s was more fundamental than before: it addressed such questions as the nature of mental illness and the definition of normality.

Nowadays, the anti-psychiatry movement of that period is often depicted as a result of the anti-authoritarian sentiment of the 1960s.[4] It is seen as a temporary fad for marxist academics, sensationalist journalists or hippies identifying with the allegedly repressed spirituality of psychiatric patients. According to the Canadian historian Edward Shorter, for example, 'the works of Foucault, Szasz, and Goffman were influential among university elites, cultivating a rage against mental hospitals and the whole psychiatric enterprise'.[5] Certainly, anti-psychiatry was part of the spirit of its time. However, its influence in the Netherlands was not limited to the media, the academic world, or psychedelic youth culture. Nor was it a plea for the abolition of the 'whole psychiatric enterprise'. On the contrary, the 'anti-psychiatric' critique in the Netherlands was actually, and paradoxically, a plea for an *intensification* of psychiatric treatment. Psychiatry should finally start doing its job and try to cure its patients, using various forms of psychotherapy, instead of merely calming the patients down and patching them up with pills.

Of course, some radical critics wanted to abolish psychiatry altogether, claiming that the only effective therapy was 'freedom', including freedom from any kind of psychiatric intervention. Most critics of the medical model in the Netherlands, however, worked in psychiatric hospitals themselves. Building on the criticism expressed by Laing and others, they proposed not an abolition but rather a reform of psychiatric care. In 1970, for instance, the Dutch psychiatrist Joost Mathijsen, a strong supporter of Laing, stated that 'traditional psychiatry' was immature. It had nothing to offer except 'adjustment pills' and reassuring 'pats on the back'. More mature psychiatrists, Mathijsen thought, would search together with the patients for the psychological and social reasons of why they had become stuck in their lives. Mature psychiatrists would reveal problems, using psychotherapy, instead of covering them up with psychopharmaceuticals.[6]

This essay will thus try to offer a new perspective on the phenomenon of anti-psychiatry by taking a look at the impact of the anti-psychiatric critique on actual therapeutic practice in Dutch clinical psychiatry during the 1970s. It was then that psychiatric nurses, psychologists and psychiatrists cooperated to replace the 'medical model' of treatment by a 'social model'.

Emancipating the Patient

During the 1970s, the ideas of Laing, Szasz, Cooper and their Dutch counterpart Jan Foudraine[7] were eagerly received in the Netherlands by psychiatrists, psychologists and – most of all – psychiatric nurses. They blended well with the writings of other psychotherapists, such as the humanistic psychologist Carl Rogers or the family therapist Jay Haley. They all criticized the medical model of mental illness and stressed the importance of self-realization in generating mental health. 'Madness', according to many of these psychotherapeutic authors, was the result of a systematic obstruction of self-realization, for instance by the parents. To quote the humanistic family therapist Virginia Satir: 'Behaviour labelled by society as "sick" or "crazy" is in fact an attempt of an individual to reveal existing problems and ask for help.'[8] The ideas of anti-psychiatrists, humanistic psychologists and family therapists together inspired Dutch mental health care workers to formulate a new ideal, which in retrospect can be characterised as 'emancipatory psychiatry'. This aimed at liberating the individual's authenticity or 'true self' and was based on the Laingian notion that 'breakdown' could be a 'breakthrough'.

This kind of thinking was the radical outcome of two important influences. The first was the Freudian notion that psychological symptoms were functional. Freud and his followers argued that neurotic symptoms such as obsessive and compulsive behaviour, restlessness, or melancholy served to protect the individual from a confrontation with his or her deeper fears, feelings of aggression, or sexual desires. The radical psychoanalyst Georg Groddeck argued that *all* illnesses had a purpose, even physical ones. From the 1930s onwards, neo-freudians like Harry Stack Sullivan, Frieda Fromm-Reichman and John Rosen, as well as family therapists such as Haley and Carl Whitaker, carried this notion to a new extreme. They stated that not only neurotic, but also psychotic symptoms were functional. When psychotic symptoms were viewed within the social context of the patient, especially his relationship with his parents, the seemingly crazy behaviour became more understandable: it was an escape reaction to a systematic effort to undermine a person's autonomy and self-confidence. Psychotic symptoms were thus essentially considered to be defence mechanisms.[9]

Another influence on the notion of mental illness as being functional was existentialism. Sartre was an important influence on Laing, Cooper and Szasz. Vice versa, Sartre strongly sympathised with critical psychiatry. As he put it in 1964: 'I regard mental illness as the "way out" that the free organism, in its total unity, invents in order to live through an intolerable situation.'[10] Elsewhere, Sartre explained his sympathy for the critical psychiatry of Laing as follows:

> 'I think Laing was looking for a theory which would put freedom first [...] I think what he meant is that within society [...] one could understand the nature of an aberrant but persistent attitude which at present is known as madness, an attitude that prevents a real contact with others and which is nevertheless a consequence of freedom. That's to say, a new conception of mental illness seen as a mode of life as valid as our own but which, however, is likely to lead to total inertia, for instance, or unbearable pain. He takes men as they are, not as mad men versus sane men but as men; some reaching a certain stage of distress, others avoiding that stage.'[11]

This notion of madness as an attempt of the free individual to safeguard one's autonomy resulted in the ideal to emancipate and liberate the 'psychiatric patient'. This emancipatory psychiatric treatment took on different forms, which can be rougly divided into two varieties. One was the model of the therapeutic community, where people often stayed for quite a long time, and psychoanalytical group therapy and psychodrama were the most important forms of treatment. As both ideal and practice, the therapeutic community became widespread in Dutch clinical psychiatry from the late 1960s onwards. A second variety of psychotherapeutic renewal was based on the notion of crisis intervention. Here, the aim was to keep people in care as short a time as possible, and to try and use their crisis to quickly get to the bottom of their social problems, e.g. using family therapy.

Of course, this is a very rough scheme and in many places, like Conolly ward, elements of both varieties were mixed. Moreover, the extent of this psychotherapeutic renewal should not be exaggerated. On many wards, especially those for chronic patients, hospital life continued much as it had before. However, psychotherapeutic practices and initiatives were held in high regard, and they attracted a lot of attention, energy, money and personnel who had a mind for the renewal of psychiatric treatment. In many psychiatric hospitals, one or two wards were transformed into therapeutic communities – this happened, for instance, at Conolly. Moreover, both inside and outside psychiatric hospitals, separate crisis intervention units were created.

In all these progressive new wards, the 'medical model' was criticized and replaced by a 'social model' of madness. Psychiatrist Jan Prins, head of treatment at Conolly, explained the difference between the two models as follows.

Madness and Autonomy

'The traditional way of thinking [in psychiatry] is: "Pete is acting crazy because he has an illness." This is the easiest viewpoint, both for Pete himself and for his family, neighbours, and those who treat him. Pete is not held responsible for his actions: pathological impulses and thoughts make him act the way he does. His parents are not "guilty" either. Everyone can wash their hands in innocence. According to the social model, however, everyone should accept responsibility for his or her own actions. Pete's parents, or his wife, should realize that their behaviour influenced that of their son or husband. Pete himself had to face the fact that, in the end, he was the one giving shape to his own life.'[12]

A central theme in the new 'social model', as it was defined both at Conolly and elsewhere, was the emphasis on self-determination and the personal responsibility of the client. In the words of the psychiatrist Peter van den Hout, head of a therapeutic community in the south of Holland, all psychiatric problems were in fact 'forms of resistance, meant to escape or repress problems of living and the pain of life.'[13] The goal of therapy at his therapeutic community, at Conolly and elsewhere, was to break through this resistance to 'change' and to point out to the clients that they were responsible for their own mental health. A woman who was in a therapeutic community during the 1970s remembers: 'The view of the psychiatrists and nurses working there was that a psychosis is an escape from reality. As a patient, you were the one who had to change, since other people wouldn't. That was the slogan.' In her experience, the goal of group therapy was to 'break people down, make you mad or scared, ridicule you a bit, and then see what you would do. To provoke a crisis, and then when the emotions come out, make you realize how you feel and behave.'[14] Another former client of a therapeutic community stated in retrospect that the leading principle of personal responsibility was so strictly followed that clients were regularly severely neglected.[15] One woman, looking back on the therapeutic community where she was treated during the 1970s, called it a 're-education camp'.[16]

The therapeutic climate of the 1970s thus contained a strong, albeit often implicit, moral agenda. The ideal was to change the clients and their family members into emotionally mature, independent, open and honest individuals who did not play 'games', but instead took responsibility for their own choices in life. This ideal, however, created a difficult paradox for the therapists and nurses working in therapeutic communities or crisis centres. In the anti-authoritarian 1970s, taking a directive attitude could easily lead to accusations of being paternalistic or arrogant. So therapists were torn between the urge to cure their clients and re-educate them on the one hand, and the ideal to not put pressure on people and let the clients heal themselves on the other hand.

A scene from a Dutch film called *Kind van de zon* (1975; *Child of the sun*) is revealing about this struggle. In one scene – which was based on real events and used real-life psychiatrists as actors – a patient, Anna, breaks down in group therapy. When she finally finishes crying, the therapists asks her quietly, but with a pressing undertone: 'Well, it is very beautiful that this has all come out now. But it would also be great if you could talk to us a bit now; if you could tell us something about you and your parents.' Sometimes clients were stimulated to talk about their feelings in a more direct way. At Conolly, residents were rewarded when they showed a willingness to co-operate with the psychotherapeutic programme and were punished if they did not. They got derogatory remarks from the therapists and nurses – in one extreme case, a client who remained impassive and refused to change was called a 'weak arse-hole'. Others were refused permission to go outside during the day or to go home during the weekends, until they had started talking or writing down their feelings.[7]

Psychiatry in Debate

Why did this attack on the medical model and the accompanying psychotherapeutic optimism become so widespread on the 'shop floor' of Dutch clinical psychiatry during the 1970s? One reason was that the attack did not yet have the unscientific, radical, unsound image it has today. Within the scientific culture in Dutch psychiatry of the 1970s, the ideas of Laing, Foudraine and others were seen by many as very legitimate. Influential professors of psychiatry such as Kees Trimbos and Piet Kuiper openly sympathised with the criticism of the medical model. Furthermore, psychiatric advisors working for the Dutch government invited Laing to give a lecture on family therapy and conduct a workshop for Dutch therapists and social workers, which he did in 1965.[8]

Psychotherapy was quite dominant in Dutch psychiatry in general during the 1960s and 1970s. Psychoanalytic journals and organisations had existed from the 1920s onwards, and after the Second World War, the influence of psychoanalysis grew fast. By the middle of the 1960s, many Dutch professors of psychiatry and other leading psychiatrists were psychoanalysts, and psychoanalytic thinking and jargon were widespread. Moreover, from the 1950s onwards, many new forms of psychotherapy like group therapy, Rogerian psychotherapy, Gestalt therapy and family therapy were introduced. In many ways, these new forms of therapy were different from classical analysis. They focused less on early childhood and sexual desires and more on the importance of human relationships and communication in the 'here-and-now'. Also, these new forms were more suitable for use in a clinical setting. Outside psychiatric hospitals, psychotherapy was booming from the late 1960s onwards, for instance in a rapidly rising number of institutions for medical psychotherapy.

The 1972 spring meeting of the Dutch Psychiatric Association was dedicated to the theme of 'psychiatry in debate', which gave rise to heated arguments about the nature of mental illness and the value of medication versus psychotherapy. Finally in 1974, the Dutch Association for Psychiatry & Neurology was officially split in two. During the 1970s, a psychotherapeutic orientation came to dominate Dutch psychiatry, judging for example by the themes of the articles published in the *Tijdschrift voor Psychiatry (Journal of Psychiatry)*. In fact, in 1975, this leading psychiatric journal nearly fused with the *Tijdschrift voor Psychotherapie (Journal of Psychotherapy)*. This was the wish of the psychiatrists, but the editorial board of the *Tijdschrift voor Psychotherapie* refused – they were afraid of becoming 'contaminated' with psychiatry.

Another background for the attack on the medical model was the growing unease of psychiatrists and nurses with medication and the fact that biological psychiatry, as a separate field of theory and research, was still in its infancy. During the 1950s, enthusiasm about the new anti-psychotic and anti-depressive forms of treatment had prevailed. Psychiatrists, nurses and family members were stunned to see how confused and delusional people became approachable. The use of force was necessary less often. An old ideal in clinical psychiatry – to send patients home again as soon as possible – suddenly seemed more achievable than ever before. Social-psychiatric services blossomed during the 1950s and 1960s.

However, the success of this 'bio-social' approach of psychiatric care was hindered by the disadvantages of the new forms of medication, which came to be discussed extensively in the Netherlands during the 1960s. First of all, there were the many physical side-effects, like parkinsonism, weight gain or loss of libido. Not only were these very hard for the patients to deal with, they caused new problems for the nurses as well. They were faced with a problematic new task: convincing patients to take their medication in spite of these disadvantages. Thus, the new pills became a new source of tension between nurses and patients. On top of this, there was a shortage of nursing personnel in many of the Dutch psychiatric hospital during the 1950s. Some hospital directors explicitly stated that because of this shortage, patients were given more medication than strictly necessary.

Possibly, as Edward Shorter argues, 'the advent of effective new medications for psychosis and neurosis [...] induced a certain insouciance toward the patient's need to feel cared for'.[19] In any case, the need of psychiatrists, nurses, and psychologists to have more emotional contact with their patients was strongly put forward from the late 1950s onwards. And vice versa as well; during the 1970s, several ex-patients wrote books in which they complained about the lack of personal attention paid to them by their psychiatrists.

Meanwhile, the legitimisation of the use of psychopharmaceuticals was not yet very strong. Not much was known about their specific workings. What did they do in the brain and in the body? Biological psychiatry as we know it today, with its own journals, conferences, university chairs, theoretical framework and jargon, was still in its early stages.[20] Influential theories concerning the role of neurotransmitters like dopamine in schizophrenia and monoamine in mood disorders were not formulated until the middle of the 1960s. From that time onwards, special units for biological psychiatric research were founded in the Netherlands, as well as university chairs. By 1970, however, biological psychiatry in the Netherlands was still much less established than psychoanalysis and other forms of psychotherapy.

The strong optimism radiated by proponents of intensive psychotherapy, the therapeutic community, or family therapy – some of whom even claimed to be able to cure schizophrenia – was eagerly received by many people working in mental health care. Many of them had grown frustrated during the 1950s and 1960s with 'revolving door-psychiatry'. The social-psychiatric approach did not result in an emptying of psychiatric hospitals, but rather in a change of the pattern of admissions. Admissions did grow shorter, but they also became more frequent. As one critic put it in 1970, he was tired of patching up soldiers (read: patients) before sending them back to the front (read: Western society), only to see them soon back in the hospital, wounded again.[21] The criticism of the medical model, as expressed by Laing and others, thus had much to offer those working in clinical psychiatry: therapeutic optimism and new hope, as well as a means to achieve a more personal relationship with patients.

On a more practical level, psychotherapy and the democratic organisation of the therapeutic community offered an ideal opportunity for ambitious psychologists and psychiatric nurses to become therapists. Many nurses at the time longed for more interesting work than cleaning the wards, handing out medication, and regulating daily life on the ward. Many psychologists were tired of conducting psychological tests. And last but not least, psychotherapeutic experiments were made possible around 1970 by an explosive growth of money and personnel in psychiatric hospitals. In Brinkgreven, for example, the number of nurses doubled between 1964 and 1974; elsewhere, a similar explosion of personnel took place. Moreover, governmental funding for clinical psychiatry tripled between 1963 and 1970.[22]

A Psychologisation of Ethics

However, people working in mental health care during the 1970s were not just influenced by these internal processes within clinical psychiatry. The popularity of psychotherapy and the 'social model' of madness were also a result of cultural changes. To use a phrase of the English professor of sociology Nicolas Rose, during the late 1960s and 1970s a 'psychologisation of ethics' took place in the Netherlands.[23] Quite suddenly around 1970, books written by psychiatrists and psychologists like Laing, Szasz, Foudraine, Erich Fromm, Rogers, and the

Madness and Autonomy

transactional analyst Thomas Harris became bestsellers. Apart from promoting psychotherapy and emotional openness as beneficial to human happiness and tolerance between people, all of them vehemently attacked Christianity, presenting it as an obstruction to personal growth. They also turned against capitalism and traditional social hierarchies, while defending individual freedom and self-realization.

The sudden popularity of these anti-psychiatrists and psychotherapists can be explained, I believe, by the fact that many Dutch people around 1970 were looking for a new set of values to justify their rapidly changing lives. As the Netherlands quickly became more prosperous during the 1960s, fundamental changes in lifestyle were taking place. Divorce became more common, and birth rates were dropping. Religious institutions lost much of their respect and following. The political Katholic Party (KVP), for example, still had 260,000 members in 1965, but only 120,000 were left in 1968.[24] The churches emptied, and belief in God and Christian values diminished. Although certainly not all Dutchmen became atheists, many started to consider religious belief a personal matter.[25] In politics, left-wing parties got a lot of support. The Dutch Socialist Party (PvdA) won the elections of 1973, while smaller and more radicalist 'green' or Marxist parties gained popularity. New social movements aimed at environmental issues or at the emancipation of women or homosexuals abounded.

As a survey from 1970 shows, many Dutchmen had by then distanced themselves from traditional values like obedience, hard work and decent behaviour.[26] Generally speaking, Dutch people started to place more priority on 'post-materialist' values like quality of life and well-being, individual freedom, and self-expression.[27] As the historian James Kennedy concludes, from the 1960s onwards, a revolution in morals was taking place in the Netherlands.[28]

New and secular morals were found, for example, in the ideas of psychotherapists. One central element in their moral agenda was the notion of man as essentially a free agent – an autonomous being naturally directed towards 'self-actualisation'. According to Erich Fromm, the main pathogenic element in Western society was that man had been robbed of the awareness of this basic inner freedom and of his own responsibility for his life and well-being. A lot would change for the better, Thomas Szasz agreed, if people would start taking responsibility for their own lives and actions.[29]

Although many of these authors strongly criticized authority, between the lines, their own writings read like a programme for a moral re-education of the Western citizen. The words they used are significant. People in the West supposedly felt 'small' and 'dependent', or were portrayed as if they were in a 'regressed' or 'childish' state of being. They should become more independent, self-assured, and 'mature' – they should grow up. The 'ideal' state of man was expressed very clearly, for instance, in a book which combined transactional analysis and Gestalt therapy, called *Born to win*.[30] The losers in life, according to this, are those who are scared of their autonomy, and who go through life hiding their true selves behind a mask. Winners, on the other hand, do accept responsibility for their own life; they know their own feelings and opinions, and do not let others determine or bind them. They are respectful to others and know how to listen, but go their own way. They are flexible and spontaneous. Their autonomy allows them furthermore to have equal and truly intimate contact with other people.

Conclusion

Anti-psychiatry in the Netherlands was not a pessimistic call for the abolition of the whole psychiatric enterprise. In fact, it was quite the contrary: an extremely optimistic reform movement aimed at an intensification of psychiatric treatment, using various forms of psychotherapy, and regarding the psychological breakdown as a possible breakthrough. Ironically, though, this optimistic reform movement itself became a new and sometimes oppressive regime, with a strong moral agenda. Critics such as Laing and Foudraine attacked Western psychiatry for its implicit morality, arguing that psychiatrists were the guardians of the established social order. Paradoxically, the result of their critical psychiatry on the shopfloor of psychiatric hospitals – at least as it was picked up by many people in the Netherlands – itself led to a very moralistic therapeutic climate.

The personal liberation of psychiatrists, psychologists and psychiatric nurses often went hand in hand with their efforts to emancipate psychiatric patients. As they themselves were breaking away from the values and lifestyle of their patients and exploring their feelings in psychotherapy, they believed patients could benefit from the same process. Thus, the revolution in morals which was taking place in Holland at the time was clearly reflected in the movement to reform psychiatric treatment.

Ever since the beginning of the psychiatric enterprise, therapists have tried to instil certain contemporary ideals of citizenship through their care of patients. Educational and therapeutic values have always been closely intertwined. For a long time, starting in the era of moral treatment during the first half of the nineteenth century, this ideal of citizenship was based on the then current bourgeois-Christian values such as moderation, calmness, self-denial and self-control.[31] In the 1970s, following the ideas of anti-psychiatrists and other psychotherapists, a new and psychological ideal of citizenship was formulated: one based on traditional humanistic values such as autonomy, human solidarity and personal responsibility, combined with a new call for openness, spontaneity and honesty. During the 1970s, psychiatric nurses and psychotherapists tried to raise their clients to become emotionally 'mature' individuals. In this sense, the anti-psychiatric period was but a new phase in psychiatry's long-standing tradition of a moral re-education of patients.

Madness and Autonomy

The therapeutic optimism of the 1970s clearly had some negative side-effects. Many parents of patients – mostly their mothers – felt like they were being blamed for the illness of their children. During the 1980s, they started to protest against this situation and tell their stories in books and in the media. Patients sometimes suffered from anti-psychiatry as well, when they were neglected, denied medication, or scoffed at for not co-operating with psychotherapy and 'changing' themselves. However, the psychotherapeutic optimism of the 1970s also had positive effects. Many patients, then and now, feel like they benefited from intensive psychotherapy. The criticism of the 1970s stimulated the awareness of therapists and nurses of the need to treat patients with respect and to pay attention to their personal biography and social situation. Moreover, partly as a result of the 'social model' of the 1970s, the family of patients is involved in psychiatric treatment nowadays much more than they were before – although psychotic disorders such as schizophrenia are now not considered functional any longer. Finally, in clinical psychiatry, the collaboration between psychiatrists, psychologists and psychiatric nurses has become much more equal. In short, like all periods of therapeutic optimism in the history of psychiatry, the period of anti-psychiatry also has both known excesses and led to a positive legacy.

Notes

1.   The case of Piet (a fictional name) is based on an analysis of his patient file and is described in more detail in my dissertation: G. Blok, *Baas in eigen brein. 'Anti-psychiatrie' in Nederland, 1965-1985* (Amsterdam: Nieuwezijds, 2004).
2.   R.D. Laing, *Het verdeelde zelf. Een existentiële studie in gezondheid en waanzin* (Meppel: Boom, 1969; Dutch translation of *The divided self*, 1960), 164.
3.   On this first 'anti-psychiatric' period, see: I. Dowbiggin, *Inheriting Madness. Professionalisation and Psychiatric Knowledge in Nineteenth Century France* (Berkeley: University of California Press, 1991), 76-93; A. Goldberg, 'The Mellage Trial and the Politics of the Insane Asylums in Wilhelmine Germany', *The Journal of Modern History*, 74 (2002), 1-32; G. Grob, *The Mad Among Us. A History of the Care of America's Mentally Ill* (New York: Free Press, 1994), 129-38; N. Reisby, 'The Anti-Psychiatry Debate of the 1890's, *Acta Psychiatrica Scandinavica*, 15 (1975), suppl. 261, 14-21; H.P. Schmiedebach, 'Eine "antipsychiatrische Bewegung" um die Jahrhundertwende', in M. Dinges (ed.), *Medizinkritische Bewegungen im Deutschen Reich (ca. 1870-ca. 1933)* (Stuttgart: Steiner, 1996), 127-59.
4.   See, for instance: C. Jones, 'Raising the Anti', in M. Gijswijt-Hofstra and R. Porter (eds), *Cultures of Psychiatry and Mental Health Care in Postwar Britain and the Netherlands* (Atlanta & Amsterdam: Rodopi, 1998), 283-95; R. Isaac, *Madness in the Streets. How Psychiatry and the Law Abandoned the Mentally Ill* (New York: Free Press, 1990).
5.   E. Shorter, *A History of Psychiatry. From the Era of the Asylum to the Age of Prozac* (New York: Wiley, 1997), 275.

6. Blok, *op. cit.* (note 1), 14.

7. On the Dutch 'anti-psychiatrist' Jan Foudraine, see: G.Blok, '"Messiah of the Schizophrenics": Jan Foudraine and Antipsychiatry in the Netherlands', in Gijswijt-Hofstra and Porter (eds), *op. cit.* (note 2), 151-69.

8. Blok, *op. cit.* (note 1), 65.

9. On the history of neo-Freudian thought and family therapy, see: E. Dolnick, *Madness on the Couch. Blaming the Victim in the Hey-Day of Psychoanalysis* (New York: Simon and Schuster, 1998).

10. Sartre quoted in D. Burston, *The Wing of Madness. The Life and Work of R.D. Laing* (Cambridge, MA/London: Harvard University Press, 1996), 62.

11. Sartre quoted in D. Jopling, 'Antipsychiatry in Sartre's "The Family Idiot"', *Review of Existential Psychology and Psychiatry*, 19 (1984-1985), 161-87: 163.

12. B. Boersma, G. van Florestein, R. Muller and J. Prins, *Conolly 1969-1976. Ervaringen met systeemtheoretische en gezins therapeutische behandeling in een intramurale situatie* (Deventer: Psychiatrisch Ziekenhuis Brinkgreven, 1977).

13. P. Van den Hout quoted in G. Blok and J. Vijselaar (eds), *De weg van Welterhof. Vijfentwintig jaar psychiatrie in Oostelijk Zuid-Limburg* (Utrecht: Matrijs, 1999), 71.

14. Quote from an interview with Ad Barendregt, conducted by journalist Michiel Louter. This interview will be published in 2005, in Louter's forthcoming book on the history of Dutch clinical psychiatry as experienced by its clients.

15. W. de Graaf in M. van der Kerkhof, 'Kritische psychiaters of toch bittertafel revolutionairen?', *Psy. Tijdschrift over geestelijke gezondheidszorg*, 8 (20 Febr. 2004), 22-6: 25.

16. Blok, *op. cit.* (note 1), 137.

17. *Ibid.*, 55-103.

18. *Ibid.*, 61.

19. Shorter, *op. cit.* (note 3), 273.

20. D. Healy, *The Creation of Psychopharmacology* (Cambridge, Mass./London: Harvard University Press, 2002).

21. Blok, *op. cit.* (note 1), 155.

22. *Ibid.*, 113.

23. N. Rose, 'Assembling the Modern Self', in R. Porter (ed.), *Rewriting the Self. Histories from the Renaissance to the Present* (London: Routledge, 1997), 224-49: 246.

24. P. de Rooy, *Republiek van rivaliteiten. Nederland sinds 1813* (Amsterdam: Mets & Schilt, 2002), 249.

25. *Ibid.*, 238-9.

26. J. Kloek and K. Tilmans (eds), *Burger. Een geschiedenis van het begrip 'burger' in de Nederlanden van de middeleeuwen tot de 21e eeuw* (Amsterdam: Amsterdam University Press, 2002) 342-3.

27. R. Inglehart, *Modernization and Postmodernization. Cultural, Economic and Political Change in 43 Societies* (Princeton: Princeton University Press, 1997), 360.

28. James C. Kennedy, *Nieuw Babylon in aanbouw. Nederland in de jaren zestig* (Amsterdam: Boom, 1995), 101.

29. J. Pols, *Mythe en macht. Over de kritische psychiatrie van Thomas Szasz* (Nijmegen: SUN, 1984), 86.

30.   M. James and D. Jongeward, *Born to Win. Transactional Analysis with Gestalt Experiments* (Reading, MA: Addison-Wesley, 1971).

31.   See: Anne Digby, *Madness, Morality and Medicine: A Study of the York Retreat, 1796-1914* (Cambridge: Cambridge University Press, 1985); J. Vijselaar, 'Zeden, zelf-beheersing en genezing (1849-1884)', in J. Vijselaar (ed.), *Gesticht in de duinen. De geschiedenis van de provinciale psychiatrische ziekenhuizen van Noord-Holland van 1849 tot 1994* (Hilversum: Verloren, 1997), 41-74: 49.

CHAPTER 4

Psychiatry and the State in Britain

Hugh Freeman

The focus of this paper is on the relationship between the British state and the mentally ill, primarily in the second half of the twentieth century. To a large extent, this is the story of the National Health Service – the NHS. This relationship with the state has inevitably involved politics – but generally not party politics, along the usual left-right dimension.

Origins

Until the 1940s, the British state did not acknowledge responsibility for providing general health care to the population. In the early modern period, the functions of the national government, embodied in the Sovereign, were very few. Everything else was a local responsibility, controlled by the lay magistrates in each county and major borough, who represented the elite of each area. They were both the judicial and the executive authorities. The counties were divided into parishes, which formed the basic organisation of the established Church of England. It was only in the 1880s that elected local government began in the counties. In the later nineteenth century, the responsibilities of the national government did enlarge gradually, but not yet to the extent of supplying health or welfare services directly.

In 1601, almost at the end of the reign of Elizabeth I, a comprehensive Poor Law was enacted. It was economic difficulties at the end of the sixteenth century, including substantial unemployment, that are said to have been largely responsible for this Elizabethan Poor Law. The unemployment was a fairly new phenomenon, and it produced the category of indigents known then as 'sturdy beggars'. These people – mostly men – were mentally and physically capable of work, but had no employment. Through the Poor Law, they could then be given relief from local funds, but only in their 'parish of settlement'. The parish could also support local people who were not capable of working, whether for bodily or mental reasons. The geographical responsibility for a local population that was then given to the parishes is a theme that will run through much of the subsequent story. It was, in fact, a form of 'community care'.

In the eighteenth century, the expansion of Britain's trade and wealth led to the evolution of a bourgeois, civil society which was largely independent of aristocratic patronage. This new society, much influenced by evangelical and Dissenting religious groups such as the Quakers and Unitarians, took up a number of humanitarian causes. One of these was to establish charitable general hospitals, which were constructed in practically every large provincial town. The primary clientele of these institutions were people who were physically ill, but in many cases, a 'lunatick ward' or annexe for the mentally ill was added to the hospital. At Manchester Royal Infirmary – where I was both a student and a house surgeon – the annexe grew to be almost as large as the main hospital. There were also three charitable hospitals wholly for the mentally ill – Bethlem and St Luke's in London and St Patrick's in Dublin.

But for reasons which so far remain unexplained, all these psychiatric additions to voluntary general hospitals had ceased to exist by the early nineteenth century.[1] It may have been that the particular problems of caring for the mentally ill were simply too different from what the hospitals saw as their primary task – caring for medical and surgical cases. Hardly any of their doctors specialised in the care of mental illness. Had this closing of psychiatric annexes not happened, the whole subsequent history of mental health care in Britain would have been quite different.

All this took place purely on a charitable basis, without any involvement of the state or of local government. But about the same time, another development was happening, though for commercial reasons – what William Parry-Jones called 'The trade in lunacy'.[2] These private madhouses were run for profit, and varied in size from a few people taken into the home of a doctor or clergyman to quite a large institution.

It was this development, in fact, which first provoked the active intervention of the state as a regulator of mental health care. Where money was involved, abuses were likely – particularly in the largely ungoverned world of the eighteenth century. As a result, Parliament passed several Acts to try and prevent the exploitation of the mentally ill by these entrepreneurs.[3] These laws had very little effect, though, because the administrative structure needed to enforce them simply didn't exist then. But on the basis of the general humanitarian concern of that period, the care of the mentally ill had become acceptable as a legitimate subject for the involvement of the state. This feeling was increased by the psychotic illnesses of King George III, which were a threat to the whole stability of the government. For the same reasons, treatment of the mentally disordered by deliberate cruelty had ceased to be an acceptable practice by this time, largely through general cultural and intellectual changes associated with the Enlightenment.

It would be wrong, though, to omit from the Georgian period a description of its most important voluntary initiative – the establishment by the Quakers of their mental hospital known as The Retreat at York.[4] In an unpublished lecture,

Leon Eisenberg has pointed out that every therapeutic use in psychiatry of the milieu in the subsequent two centuries has really been a rediscovery of the 'Moral Treatment' that was developed at The Retreat. This principle – which was the opposite of much previous practice – was to provide a quiet, supportive and encouraging environment in which natural recovery could occur. Moral Treatment was the inspiration for the non-restraint movement in early nineteenth century English mental hospitals, and even for the Therapeutic Community of the 1940s. The Retreat's methods were based on a shared religious ideology between staff and patients – a principle which Michel Foucault notably failed to understand.[5]

The first hesitant step towards publicly provided – rather than charitable – mental health care was an Act of Parliament of 1808. This was a permissive law, which allowed counties to establish asylums through their local property taxes, known as 'rates'. The Act did not actually require them to do *anything*, though, and most of them did nothing, in some cases claiming that there were 'no lunatics' within their boundaries. The real importance of this legislation was in establishing the principle that public funds could be used to provide a form of health care in hospitals.

The mid-nineteenth century, though, is the crucial period in this account. One of the changes of that time may seem at first to have nothing to do directly with the care of the mentally ill. The Elizabethan Poor Law had provided relief mainly in the form of money given to destitute people at home. But with a rapidly growing and more urbanised population, these payments caused a steadily increasing burden on the local rates. Since that growth of local taxation alarmed the wealthier classes, in 1834, the Poor Law Amendment Act tried to control this cost by providing relief only in institutions – the workhouses.

A workhouse was built for each group of parishes, known as a 'Union', and the geographical responsibility for a population that began with the Elizabethan Poor Law still continued. The capital investment that constructed workhouses in every part of the British Isles in the mid-nineteenth century now seems enormous, particularly as it was all done from local funds. Compared with the lack of hospital building a century later, the contrast is striking.

The Amendment Act was a utilitarian solution to the need that was felt for reducing the costs of poor relief. Conditions in workhouses were required to be 'less eligible' – which means worse – than those which a poorly paid labourer would experience outside. But the people who flooded into the workhouses were not 'sturdy beggars', who should have been working. They were mostly orphaned children, abandoned mothers, frail old people, and the sick and disabled of every kind – including the mentally ill. They could not be deterred from entering by bad conditions.

Ten years later, an even more important step was the Lunacy Act of 1845, passed through the initiative of the great reformer, Lord Shaftesbury. This required every county or group of counties to provide an asylum for the insane from its own locally raised funds. Every asylum had to have a medical officer, and this was the beginning of the psychiatric profession, though they were really general practitioners then. Except for a few private patients, all residents of asylums were classified as 'paupers'. In this way, the Poor Law system and the asylum system were closely involved with each other. The procedures for admission to an asylum were regulated by law, and a national inspectorate was set up for these institutions, as it was for the Poor Law. These two inspectorates were the first examples of direct government intervention in local responsibilities. Paradoxically, the asylums followed a humanitarian agenda, while the workhouses had a primarily utilitarian, financial purpose, so that the two could sometimes be at cross-purposes. There is no evidence to support the Marxist view that the purpose of the asylums was simply to remove unproductive people from society.[6] It is clear that the patients admitted were severely ill and that their relatives had done as much as they could.

Once the asylums existed, mentally ill residents of workhouses were supposed to be transferred to hospital care. But the Guardians of the Poor had to pay more for a patient in an asylum than for a resident of a workhouse. As a result, the Poor Law authorities resisted making these transfers. The consequent mix-up between the mentally ill, needing medical care, and the indigent, who needed social care, was not resolved until a century later; since then, that problem has re-occurred.

In the workhouses, the proportion of residents who were ill or decrepit grew so large that these institutions were becoming like hospitals. Poor Law Guardians responded to this situation by building their own hospitals, known as Union Infirmaries. This development began in the 1860s and continued so that, eventually, these infirmaries were provided in every major centre of population. The particular relevance of this development to the present theme is that when the NHS began in 1948, the largest proportion of hospital beds that it took over then were in the former Poor Law infirmaries.

Also, because a proportion of admissions to the infirmaries were mentally ill, most of these institutions included a special observation unit for these cases. If such individuals settled down quickly, they would be discharged, but otherwise, they would be transferred to an asylum. Sometimes, though, neither of these disposals happened, and the patients simply remained in what was called the 'mental block'. From the 1950s, many of these facilities developed into general hospital psychiatric units.

While all this was going on under the Poor Law, the asylum system was extending throughout the British Isles, and the mental institutions were becoming much larger. Admission rates, though, didn't change much, allowing for the growth in population. Why the resident numbers in asylums increased so much is an important question in itself. Torrey & Miller have argued that schizophrenia was a new disease in the early nineteenth century, and that its frequency in the population then increased steadily.[7] What is certain is that a high proportion of the patients in asylums were also physically ill – from disease, malnutrition, or alcohol. Much of the mental illness there had an organic basis, particularly tertiary syphilis, so that the medical work in asylums was still largely general practice. At the same time, there were many mentally ill paupers still in work-houses, who had not been transferred to asylums for financial reasons; this factor complicates estimates of the total numbers of people suffering from severe mental illness.

The organisation and culture of the mental hospitals – similar to that in other industrialised countries – then existed largely unchanged for almost a century. But one innovation which was very significant for the future occurred in 1874. The national government decided to pay counties a small weekly subsidy for every pauper patient in their asylums. This was the first time that any payment had been made from central taxation for any health or welfare purpose. Just why this happened has not so far been well explained.

Political considerations became important again in 1890, when another Lunacy Act made it more difficult for patients to be admitted to asylums. The new law required the agreement of a magistrate, except in emergencies; it was the result of a long campaign by pressure groups, who alleged that sane people were being illegally confined in asylums. There was little evidence for this view, and they were mainly playing on atavistic fears in the public's mind. Asylums were now required to observe a mass of legal restrictions, which were a major barrier to progress. Though the medical superintendent had a powerful role within the institution, individuals outside decided who should be admitted, and the budget was controlled by local politicians in the county or city.

In the twentieth century, the highest ever recorded rate of mental hospitalisation in relation to population was in 1915. World War I then produced a huge number of psychiatric casualties, described as suffering from 'shellshock'.[8] This phenomenon upset psychiatric orthodoxy, by discrediting theories of 'degeneration' as the cause of mental illness. It also encouraged some acceptance of Freudian theory, but the long-term effects of the war on mental health care in Britain were in fact surprisingly small. Within a few years, mental hospitals were functioning much the same as before 1914, though malarial treatment for tertiary syphilis and continuous narcosis were introduced as the first specific therapies. An *exposé* by one medical officer of poor conditions in a mental hospital in Manchester attracted some attention, but political and public interest in the subject was only brief.[9] Outside the public system, a few small institutions such as the Cassel Hospital and Tavistock Clinic provided psychotherapy on a charitable basis, but the numbers of patients involved in this were very few. The Ministry of Pensions established some patient clinics for veterans with psychiatric disabilities, which offered a form of psychotherapy; little has been recorded about these

Psychiatry and the State in Britain

facilities, and they did not last for more than a few years. Some voluntary hospitals in cities established a psychiatric outpatient clinic, usually staffed by psychiatrists in private practice, who were few in number nationally. The number of patients seen must have been very small, though there are few reliable records of these activities.

The general point made above that political differences did not follow party lines was not entirely true. The brief Labour government of 1924 set up a Royal Commission to examine the law on mental illness. Its report was very progressive, but nothing happened then until 1930, when the second Labour government passed the Mental Treatment Act. This had two important provisions – it provided for voluntary admission to mental hospitals, and it allowed their medical staff to see psychiatric outpatients at other hospitals. This indicated the beginning of a retreat from the custodial and authoritarian principles that had governed both the asylums and the Poor Law during the previous century. This government also abolished the Poor Law and brought its functions under the control of local government – a symbolically important step in reducing stigma.

My examination of government records from the 1930s about these new outpatient clinics has not revealed very much as to what went on in them.[10] There is little doubt, though, that this outpatient work was all on a very modest scale. Compared with the USA at that time, psychiatry in British general hospitals hardly existed at all. In the few years before the war began in 1939, new physical treatments were just beginning to be introduced, and refugee psychiatrists from Europe played a very useful part in this.[11] Academic psychiatry was also in its infancy, and virtually nothing would have happened but for the practical support of the Rockefeller Foundation.[12]

'Social Psychiatry' in this period was no more than a few small voluntary initiatives, again owing much to American help. The first Child Guidance Clinics were established, and the first psychiatric social workers (PSWs) were trained, in very small numbers; in both cases, the theoretical orientation of their work was derived from psycho-analysis. A few psycho-analysts were in private practice – almost all in London. The Mental After-Care Association provided some convalescent homes, and there was also one for ex-servicemen. Local government was responsible for the care of the mentally retarded, helped by some voluntary societies. Just before World War II, a number of voluntary welfare bodies combined to form the National Association for Mental Health (NAMH), which provided casework and educational services. All this took place in almost complete isolation from the mental hospitals.

However, by far the most significant event in this whole story was the establishment of the National Health Service in 1948. Attempts to reorganise general health care in Britain between the two World Wars had achieved relatively little, partly as a result of the world economic Depression, and partly because the political and cultural climate was strongly conservative.

Once war began, though, the whole political atmosphere changed, particularly after Churchill formed his coalition government with Labour in 1940. To cope with wartime needs, an Emergency Medical Service had been set up, financed by the central government, which was an addition to the existing hospitals. Its experience showed that medical services could be run by the state, and not just by the existing local governments or by voluntary (charitable) hospitals. The general idea of a national health service was accepted in principle as early as 1942, and lengthy discussions about it went on behind closed doors. These were held between representatives of the doctors – mainly the British Medical Association (BMA) – and staff of the Ministry of Health. There was no attempt to consult the public about this.

This whole situation was enlivened in late 1942 by the appearance of the Beveridge Report on social security, which set out the basic structure of a postwar welfare state. Going far beyond his terms of reference, Sir William Beveridge created a vision of a better society, in which free and comprehensive health care would be one of the fundamental rights of its citizens. His big failure, though, was calculating the financial projections for this development in a completely wrong way; that mistake had an unfortunate influence for many years to come. What he clearly understood, though, was that the different aspects of health and welfare services were closely related to each other; they couldn't be developed in isolation. People had often gone into mental hospitals for social reasons, rather than for medical and nursing care. But these needs could now be provided outside the hospitals by other services which were more appropriate. The Beveridge Report stirred up enormous public interest, as a result of which the government was obliged to respond to it in a generally favourable way.

Early plans for the NHS left out the mental hospitals. The rationale for this omission was that the administrative and legal arrangements of mental institutions were so different from those of general hospitals that the two couldn't be fitted within a single system.[13] To change these peculiar arrangements of the mental hospitals would have needed legislation, and this was impossible in wartime.

However, the BMA argued strongly against this separation. From long experience, they were opposed to any hospitals being run by local government, as the mental hospitals were then. The BMA wanted all hospitals to be independent of local government, with its political influences, and their arguments were successful. This was a critical point, because a continued separation between the two kinds of hospitals would almost certainly have prevented much of the progress that occurred in later years. A separate mental hospital system from the NHS general hospitals would inevitably have been an inferior one – as experience world-wide has shown. It would have inhibited the growth of psychiatry in general hospitals and would have made it difficult for staff to operate between different parts of the mental health service.

By the end of the war, both main parties were publicly committed to the principle of the NHS, but the Conservatives had a much more modest idea of what it should be like. What happened next would depend on the result of the 1945 general election. This was won by Labour, and the new Minister of Health was Aneurin Bevan, a major political figure on the left of the party. His responsibilities also included housing and local government, so that he played an important role in the Cabinet, and in the evolution of the Welfare State.

In spite of all the wartime discussions, plans to set up the NHS remained extremely vague in 1945 and 1946, apart from the decision to include the mental hospitals. Bevan described the separation of mental from physical care as 'a source of endless cruelty and neglect'.[14] The principles of the NHS were to be very important for the future management of psychiatric disorders, providing care that was free and comprehensive for all patients.

Bevan made a bold decision to nationalise all the hospitals in the UK, apart from a few small private ones. This provoked relatively little argument in the end, compared with the arrangements for general practice, where bitter disputes were settled only just before the NHS was due to start. All referrals to specialists were now to go through GPs, and patients were not to go directly to hospitals, except in emergencies. This was a 'filter', which had the effect of reducing the pressure on specialist services, including psychiatry.[15] Of all the hospital beds in the country, nearly half – 44 per cent – were in mental illness or mental retardation hospitals in 1948. A high proportion of their patients were then chronic or long-stay.

In NHS general hospitals, medical superintendents, where they existed, were now abolished. Instead, the arrangements of the voluntary teaching hospitals were introduced everywhere. All the medical consultants formed a committee, which decided the hospital's medical policy collectively. Its practical implementation, as well as that of the policy of the nursing staff, was then the responsibility of the Hospital Secretary or Administrator. There was thus a tripartite arrangement, rather than a hierarchical one. Before 1948, the voluntary hospital consultants were not paid for their hospital work, deriving their income from private practice, but now they received a salary – usually on a part-time basis.

The Ministry of Health controlled the NHS through 14 Regional Hospital Boards (RHB), each related to a university with a medical school. In turn, the RHB supervised groups of hospitals, each under a Hospital Management Committee (HMC). Mental hospitals, though, were not part of a group, like the rest, but each had its own HMC. Mental hospitals were mostly much larger than general hospital groups, and this was one of the ways in which the psychiatric institutions still remained different.

Although hospital medical directors in general hospitals were abolished, the law still required every mental hospital to have a medical superintendent. However, some senior doctors in mental hospitals were also designated now as consultant psychiatrists, and under the NHS, they were supposed to be completely autonomous clinically, like consultants in general hospitals. How this impasse of responsibility was resolved depended on the influence of local personalities in each hospital. But as time went on, consultant psychiatrists became increasingly rebellious about the role of the medical superintendent.

After the end of the war, the demand for admission to mental hospitals grew rapidly, and in most cases, people came in as voluntary patients. Over the next 20 years, total admissions increased nearly ten times, and first admissions trebled in number.[16] The growth in admissions was seen then as a positive trend, since it was believed to be better for patients to be admitted at an earlier stage of their illness. From about the mid-1950s, though, this view of hospitalisation was completely reversed, and *reducing* admissions was seen – not always logically – to be the main criterion of success.

However, because of the greater acceptability of mental hospitals to the public at this time, serious overcrowding resulted. There had been no new building or redevelopment of hospitals during the war, and even repairs had been neglected. Living conditions for patients were generally poor, and there were serious shortages of staff. Full employment nationally then meant that it was relatively easy for mental nurses to earn more in other jobs. Psychiatrists were also in short supply, but on the positive side, ECT had come into general use and many schizophrenic patients were being treated with insulin coma. Though this latter treatment was eventually found to have no specific therapeutic effect, it encouraged a more active and optimistic regime in mental hospitals.[17]

Overcrowding in mental hospital wards now became a big problem for the Ministry of Health, which had taken over these hospitals from local governments. For about ten years after the end of the war, there continued to be practically no building of new hospitals. Public housing and schools were given the greatest priority for capital spending, while total investment was limited by the country's critical economic situation and by the effects of the Korean war. But why hospital building in Britain should have been so minimal for so long is a political question that is still unanswered.

One medical event of the late 1940s which was surprisingly important here was the treatment of tuberculosis. Between the wars, special sanatoria and clinics for this condition had developed in the UK on quite a large scale, mostly run by local governments. But there were never enough beds available in them, and just after the war, waiting lists of tuberculous patients for admission to sanatoria represented a major health problem. In 1948, though, streptomycin was discovered in America, and within a surprisingly short time, the need for hospital beds for tuberculosis got rapidly less. Far from building new accommodation for these patients, the Ministry of Health was now reducing beds and then closing them down.

In my research on the subject, I found that the example of tuberculosis made a big impression on senior medical figures in the Ministry.[18] I believe that it affected their view of the very large number of beds then occupied by patients with mental illness – 154,000 in 1954. Yet in spite of the size of inpatient provision, direct public expenditure on mental health amounted to less than 0.2 per cent of the Gross National Product, because the cost of each inpatient was relatively low.[19] Outpatient services, which did not need much accommodation, grew rapidly, and the treatment of outpatients with ECT made a big contribution to the care of major depression. Patients also began to be visited at home by both psychiatrists and social workers; PSWs were appointed to the staff of mental hospitals, though the number trained each year remained small for some years.

However, politics cannot be forgotten for long. Bevan had been outstandingly successful in establishing the NHS, in spite of the enormous upheaval involved. Within the government, though, his political position was diverging strongly from that of the central figures – Clement Attlee, Ernest Bevin, and Herbert Morrison. In 1950, he was moved to a lesser position – Minister of Labour – and responsibility for housing and local government was separated from the Ministry of Health. The new Minister of Health was not in the Cabinet, and so the NHS moved sharply downwards in the political agenda. Another consequence was that the new Ministry, which was quite small, would be avoided by the more able and ambitious civil servants – which would also reduce its influence in the competition for resources.

Meanwhile, the very misleading financial estimate made earlier by Beveridge, with the prediction that the cost of the NHS would actually *fall* after a few years, began to have unfortunate effects. When the cost of health care proved to be much more than had been budgeted, and when it increased year by year, instead of falling, there was panic in the government. This was quite irrational, since the total cost was actually quite low, compared with similar industrialised countries, and from the administrative point of view, the NHS was extremely cheap. But thinking in the Treasury didn't change much over the next 50 years. They went on insisting that 'demand' for health care was too high and that the only real problem was the public's 'perception' of what needed to be provided. In fact, it was the Treasury whose perception was wrong, and they confused 'demand' with need.

At this time, one of the ways in which the UK differed from both Continental Europe and the USA was the almost complete failure of academic psychiatry to take root. There was one university chair in London, and one in Edinburgh, but hardly anything at other medical schools. The London chair was based at the Maudsley Hospital, which had opened in 1925 as a psychiatric unit outside the restrictions of the Lunacy Acts. Systematic teaching was developed there, as well as some research, while the same developments occurred, on a smaller scale, at the Royal Edinburgh Hospital. Why there should have been such a difference from, say, Munich or Paris or Baltimore has never been well explained. In the Netherlands, a much smaller country than the UK, there were six chairs of psychiatry at this time. Most doctors working in British psychiatry simply picked up their working knowledge in mental hospitals on the old apprenticeship system. There was a Diploma in Psychiatry, but it was considered very inferior to the higher qualifications in medicine or surgery.

An organisation of doctors working in mental hospitals had been started in 1841, but a century later, when it had become the Royal Medico-Psychological Association, it was still quite small and had little influence. The two most powerful bodies in British specialist medicine – the Royal Colleges of Physicians and of Surgeons in London – were opposed to the growth of new specialist organisations. The Physicians believed that in so far as psychiatry had any right to be represented to the government, this should be done through their College.

Frankly speaking, the standard of doctors working in mental hospitals then was generally low, though it had been improved by the arrival of refugee psychiatrists from Europe and by others who had been rapidly trained by the Army during World War II. These two categories of specialists had not grown up professionally within the culture of mental hospitals and were more resistant to its authoritarian habits. Whereas the NHS had a surplus of trained physicians and surgeons for the available consultant posts, it was desperately short of competent psychiatrists as well as of other specialists such as anaesthetists and pathologists. At the end of 1949, there were only 405 consultant psychiatrists in England and Wales, whereas the planned number – still very modest – was 670.[20]

One very positive factor, though, from the medical point of view was that through the NHS, the psychiatric profession remained united. In many countries, particularly the USA, most trained psychiatrists worked exclusively in private practice, leaving the public mental hospitals with few competent doctors. In Britain, hardly any specialists stayed completely outside the NHS. In fact, a part-time appointment as a hospital consultant was virtually a *sine qua non* for a doctor to be recognised as a specialist. So Bevan's compromise, leaving consultants with a large degree of freedom, prevented a split between those working in the public hospitals and specialists seeing only private patients. Had this not been the case, the development of a significant psychiatric profession within the NHS would hardly have been possible.

Changes of the 1950s

For about ten years after the end of World War II, there was little sign of significant change in mental health care. Outpatient ECT, offered mostly at general hospitals, was the first effective treatment that did not require admission to hospital, and a few experimental day hospitals showed the possibility of a more flexible kind of care.[21] Practically all psychiatric accommodation then dated from before 1910. The total number of patients resident in mental hospitals increased every year up to 1954. But from then on, it reduced year by year, as it did in the USA, though not in other countries. There was no change in national policy on health at this time, but there was a change in the *zeitgeist* of society, with large institutions becoming less desirable as a response to society's problems.[22] This suggests that the steady reduction in the role of mental hospitals within the general provision of psychiatric care, occurring over the next four decades, had a primarily ideological basis. It included an explosion of new ideas – broadly described as 'social psychiatry' – which originated to a major extent in the UK.

In 1952, however, there was an important therapeutic development – the discovery in France of the first neuroleptic, chlorpromazine. Since then, opinions have been divided as to how much the neuroleptics contributed to the steady decline in the numbers of mental hospital residents. Writers hostile to conventional psychiatry have claimed that the drugs made little difference, but this seems quite illogical. Together with outpatient ECT, the neuroleptics made it possible, for the first time, to treat severe psychiatric disorders in a wide variety of settings: outpatient clinics, day hospitals, hostels and general practice. That must inevitably have reduced the numbers in hospital. Another factor operating in the same direction was the steady growth of treatment and care on a day basis, for those who did not need full-time medical and nursing provision. By 1959, there were 65 such units in the UK, mostly for the adult mentally ill.[23]

In 1954, the Conservative Prime Minister appointed a second Royal Commission to examine the law on mental illness and mental deficiency. It is not at all clear, though, why the government decided to take this step at that particular time. The Ministry of Health had been having some trouble over the compulsory detention of a few people diagnosed as 'mentally deficient', and this may possibly have been the provoking factor.

It was also in the mid-1950s that official reports on the mental hospitals in the NHS began to change their language. References to overcrowding disappeared, and the possibility of alternative ways of managing psychiatric disorders began to be mentioned. Within a few years, the phrase 'community care' was to be seen for the first time. When new hospital building was being considered again, the Ministry made it clear to the regions that they would not agree to the construction of any new mental hospital. Yet even though mental hospitals had then been the foundation of mental health care for over a century, this reversal of policy was never announced publicly. I have been unable to find any document in the government archives stating that such a decision had ever been made.

In 1959, the government was truly conservative in having very little legislation in mind. They filled the gap by embodying the report of the second Royal Commission in a Mental Health Act. This swept away a whole jungle of legislation on lunacy, some of it going back for centuries. People could now go into any hospital for psychiatric treatment, with or without compulsion. Magistrates were removed from the compulsory admission process, which was now to be undertaken only by doctors, assisted by social workers. Voluntary admission was abolished and psychiatric patients would be managed legally in exactly the same way as medical or surgical cases – described as 'informally'.

The results were dramatic in that within a year or so, the proportion of psychiatric patients who were compulsorily resident in hospital had fallen to only 7 per cent. Before 1930 it had been 100 per cent. It has often been said that the 1959 Mental Health Act legislated a policy of community care, but in fact this was not so. The Royal Commission had recommended that local health authorities – counties and cities – should be given a positive duty to provide community care services, and that they should receive specific government grants for doing so. But the Treasury fought successfully against these proposals, and it managed to delay special community care funds for 30 years. The Mental Health Act did in fact remove any legal barriers to community care, and it expressed general approval of a non-institutional approach. But that was all. The local health authorities had had their hospitals removed from their ownership by the NHS in 1948, but they were still responsible for employing mental health social workers, who were mostly untrained then.

While all this was happening, an important development was going on in Lancashire, in the north-west of England.[24] A group of influential specialists in Manchester – none of whom had previously been involved in psychiatry – decided that the mental hospitals in the region had become obsolete. With the very small amounts of money available for developments, they created a number of local services for medium-sized towns which had autonomous local governments. Each was headed then by only one consultant psychiatrist and was based in the 'mental block' of a former Poor Law infirmary. One of the units had as many as 220 beds, but these were mostly filled by patients with chronic psychoses.[25] The population served by each unit was 200,000 – 250,000.

The new district consultants were given access to beds in the nearest mental hospital, but to everyone's surprise, they made practically no use of these facilities. By close co-operation with the local health authority and the general practitioners, they were able to run an efficient service for their catchment population. The administrative autonomy of consultants in the NHS allowed for such experiments in the provision of services, provided that many new resources were not needed. The service provided was, of course, a fairly basic one, but it did respond to the needs of the most serious cases – particularly of schizophrenia. Though not many people recognised it at the time, this was the basic model on which future mental health policy would be based.

Developments of the 1960s

In 1961, I became a consultant for the city of Salford, next to Manchester.[26] Here, circumstances were rather different from the other cities because the 'mental block' of the former Poor Law infirmary had been completely destroyed by a bomb in 1940. Only a few beds could be obtained for psychiatry in the two general hospitals, and so most of the inpatient accommodation had to be in the nearest mental hospital. However, an autonomous unit was developed there, and its work was integrated with that of the general hospitals and community services. The fundamental principle was to make all staff involved feel part of a single organisation, wherever they were based. In this way, the wasteful and often hostile processes of negotiation and bargaining over matters such as admission to hospital could be largely eliminated. The individual patient still remained the responsibility of the same team, wherever this person was. An important principle of these developments was that the hospital unit was part of the comprehensive service.

On the political side, following the Conservatives' return to office in 1951, there had been six successive Ministers of Health in the subsequent nine years. None of them made much impression until Enoch Powell came into office in 1960. Like Bevan, Powell was a highly intelligent and articulate politician, though at the opposite end of the political spectrum. He saw an analysis of total mental hospital patients for the five years following the peak total in 1954. This showed a steady downward slope in resident numbers, and if that was projected onwards, it theoretically reached nil in 1975.[27] He concluded that the size of mental hospitals would have to be drastically reduced. This was not a value judgement; it was simply a response to what seemed an inevitable trend.[28]

Powell also produced the first national plan for general hospitals.[29] From the psychiatric point of view, the most important part of this plan was that it included psychiatry as one of the basic specialties of the district general hospital (DGH). So as the mental hospitals would be declining, a new network of general hospital psychiatric units would be evolving. For the first time, day care was given a specific role in the planning of psychiatric services. It has been argued that the biggest motive for this change was financial – that the cost of bringing the mental hospitals up to date would have been prohibitive. My research has been unable to find any evidence for this view. In any case, the cost of building a new system of psychiatric units could hardly have been less than that of modernising the mental hospitals. One of the biggest problems of the mental hospitals was that, a century or so after their foundation, most were in the wrong place to act as the centre of a district psychiatric service. In London, they were mainly in the outer suburbs, far from the population they served. The 1962 Hospital Plan also assumed that psychiatry ought to be in the district general hospital, so that it could co-operate with the other major specialties. At the time, this was still a fairly revolutionary concept, however, there was still very little capital for building new hospitals.

While this was going on in the UK, there were big developments in the USA, where the national plan for comprehensive community mental health centres was inaugurated in 1963. But 'community mental health', as it was understood there, was very different from 'community psychiatry', as it was developing in Britain. The former was a very broad concept which assumed that early intervention in the crises of individual lives would prevent the later development of mental illness. The British approach was to provide an integrated service for identified psychiatric disorders, related to local communities. Freeman & Bennett described it as an 'eclectic, non-ideological, and largely atheoretical discipline [...] open to and capable of absorbing ideas or data from any school, provided that these are found pragmatically to be capable of reducing disease, distress, or disability'.[30] I believe it is true to say that the British model has stood the test of time much better than the American one. Yet the official commitment in Britain to 'community care' of psychiatric disorders, which gradually emerged, was not supported by the necessary central funds.

In the 1960s, the *practical* question of *where* a patient should be cared for at any particular time began to be changed by anti-psychiatry into a *moral* question. All hospital care was then labelled as 'oppressive', and reducing admissions rather than providing the most appropriate care for a person at any particular time became a principal objective. In fact, through the 'Cultural Revolution' of the 1960s, the psychiatric profession in Britain then faced attacks on the whole legitimacy of its discipline. The most prominent figure in this confrontation was R.D. Laing, a psychiatrist himself.[31] Though he was for some time the most famous psychiatrist in the world, this did not last, and his long-term influence on provision for mental health turned out to be small. The *événements* of the 1960s, though, made it clear that the power of the mass media was a new factor that professionals would have to be aware of.

Two other critical questions emerged in Britain over the course of time. Firstly, could *all* the functions of the mental hospital – including the care of chronically ill patients – be reproduced by a 'dispersed institution'? This would have to include management of the small proportion of psychiatric patients who showed severely disturbed behaviour. Secondly, would there ever be enough money to provide effective community-based services throughout the country?

Logically, the mental hospitals should have been starved of resources, to help pay for new services. Yet in fact, the 25 years from 1960 were the best period they ever had in Britain. Following a series of public scandals – most of which con-

　　　　　　　　　　　　　Psychiatry and the State in Britain

cerned psycho-geriatric or mentally retarded patients – successive governments became very sensitive about conditions in these institutions. As total numbers fell, the living conditions of patients were enormously improved, staffing ratios increased, the quality of the psychiatric profession was enhanced, and a whole series of psychiatric sub-specialties developed services of their own.

These sub-specialties were: psycho-geriatrics, forensic psychiatry, rehabilitation, liaison psychiatry, child and adolescent psychiatry, and substance abuse. Without the accommodation and space that mental hospitals could provide, it is very unlikely that these developments could have occurred. As well as psychiatrists, nurses, social workers and psychologists also developed similar specialist skills. The most important of these groups were community psychiatric nurses (CPNS); their profession constituted a particularly British contribution to psychiatric care. In a typically British way, this innovation was never planned but grew out of informal experiments at several hospitals in the late 1960s. Formal training in community work for registered mental nurses developed during the next decade. In 1985, there was a ratio of about one CPN to 24,000 of the population, but with wide regional variations.[32] By the 1990s, CPNS had become an essential element in community-based psychiatric services, taking over much of the supervisory work that social workers had undertaken with patients at home. This was because a 'generic' unification of social workers in 1971 largely destroyed the skills developed by specialised groups such as PSWS and the Mental Welfare Officers of local authority health departments. Where these staff had been integrated into mental health services, the integration often came to an end. As Kathleen Jones pointed out, the 'integration' of social work meant the *dis*integration of mental health services.[33]

Social Psychiatry

At this point, it is worth considering the place of 'social psychiatry' in the evolution of British mental health services up to the 1960s. There have been varying definitions of this phrase – as there have been of 'community psychiatry' – but such semantic arguments are best avoided. In the UK, the views taken of the subject were essentially practical, induced mainly from clinical experience, rather than deduced from some theoretical principle. In this, professionals in the mental health field were largely following a tradition that had long been influential in British politics and administration.

First of all, it came to be accepted that social factors were very important both in the evolution of psychiatric disorders and in their management. Such views were then unusual in the rest of medicine, except for public health, but that specialty had gone into decline as infectious diseases became less important. Child guidance (which evolved into child and adolescent psychiatry) was the first aspect of the psychiatric discipline to focus on family and environmental influences.[34] Its initial Freudian orientation, however, was modified in the UK by a more clinical approach, which would later give birth to scientific child psychiatry. In adult psychiatry, the importance of housing conditions began to be recognised even before World War II; when the NHS began, home visits by both psychiatrists and social workers (then mostly untrained) made mental health staff constantly aware of the influences of everyday life.[35] In this, they were following the tradition of British general practice, which was heavily focused on domiciliary work. The fact that Britain in the mid-twentieth century was the most urbanised country in the world may well have been relevant to this tradition. From the late 1950s, research into the family environment of schizophrenic patients, begun by Morris Carstairs and George Brown at the Maudsley Hospital, was to lead over more than 30 years to important scientific and clinical developments.

Secondly – and probably more important in the long run – was the emergence of a whole range of clinical initiatives, which first modified and then eliminated the previously monolithic structure of mental hospital practice. As mentioned earlier, it began in 1930 with voluntary admission and outpatient consultations. After World War II, the process continued with extramural ECT and rapidly growing outpatient consultations, which began to extend into general hospitals. By the early 1950s, 'part-time hospitalisation' had emerged in the form of the first day hospitals. During the War, military hospitals had been the setting for the early development of 'therapeutic communities', and their principles influenced institutions of all kinds, particularly mental hospitals.[36]

There, attention to the social environment and to institutional habits led to a climate of liberalisation, in which patients were encouraged to make the most of their capacities for normal living. A leader in this development was Dr D.H. Clark at Cambridge, who described it as 'Administrative Psychiatry' because all the resources of the hospital were co-ordinated in the process of rehabilitation.[37] Weekend leave became common, family visiting was encouraged, and patients increasingly went outside hospital for recreation or even work. As a result, many long-stay patients were found not to need the permanent medical and nursing care of a hospital, though they were not yet ready for independent life outside. To fill this gap, a variety of forms of 'sheltered accommodation' were developed – staffed hostels, unstaffed group homes, supervised lodgings in private homes, and individual apartments with visiting staff. For some time, it was assumed that these residents would eventually graduate to independent living, but as experience accumulated, it became clear that a significant number would need some degree of shelter permanently. That lesson was not popular with administrators and funders.

These different forms of accommodation could be seen as a 'ladder', which people moved up towards independence, as they improved. But equally important was the question of occupation. Occupational therapy had arrived in the UK

Psychiatry and the State in Britain

from Germany, via the Netherlands, in the 1920s; it only ever served a minority of mental hospital patients, though. After the War, the idea arose that actual work was more therapeutic than mere occupation; it also allowed patients to earn some money. Although there was a national system of rehabilitation units and sheltered workshops, these overwhelmingly served the physically handicapped. Within psychiatry, therefore, a new movement of 'industrial therapy' brought workshops into the hospitals, mainly undertaking sub-contract work for industry. The leading figure in this was Dr Donal Early of Bristol.[38] He emphasized that a second 'ladder' of work was needed, in collaboration with that for accommodation. This consisted of a series of increasingly complex tasks; patients would move on to a more difficult one, as their condition improved. Until the mid-1970s, the volume of economic activity in the UK allowed many people with psychiatric problems to be usefully employed.

One further aspect of the social approach was public education. As in other countries, prejudice, ignorance and feelings of rejection towards the mentally ill were common in the UK. The NAMH and other voluntary bodies did their best to combat this antagonism, emphasising how much had changed in the mental health services. These efforts had only modest success, though in the late 1950s, there were some useful television programmes. In the next decade, however, things were to get much worse with the emergence of anti-psychiatry, often linked with political extremism. The film 'Family Life' was a notable expression of these views; it made a big impression on the British public, encouraging the view that parents and 'capitalism' were the causes of schizophrenia.

From today's standpoint, it may seem surprising that all these 'social' approaches were conceived and introduced on an entirely intra-professional basis, with psychiatrists taking the leading roles. As with the negotiations leading to the NHS, there was virtually no involvement with other influential groups. Voluntary organisations and most politicians saw it as their role to support the professionals, not to undermine them. Yet the psychiatrists who achieved all these changes would soon be denounced as 'reactionary' and practising 'social control'. In Britain and other West European countries, Marxism became dominant in both the universities and the media, establishing a form of academic totalitarianism. This particularly affected the training of social workers, whose numbers were growing rapidly. Amongst other developments, the word 'social' would become hijacked to suit a Marxist paradigm. This involved a denial of the reality of mental illness and its treatment that has remained influential.

A Mental Health Policy?

At various points, one could have asked the question – is there a national mental health policy? – and the answer would have been uncertain. But in 1975, an official white paper was published which clearly set out such a policy.[39] Preparation of it had been started several years before, under a Conservative government, but by the time it was actually published, Labour was again in office. At this period, differences between the two main parties on health policy were relatively small, and for all its faults and deficiencies, the NHS was enormously popular with the public. This national mental health policy laid down a provision of inpatient beds at the rate of 0.5 per 1,000 of the population; most psychiatrists regarded this as too low, but with the passage of time, political and financial pressures were to reduce it further.

During this period, there had been very considerable growth in the numbers and quality of the psychiatric profession. The inauguration of the Royal College of Psychiatrists in 1971 symbolised that the specialty had come of age.[40] Medical superintendents were finally abolished in mental hospitals, though 20 or 30 years later, the role was to be reinvented in a changed NHS. Academic psychiatry finally expanded to serve every medical school, and research activity increased enormously.[41]

The run-down of mental hospital numbers up to then had been relatively easy. Only the least ill or disabled long-stay patients were resettled outside – in hostels, group homes or even independent accommodation. Their medical care was transferred to local GPs, and they were reviewed periodically in psychiatric outpatient clinics, with occasional visits from a CPN. Their financial support came from Social Security. By 1981, the number of occupied psychiatric beds had fallen from a peak of 3.4 per thousand in 1954 to 1.58 per thousand.[42]

But as this process went on, the level of morbidity among the remaining patients in mental hospitals steadily increased. At the same time, the new general hospital services were having to be paid for, and there were managerial complaints that as long as the mental hospitals still existed, very little money could be saved. It was said that although 80 per cent of the patients were in the community, 80 per cent of the money was being spent on hospitals. Yet the question I raised above – could *all* the functions of the mental hospital be reproduced in other ways? – was still largely unanswered. While British psychiatry had by now grown into a fairly large and well trained profession, the best one could say of community services was that they were patchy, though quite good in some places.

The answer to the second question was that although the rhetoric of community care had been officially spoken then for about 20 years, the money that it required had never existed in the budgets of the local authorities who were mainly responsible for it. It would have been reasonable to say that, up to then, 'community care' as a comprehensive national system was never much more than a shared myth.[43]

'No Such Thing as Society'

However, worse was to come. The year 1979 was a political watershed, with the return to office of the Conservatives under Mrs Thatcher. Their monetarist ideology, with the slogan that 'There is no such thing as society', was to cause profound economic, social and cultural changes. Whereas doctors had always been by far the most influential group in the planning and delivery of health services, they were quickly replaced by managers, some of whom had little knowledge of hospitals or health care. The multi-disciplinary management that had existed since the beginning of the N H S was now abolished and was replaced by a hierarchical system, directed by a Chief Executive. Both managers and politicians were very unwilling to face the reality of severe, chronic mental illness, because of the alarming cost implications of caring for these people in an acceptable way over a very long time. Two experiments to care for groups of them in a domestic environment – 'hospital hostels' – were very successful, but they were eventually closed down by managers, because of the cost of the trained staff they required.[44] This was one of the very few examples of a form of service provision being tested empirically, yet the clear results were ignored in the prevailing political climate.

In both the U K and the U S A, there had been big falls in the mental hospital population, but that in the U S A had been much more rapid and had been largely driven by financial motives. In the U K, it had always been accepted officially that mental hospital accommodation should not be closed until an adequate alternative was in place. But in the early 1980s, the Government made it clear that they wanted the process to be speeded up, so that mental hospitals could actually be closed and their buildings and land sold. At the same time, all hospitals were having their numbers of beds reduced because of financial pressures.

By 1982, the number of psychiatric hospitals with over 1,000 beds had fallen to 23, compared with 65 in 1972.[45] Total psychiatric beds in the U K were then 120,678, of which just over 11,000 were in general hospital units; compared with other West European countries, the provision of beds was lower, in relation to population, but that of qualified psychiatric nurses was the highest.

A long and detailed research study by the Medical Research Council of two mental hospitals in outer London showed that when there was plenty of time and money, most of the residual long-stay patients could be resettled outside. Most of them did well there and were happier than in hospital. But there was still nearly a fifth who had to be transferred to other hospitals, and government plans took no account of this group, known as the 'Difficult to Place' patients. Nor did the re-provision of beds allow for the new long-stay patients who would continue to accumulate indefinitely, in small numbers.[46] Furthermore, in most parts of the country, there was neither plenty of time nor plenty of money for the resettlement process, as there had been in this London scheme.

In 1983, with a new Mental Health Act, the lawyers had their revenge for the previous Act of 1959. More legal restrictions and bureaucracy were imposed in relation to compulsory admission or treatment, making the work of health professionals more difficult, and often having bad effects on patients. Once again, a vocal lobby had been successful, through an unholy political alliance of elements from both Left and Right.

What happened next was a return to the 'Trade in Lunacy' of 200 years earlier. Without any public discussion or even a public announcement, the NHS withdrew from providing long-term care, for either physically or mentally disabled patients. Instead, the social security system began to pay for these people to go into privately run nursing homes. In the case of patients with chronic mental illness, they were transferred into units that were similar to the hostels that had formerly been provided by local authority social services. In response to this unannounced change of policy, an enormous number of private institutions commenced business, mostly in large old houses.

Correspondingly, the long-stay accommodation in hospitals which was part of psychiatric and geriatric services was steadily reduced, so that the closure of mental hospitals became easier. Local authority social services had the responsibility of inspecting these new private homes regularly, but they often lacked the resources to do this effectively. If they wanted to close a home because the conditions were bad, there was nowhere that the residents could go: the hospital beds they came from had ceased to exist. Now, the question was raised whether these smaller units were simply re-creating the asylum in a new form. The Government claimed that the number of places for the mentally ill was no less than before, but a high proportion of these were now in small, private facilities which had no trained staff. This presented a much greater problem than before of monitoring their standards of care because of the vastly increased number of places in which patients were resident.

Nonetheless, in the decade between 1976 and 1986, the number of consultant psychiatrists increased by over one-third in England to a level of 3.1 per 100,000, although this was still much lower than in some other European countries.[47] However, the work of psychiatrists was now much more dispersed than it had been with the mental hospital system.

In 1993, local authority social services ceased to be providers of old people's homes or psychiatric hostels, and became simply the funders for private or charitable operators. For local authorities, it was a partial return to the situation before the Poor Law Amendment Act of 1834, when they simply subsidised poor people in the community. Psycho-geriatric services which had integrated hospital facilities with social services accommodation often found their arrangements disintegrating.

Even acute psychiatry, which was supposed to remain entirely within the NHS, was unable to function fully, because managers had closed down so many

beds. By the end of 1993, 89 of the 130 mental hospitals that were open in England in 1953 had closed, and the total number of psychiatric beds had fallen to a
little over 50,000.[48] This was to keep within unreal financial targets. In the five
years from 1996, nearly 10 per cent of all acute psychiatric beds were closed
– nearly always against psychiatric advice. As a consequence, private beds often
had to be used – at enormous cost to the NHS; this was particularly true for
patients requiring secure accommodation.

One of the strengths of the NHS had been that it did not have to collect money
or charge for transactions between different units within it. This advantage was
thrown away, and a huge accounting system set up by the Conservative 'Internal
market'. The cost of this and of endless administrative changes was enormous,
but this financial burden was concealed from the public, and the full amount is
still not known. Yet this and the endless bureaucracy it created was described as
'reform'. The NHS had succeeded to a significant extent because of the idealism
and commitment of those who worked in it, most of whom were badly paid.
Now, the change in culture and habits of thought that percolated down from the
government included a contempt for these feelings, for the ideal of public service, and for the expertise of health professionals. The only thing that mattered
now was money.

With the great reduction in psychiatric beds, there was a decentralisation of
the mental health services. Many of these now operated from small centres,
which had no accommodation for inpatients. This made them more accessible
geographically for patients and often more acceptable than a large institution.
On the other hand, it partly removed psychiatrists and other staff from the district general hospital, which is the focus of all other specialist health care. Yet the
move of psychiatric inpatient work into general hospitals, which had seemed to
be such a sign of progress, was now raising serious doubts. Acute psychiatric
wards in general hospitals were often proving unable to provide the therapeutic
milieu which was supposed to be their main purpose. Accommodation was
unsatisfactory, staffing was inadequate, and a high proportion of beds tended to
be occupied by patients who really needed either more secure accommodation
or its opposite – a more domestic setting. General social changes – which included widespread drug abuse, extreme cultural diversity, and a loss of respect
for health professionals – added to the problems of general hospital units, particularly in inner cities.

In a return to the 1940s and 1950s, overcrowding re-emerged as a regular
feature of psychiatric units. It was partly due to ill-considered reductions in beds
by managers and partly to the presence of patients waiting to go to other accommodation that would have been more suitable for them, such as a secure unit.
In London particularly, wards occupancy levels of 120 per cent were regularly
recorded. Deteriorating morale was seen in 14 per cent of posts for consultant
psychiatrists being unfilled in England, though this situation was better in

Scotland. The recently introduced European Directive which restricts the working hours of junior doctors is likely to make the staffing of general hospital units increasingly difficult.

At the fiftieth anniversary of the NHS in 1998, a Labour government was again in office, but one so committed to financial orthodoxy that it was unwilling for some years to deal with the large gap between Britain and other West European countries in spending on health. More than anything, the NHS needed a period of quiet and consolidation, but it was about to be put through yet another enormous administrative upheaval in 2002, for uncertain reasons. The main unit of administration for health services, with the budgetary power to commission services, was now the Primary Care Trust, consisting mainly of representative general practitioners. Hospitals and some community services had become independent NHS Trusts, having to obtain their funds from the new PCTs which are more numerous (and so more costly) than the former District Health Authorities. Regional Health Authorities had first been abolished and then re-created as Strategic Authorities. It was all more confusing than ever, and the costs of reorganisation were again immense (though unpublished).

When the NHS began, there was full employment, addiction to dangerous drugs was unknown, serious crime was uncommon, there was relative cultural homogeneity, and health professionals received general respect from the public. In the succeeding 50 years, every one of these conditions changed totally. Psychiatry has had to accommodate to this changed world as well as it can. Whether it can succeed in today's economic and social climate remains to be seen.

Notes

1.   R. Mayou, 'The history of general hospital psychiatry', *British Journal of Psychiatry*, 155 (1989), 764-76.
2.   W.L. Parry-Jones, *The Trade in Lunacy* (London: Routledge & Kegan Paul, 1972).
3.   K. Jones, *A History of the Mental Health Services* (London: Routledge & Kegan Paul, 1972).
4.   A. Digby, *Madness, Morality & Medicine* (Cambridge: Cambridge University Press, 1985).
5.   M. Foucault, *Madness & Civilization* (translation R. Howard) (London: Tavistock, 1967).
6.   A. Scull, *Decarceration: Community Treatment and the Deviant, a Radical View* (New Jersey: Prentice Hall, 1967).
7.   E.F. Torrey and J. Miller, *The Invisible Plague* (New Brunswick, N.J.: Rutgers University Press, 2002).
8.   B. Shephard, *A War of Nerves* (London: Jonathan Cape, 2000).
9.   M. Lomax, *The Experiences of an Asylum Doctor, with Suggestions for Asylum and Lunacy Law Reform* (London: George Allen & Unwin, 1921).

10. H.L. Freeman and D.H. Bennett, 'Origins and development', in D.H. Bennett and H.L. Freeman (eds), *Community Psychiatry* (London: Churchill Livingstone, 1991), 40-70.

11. U.H. Peters, 'The emigration of German psychiatrists to Britain', in H.L. Freeman and G.E. Berrios (eds), *150 Years of British Psychiatry: The Aftermath* (London: Athlone Press, 1996), 565-80.

12. K. Angel, E. Jones and M. Neve, 'European Psychiatry on the Eve of War', *Medical History*, Suppl. 22 (2003).

13. C. Webster, *The Health Services Since the War*, Vol I (London: Her Majesty's Stationery Office, 1988).

14. A. Bevan, *Aneurin Bevan on the National Health Service* (Oxford: Wellcome Unit for the History of Medicine, 1991).

15. D.P. Goldberg and P. Huxley, *Mental Illness in the Community* (London: Tavistock, 1980).

16. J. Raftery, 'The decline of the asylum or the poverty of the concept', in D. Tomlinson and J. Carrier (eds), *Asylum in the Community* (1996) (London: Routledge), 18-30.

17. B. Ackner, A. Harris and A.J. Oldham, 'Insulin treatment of schizophrenia: a controlled study', *Lancet*, 1 (1957), 607-9.

18. G.E. Godber, 'Interview with Hugh Freeman', in G. Wilkinson (ed.), *Talking About Psychiatry* (London: Gaskell, 1993), 145-56.

19. Ministry of Health, *Report for the Year Ending 31 December 1954* (London: Her Majesty's Stationery Office, 1955).

20. C. Webster, *The Health Services Since the War*, Vol I (London: Her Majesty's Stationery Office, 1988).

21. W.A.J. Farndale, *The Day Hospital Movement in Great Britain* (Oxford: Pergamon, 1960).

22. K. Jones, *Experience in Mental Health: Community Care and Social Policy* (London: Sage, 1988).

23. Farndale, *op. cit.* (note 21).

24. J.V. Pickstone, 'Psychiatry in district general hospital', in J.V. Pickstone (ed.), *Medical Innovations in Historical Perspective* (London: Macmillan, 1986), 247-61.

25. H.L. Freeman, 'Oldham & District Psychiatric Service', *Lancet*, i (1960), 218-21.

26. H.L. Freeman, 'Community mental health services: some general and practical considerations', *Comprehensive Psychiatry*, 4 (1963), 417-25.

27. G.C. Tooth and E.M. Brooke, 'Trends in the mental hospital population and their effect on future planning', *Lancet*, i (1961), 710-3.

28. J.E. Powell, 'In conversation with Hugh Freeman', *Psychiatric Bulletin*, 12 (1989), 402-6.

29. Department of Health & Social Security, *A Hospital Plan for England & Wales* (London: Her Majesty's Stationery Office, 1962).

30. Freeman and Bennett, *op. cit.* (note 10).

31. R.D. Laing and A. Esterson, *Sanity, Madness & the Family: Families of Schizophrenics* (London: Tavistock, 1964).

32.   J.W. Rowlinson and A.C. Brown, 'Community psychiatric nursing in Britain', in Bennett and Freeman (eds), *op. cit.* (note 10), 463-87.

33.   K. Jones, *Experience in Mental Health: Community Care and Social Policy* (London: Sage, 1988).

34.   C.J. Wardle, 'Historical influences on the development of services for child and adolescent psychiatry', *British Journal of Psychiatry*, 159 (1991), 53-68.

35.   S. Taylor, 'Suburban neurosis', *Lancet*, i (1938), 759-61.

36.   D.W. Millard, 'Maxwell Jones and the therapeutic community', in Freeman and Berrios (eds), *op. cit* (note 11), 581-604.

37.   D.H. Clark, *Administrative Psychiatry* (London: Tavistock, 1964).

38.   D.F. Early, 'Economic rehabilitation', in H.L. Freeman (ed.), *Psychiatric Hospital Care* (London: Bailliere, Tindall & Cassell, 1965), 176-87.

39.   Department of Health & Social Security, *Better Services for the Mentally Ill* (London: Her Majesty's Stationery Office, 1975).

40.   J.G. Howells, 'The establishment of the Royal College of Psychiatrists', in G.E. Berrios and H.L. Freeman, *150 Years of British Psychiatry* (London: Gaskell, 1991), 117-36.

41.   J.L. Crammer, 'Training and education in British Psychiatry 1770-1970', in Freeman and Berrios (eds), *op. cit.* (note 11), 209-42.

42.   J.K. Wing, 'The cycle of planning and evaluation', in G. Wilkinson and H.L. Freeman (eds), *The Provision of Mental Health Services in Britain: The Way Ahead* (London: Gaskell, 1986), 35-48.

43.   R. Titmuss, 'Community care, fact or fiction?', in *Emerging Patterns for the Mental Health Services and the Public* (London: National Association for Mental Health, 1961), 1-11.

44.   T. Wykes and J.K. Wing, 'A ward in a house: accommodation for 'new' long-stay patients', *Acta Psychiatrica Scandinavica*, 63 (1982), 315-30.

45.   H.L. Freeman, T. Fryers and J.H. Henderson, *Mental Health Services in Europe, Ten Years On* (Copenhagen: WHO, 1985).

46.   N. Trieman, J. Hughes and J. Leff, 'The TAPS project 42: the last to leave hospital', *Acta Psychiatrica Scandinavica*, 98 (1998), 354-9.

47.   Department of Health & Social Security, *Statistics of Mental Illness & Mental Handicap Hospitals in England* (London: Her Majesty's Stationery Office, 1986).

48. D. Kingdon and H.L. Freeman, 'Personnel options in the treatment of schizophrenia', in M. Moscarelli and N. Sartorius (eds), *The Economics of Schizophrenia* (Chichester: Wiley, 1995), 139-48.

CHAPTER 5

The Transformation of Mental Health Policy in Twentieth-Century America

Gerald N. Grob

Introduction

In mid-nineteenth century America, the asylum was widely regarded as the symbol of an enlightened and progressive nation that no longer ignored or mistreated its insane citizens. The justification for asylums appeared self-evident: they benefited the community, the family and the individual by offering effective medical treatment for acute cases and humane custodial care for chronic cases. In providing for the mentally ill, the state met its ethical and moral responsibilities and, at the same time, contributed to the general welfare by limiting, if not eliminating, the spread of disease and dependency.

After the Second World War, by way of contrast, the mental hospital began to be perceived as the vestigial remnant of a bygone age. In its place, advocates for change struggled to create a new community-oriented policy that ultimately resulted in what became known as de-institutionalisation. In this endeavour they were not alone; other nations pursued similar policies. Indeed, de-institutionalisation of persons with serious mental illnesses has seemingly become a fact of life. The decline in inpatient populations has been striking. Between 1955 and 2000 the number of patients in American public mental hospitals declined from a high of 558,000 to 55,000.[1] The decline is even more dramatic if the growth of the population is taken into account. Had the proportion remained stable and the mix of patients constant, mental hospitals would have had about 950,000 patients in 2000. Other nations experienced similar declines in hospital inpatient populations, although variability was characteristic.

Many have criticized the consequences of de-institutionalisation and insisted that it created disasters for those intended as its beneficiaries. Few, however, have demanded a return to an institutional-based policy. Yet the intent of de-institutionalisation as a policy has not always been clear. Indeed, over time it has come to imply quite different meanings. In its origin, at least in the United States, it was synonymous with the creation of a linked and integrated system of services that would follow patients from the hospital into the community. Subsequently,

it implied the end of institutional care. More recently, de-institutionalisation referred to barriers to long-term inpatient residence. Whatever its meaning, however, there is little doubt that the outcomes have had relatively little to do with the
original intentions and expectations. Although not necessarily a complete failure,
de-institutionalisation can hardly be characterized as a policy triumph.

What were the origins of de-institutionalisation and why did it fail to achieve
goals that, at least in theory, held out the promise of a better life for persons with
severe and chronic mental illnesses? The answer to this question is anything but
simple, particularly if national differences are taken into account. A careful examination of this policy (which affected individuals with physical and developmental disabilities as well) reveals sharp differences not only between nations,
but within national borders as well. In the United States, for example, there were
extraordinarily sharp variations between states: some reduced populations gradually; some built new hospitals or replaced older ones; and others closed down
their hospitals entirely. Many of these differences reflected unique regional contexts and traditions. On the international scene, the differences were equally varied. Italy closed its mental hospitals in precipitous fashion, whereas the pace of
de-institutionalisation in Germany, Belgium, the Netherlands and France was
slower and more modest in scope. Japan, by contrast, increased its hospital
population.

That there were common forces driving de-institutionalisation that transcended national boundaries is obvious. A variety of factors played a role in creating alternatives to the institutional care of persons with mental illnesses in many
nations: humanistic and egalitarian ideologies that were so common after the
Second World War (in part a response to the perceived war against totalitarian
regimes); the emphasis on environmental aetiologies in the social and behavioural sciences; the emergence of a literature that was critical of mental hospitals
(as well as other institutions) and their dehumanizing impact upon individuals;
the spiraling costs associated with improved hospital care; and radical critiques
of capitalist societies. Yet unique circumstances created significant differences
in the manner and also the timing in which de-institutionalisation was implemented. The experiences of the USA illustrate the importance of indigenous factors that gave rise to outcomes that often varied in the extreme.

Prelude to De-institutionalisation

The drive to reduce mental hospital populations that was characteristic of the
late twentieth century did not occur in a social vacuum; it was linked with earlier
developments. Of major significance was the change in the nature of the patient
population of mental hospitals after 1890. Between the 1830s and 1880s, the
proportion of long-term or chronic cases in hospitals was relatively low com-

pared with the extraordinarily high percentage between 1890 and 1950. Funding patterns played a key role in inhibiting the increase in chronic cases. Prior to 1890 fiscal responsibility for the care of persons with mental illnesses was divided between local communities and states. After 1890, however, many states – led by New York and Massachusetts – adopted legislation that relieved local communities of any role whatsoever in caring for persons with severe mental disorders. The assumption of those who favoured centralisation was that local care, although less expensive, was substandard and also fostered chronicity and dependency. Conversely, care and treatment in hospitals, though more costly initially, would in the long run be cheaper because it would enhance the odds of recovery for some and provide more humane care for others.[2]

Although the intent of state assumption of responsibility was to ensure that persons with mental illnesses would receive a higher quality of care and treatment, the consequences in actual practice turned out to be quite different. In brief, local officials saw in the new laws a golden opportunity to shift some of their financial obligations onto the state. The purpose of the legislation was self-evident, namely, to remove the care of chronically mentally ill persons from local jurisdictions. But local officials went beyond the intent of the law. Traditionally, nineteenth-century almshouses (which were supported and administered by local governments) served in part as old-age homes for senile and aged persons without any financial resources. The passage of state care acts provided local officials with an unexpected opportunity. They proceeded to redefine senility in psychiatric terms and thus began to transfer aged persons from local almshouses to state mental hospitals. Humanitarian concerns played a relatively minor role in this development; economic considerations were of paramount significance.[3]

Faced with an opportunity to shrink expenditures, communities were more than happy to transfer responsibility for their aged residents to state-supported facilities. Between 1880 and 1920, therefore, the almshouse populations (for this and other reasons) dropped precipitously. What occurred, however, was not a de-institutionalisation movement, but rather a lateral transfer of individuals from one institution to another.

During the first half of the twentieth century, as a result, the character of mental hospitals underwent a dramatic transformation. By 1904, only 27.8 per cent of the total patient population had been institutionalised for 12 months or less. Six years later this percentage fell to 12.7, although rising to 17.4 in 1923. The greatest change, however, came among patients hospitalized for five years or more. In 1904, 39.2 per cent of patients fell into this category; in 1910 and 1923 the respective percentages were 52.0 and 54.0.[4] Although data for the USA as a whole were unavailable after 1923, the experiences of Massachusetts are illustrative. By the 1930s nearly 80 per cent of its mental hospital beds were occupied by chronic patients.[5] Chronicity, however, is a somewhat misleading term, for the group that it described was actually heterogeneous. The aged (over 60 or 65) constituted by far the single largest component. As late as 1958, nearly a third of all resident state hospital patients were over 65.[6]

The increase in long-stay patients tended to reinforce the belief that hospitals were merely serving a custodial role. This belief was strengthened by both the Great Depression of the 1930s and the Second World War; both led to a fall in the quality of institutional care because of the decline in state appropriations in the 1930s and the loss of professional personnel during the war. Yet appearances were somewhat deceiving, for a substantial number of patients were discharged after relatively short hospital stays. In a study of more than 15,000 patients admitted for the first time to Warren State Hospital in Pennsylvania during the period from 1916 to 1950, Morton Kramer and his associates found marked improvements in the release rates of the cohorts of 1936-1945 and 1946-1950, as compared with those of 1916-1925 and 1926-1935. A comparison of the earliest and latest cohorts indicated that the probability of being released within a year of admission increased from 42 to 62 per cent. Subsequent studies revealed that the experiences of Warren State Hospital were by no means atypical, suggesting that some patients continued to benefit from hospitalisation.[7]

At the same time that the nature of the mental hospital resident population was changing, American psychiatry was undergoing a fundamental transformation. Between 1890 and 1940 psychiatrists began to look beyond the institutions in which their specialty had been conceived. Nineteenth-century psychiatrists had emphasized managerial and administrative issues, and in so doing had made the care of institutionalised patients their primary responsibility. Their twentieth-century successors, by contrast, were looking beyond the institutions which had for so long defined their specialty. The rise of modern 'scientific' medicine only strengthened their desire to create a new kind of psychiatry. Under such circumstances, it was understandable that psychiatrists between 1890 and the Second World War began to redefine concepts of mental disorders and therapeutic interventions, as well as the very context in which they practised. In so doing, they began to distance themselves from traditional mental hospitals which – unlike their nineteenth-century predecessors – had large numbers of chronic and especially aged patients whose need for general care was paramount. The effort to shift the foundations of psychiatric practice seemed appropriate in view of the widespread, if inaccurate, belief that scientific medicine was responsible for the decline in mortality from infectious diseases and the increase in life expectancy at birth. By identifying with general medicine, psychiatrists slowly began to shift the location of their practice from mental hospitals to outpatient facilities, child guidance clinics, and private practice.

Perhaps the most visible symbol of change was the creation of a mental hygiene movement after 1900. Reflecting a commitment to science, mental hygienists saw disease as a product of environmental, hereditary and individual

Mental Health Policy in Twentieth-Century America

deficiencies; its eradication required a fusion of scientific and administrative action. As members of a profession that they believed was destined to play an increasingly central role in the creation of a new social order, psychiatrists began to redefine their role. The emphasis on scientific research rather than care or custody, on disease rather than patients, and on alternatives to the traditional mental hospital was merely a beginning. More compelling was the utopian idea of a society structured in such a way as to maximise health and minimise disease. The founding of the National Committee for Mental Hygiene in 1909 was a visible symbol of change. The new psychiatry, insisted Dr. Thomas W. Salmon (its first medical director), had to reach beyond institutional walls and play a crucial part 'in the great movements for social betterment'. Psychiatrists could no longer limit their activities and responsibilities to the institutionalised mentally ill. On the contrary, they had to lead the way in research and policy formulation and to develop mechanisms to promote mental hygiene goals. Their responsibilities, he added, included the care of the feeble-minded, the control of alcoholism, the management of abnormal children, the treatment of criminals, the fostering of eugenics, and the prevention of crime, prostitution and dependency.[8]

The effort to define alternative career roles, however, did not create a specialty where consensus rather than conflict was characteristic of practice and theory. Some psychiatrists emphasized brain pathology; some insisted that bacterial infections in any part of the body could lead to mental illness; some centered their attention on the role of the endocrine system; and others emphasized the importance of understanding the manner in which the individual's life history shaped maladaptive traits that gave rise to mental disorders. Therapies were equally eclectic. By the 1930s malaria fever therapy, insulin and electric shock therapy, psychosurgery, and a variety of psychotherapies existed side by side. The absence of theoretical rationales for many therapies was by no means unrecognised. 'At present,' noted the authors of a leading text, 'we can only say that we are treating empirically disorders whose etiology is unknown with shock treatments whose action is also shrouded in mystery.'[9]

Winds of Change

In 1945 there was little evidence that the mental health scene would begin to undergo radical changes. At that time, the average daily resident population was about 430,000; approximately 85,000 were first-time admissions. Nearly 88 per cent of all patient care episodes occurred in mental hospitals; the remainder were located in general hospital psychiatric units. In 1951 total state expenditures for all current operations was $5 billion. Of this sum, 8 per cent was for mental hospitals. Some states expended as little as 2 per cent on mental health care; the largest (New York) one-third.[10]

Yet within a short time American mental hospitals slowly began to lose their social and medical legitimacy as the prevailing consensus on mental health policy dissolved. The experiences of the military during the war in successfully treating soldiers manifesting psychiatric symptoms and returning them to their units led to a faith that outpatient treatment in the community was more effective than confinement in remote institutions that shattered established social relationships. The war also hastened the emergence of psychodynamic and psychoanalytic psychiatry with its emphasis on the importance of life experiences and socio-environmental factors.[11] Taken together, these changes contributed to the belief that early intervention in the community would be effective in preventing subsequent hospitalisation and thus avoiding chronicity. Finally, the introduction of psychological and somatic therapies (including, but not limited to, psychotropic drugs) held out the promise of a more normal existence for persons with mental illnesses outside of institutions. As early as 1945 Robert H. Felix (who played a major role in postwar mental health policy) argued that psychiatry had an obligation to 'go out and find the people who need help – and that means, in their local communities'. Three years later he and R.V. Bowers insisted that mental hygiene had to be concerned 'with more than the psychoses and with more than hospitalized mental illness.' Personality, after all, was shaped by socio-environmental influences, and they explicitly alluded to wartime psychiatric experiences. Psychiatry, in collaboration with the social sciences, had to emphasize the problems of the 'ambulatory ill and the preambulatory ill (those whose probability of breakdown is high)'. The community, not the hospital, was psychiatry's natural habitat.[12]

Changes in outlook and administrative practices that were transforming hospitals were already evident by the early 1950s. After the Second World War, Karl and William Menninger, in collaboration with state and federal authorities, transformed both Winter Veterans Administration Hospital and Topeka State Hospital in Kansas. Release rates at two Massachusetts institutions (Worcester State Hospital and Boston Psychopathic Hospital) and at the Butler Health Center in Providence, Rhode Island, antedated the introduction of the psychotropic drugs. Moreover, average length of stays declined as well.[13]

Perhaps the most significant element in preparing the groundwork for the emergence of de-institutionalisation was the growing role of the federal government in social welfare and health policies and the diminution of the authority of state governments. The enactment of the National Mental Health Act of 1946 and subsequent creation of the National Institute of Mental Health (NIMH) thrust the federal government into mental health policy, an arena historically reserved for state governments. Under the leadership of Robert H. Felix, the NIMH dedicated itself to bring about the demise of public mental hospitals and to substitute in their place a community-based policy. The passage of the Community Mental Health Centers Act in 1963 ended two decades of agitation. The legislation provided federal subsidies for the construction of centres which were intended to be the cornerstone of a radically new policy. The goal was to have 2,000 centers in operation by 1980. A free-standing institution with no links to mental hospitals (which still had an inpatient population of about half a million), centres were supposed to facilitate the early identification of symptoms, offer preventive treatments that would both diminish the incidence of mental disorders and render long-term hospitalisation superfluous. Ultimately, the hope was that traditional mental hospitals would become obsolete. These centres, moreover, would be created and operated by the community in which they were located.[14]

The Community Mental Health Centers Act, however, ignored the context in which persons with severe and chronic mental illnesses received care. In 1960, 48 per cent of patients in mental hospitals were unmarried, 12 per cent were widowed, and 13 per cent were divorced or separated. The overwhelming majority, in other words, may have had no families to care for them. Hence, the assumption that persons with mental illnesses could reside in the community with their families while undergoing psycho-social and biological rehabilitation was unrealistic.[15] Similarly, the goal of creating 2,000 Community Mental Health Centers (CMHCs) by 1980 was equally problematic. If this goal had been met, there would have been a severe shortage of qualified psychiatrists or a dramatic change in the manner in which medical graduates selected their specialty. Indeed, training a sufficient number of psychiatrists to staff centres would have decimated other medical specialties without a large expansion of medical education.[16] To be sure, there could have been an increase in the training of other mental health professionals. But the law as passed included no provision to facilitate training. The subsequent absence of psychiatrists at CMHCs proved significant, given the significance of drugs in any treatment program.[17] The legislation of 1963, in other words, reflected a victory of ideology over reality. Indeed, in the 1950s and 1960s mental health rhetoric often drowned out any appreciation of reality.

The ideological debates in the Kennedy Administration could have led to a significant transformation; the improvement of mental hospitals and construction of a more integrated system of mental health care was a viable option in the early 1960s. During the preceding decade the concept that the mental hospital could act as a therapeutic community had taken shape. Given concrete form by Maxwell Jones, a British psychiatrist who had worked with psychologically impaired servicemen and repatriated prisoners of war, the concept was popularised in the United States by such figures as Alfred Stanton and Morris Schwartz, Milton Greenblatt, and Robert N. Rapoport.[18] The Council of State Governments (representing the nation's governors) and the Milbank Memorial Fund sponsored studies that emphasized the potential importance of community institutions.[19] Indeed, the therapeutic innovations of the 1950s seemed to presage a policy capable of realising the dream of providing quality care and effective treatment for persons with mental illnesses. The simultaneous development of milieu therapy (employing environmental modifications as a therapeutic tool) and the deployment of the new psychotropic drugs indicated a quite specific direction. Drug therapy would make patients amenable to milieu therapy; a more humane institutional environment would facilitate the release of large numbers of patients into the community; and an extensive network of local services would in turn assist the reintegration of patients into society and oversee, if necessary, their varied medical, economic, occupational and social needs.

But those in policy-making positions in the NIMH had a public health view of mental illnesses and prevention, a strong belief in social aetiology, and a pervasive suspicion and distrust of the mental hospital system and state mental health authorities; they believed that state governments were a barrier to fundamental change and that the lead had to be taken by enlightened federal officials. That congressional legislators from some states opposed passage of civil and voting rights legislation only confirmed this negative perception.

The provisions of the Community Mental Health Centers Act (largely the work of NIMH officials who served as staff for Kennedy's interagency task force responsible for drafting a federal policy) were vague, although the goal – as President Kennedy remarked when he signed the bill into law – was to replace custodial hospitals with local therapeutic centres. The act did not define the essential services of CMHCS, but left that responsibility to the Department of Health, Education, and Welfare. In a bureaucratic struggle over who would write the regulations and standards, Felix prevailed over the Bureau of Medical Services in the Department of Health, Education, and Welfare. The regulations as promulgated in effect bypassed state authorities and gave more power to local communities. The most curious aspect of the regulations was the omission of any mention of state hospitals. In one sense this was understandable, given the belief that centres would replace mental hospitals. Nevertheless, the absence of linkages between centres and hospitals was striking. If centres were designed to provide the comprehensive services and continuity of care specified in the regulations, how could they function in isolation from a state system that still retained responsibility for nearly half a million patients with severe mental illnesses? Not surprisingly, the result was deep and bitter divisions in mental health between state and federal officials in the early 1960s.[20] These resentments continued in subsequent decades and were reflected in some of the federal-state debates over the administration of Medicaid, a programme enacted in 1965 to provide access to medical care for poor, indigent and disabled individuals. Such acrimonious federal-state relations hardly offered the best organisational framework for constructive changes in the states.

In theory, CMHCS were to receive patients discharged from mental hospitals and to take responsibility for their aftercare and rehabilitation. In fact, this did not occur. Indeed, previous studies had already raised serious questions about

Mental Health Policy in Twentieth-Century America

the ability of community clinics (as they were known in the 1950s) to deal with persons with serious mental disorders. Three California researchers found evidence that there were 'marked discontinuities in functions' of hospitals and clinics. Those who required an extensive social support network were not candidates for clinics, which provided no assistance in finding living quarters or employment or a system of social supports. In other words, patients seen in clinics were not similar to those admitted to hospitals.[21]

Such findings were largely ignored by those caught up in the rhetoric of community care and treatment. Using an expanded definition of mental illness and the mental health continuum, CMHCS served largely a new set of clients who better fit the orientations of mental health managers and professionals trained in psychodynamic and preventive orientations. The treatment of choice at most centres was individual psychotherapy, an intervention especially adapted to a middle-class educated clientele who did not have severe disorders and which was congenial as well to the professional staffs composed largely of social workers and clinical psychologists. Most CMHCs, charged Donald G. Langsley (President of the American Psychiatric Association) in 1980, were offering 'preventive services that have not yet been proved successful' and 'counseling and crisis intervention for predictable problems in living'. 'A critical consequence of these events,' he added, 'has been the wholesale neglect of the mentally ill, especially the chronic patient and the de-institutionalised.'[22]

Moreover, many CMHCS were caught up in the vortex of community activism so characteristic of the 1960s and 1970s, and devoted part of their energies to social reform. The most famous example of political activism occurred at the Lincoln Hospital Mental Health Services in the southeast Bronx in New York City. Hospital officials sought to stimulate community social action programmes in order to deal with the chronic problems of urban ghettos. The result, however, was not anticipated. In early 1969 non-professional staff workers went on strike and demanded that power be transferred from professionals associated with a predominantly white power structure to the poor, to African-Americans, and to disfranchised persons.[23] However laudable the intention, such activities removed centres still further from a population whose mental illnesses often created dependency. The result exacerbated discordance between the work of CMHCS and the system of mental health services administered by the states. The former's agendas were primarily focused on stress, psychological problems and preventive activities in community settings, while the latter maintained their traditional responsibility for persons with severe and persistent mental illness. It was in this context that de-institutionalisation policies proceeded.

De-institutionalisation

A major turning point in mental health policy was the decision in 1964 by the federal government to bypass the states and work directly with communities in developing CMHCs and establishing priorities. In addition to shifting the focus of services from those with more serious illness to clients with less disabling disorders, these policies and the way they were implemented left many state administrators embittered. The publication of DSM-III in 1980, which elevated many behaviours to the status of distinct pathological entities, contributed still further to the tendency to shift services away from individuals with more serious mental illnesses.[24] Indeed, after 1963 there was a dramatic expansion of services to new populations. The growth of private and public insurance for inpatient psychiatric care, an expanded definition of mental disorders and the need for treatment, a dramatic increase in the number of mental health professionals (from about 28,000 in 1947 to 600,000 in 1992), and greater public acceptance of psychiatric care all hastened the expansion of client populations and thus deflected attention from the needs of persons with serious and persistent mental illnesses. In 1955 there were about 1.7 million episodes of mental illnesses treated in organised mental health facilities; by 1983 there were 7 million.[25]

Developments during the 1970s hardly improved the condition of persons with severe disorders. The fiscal impact of the Vietnam War began to place significant pressures on the federal budget. Even if the goal of creating 2,000 centres had been reached by 1980, it would hardly have made a difference, given the fact that these institutions did not for the most part deal with persons with severe mental disorders. Nor was the Nixon Administration sympathetic to proposals to expand mental health initiatives.

The creation of Jimmy Carter's Presidential Commission on Mental Health in 1977 seemed to presage a new era. The Commission, however, was beset by pressures from all sides. Its final report represented a compromise that attempted to satisfy a variety of groups. The compromise diminished the central position of individuals with severe mental illnesses by placing them on the same plane as other clients of the mental health system despite the fact that the former had by far the greatest needs.[26] The earlier friction about the role of the states in mental health policy made it difficult to achieve a legislative consensus. The Mental Health Systems Act, which was passed just prior to the presidential election of 1980, was weakened by the need to satisfy all constituencies. Nevertheless, some of its provisions offered the hope of improving services to persons with severe and persistent mental illnesses. When Ronald Reagan came into office in 1981, however, the act was repealed, and responsibility for persons with mental disorders again devolved predominantly to the states. The NIMH retreated from services provision to focus almost exclusively on its research mission.

In the 1960s much attention was focused on preventive and community mental health. Yet the Community Mental Health Centers Act – the seeming culmination of more than a decade of ferment – played an inconsequential role in de-institutionalisation; its clientele was not drawn from the ranks of persons with severe and persistent mental illnesses. Nor did the introduction of psychotropic drugs in the mid-1950s lead to the wholesale discharge of patients from mental hospitals. Between 1955 and 1965 the inpatient population of state mental hospitals fell only by about 15 per cent. Between 1965 and 1975, by contrast, the decline was 60 per cent. The decline, however, was by no means equal. Between 1955 and 1973 the rates of reduction varied from less than 20 per cent in Nevada and Delaware to more than 70 per cent in California, Illinois, Hawaii, Utah and Idaho. The decline in New York State, which had the largest inpatient population, was 52 per cent.[27] The differences between states reflected a variety of factors, including historic social welfare policies and traditions as well as populations with different characteristics.

In some respects, the term 'de-institutionalisation' is somewhat of a misnomer. Indeed, the first wave of de-institutionalisation actually involved a lateral transfer of patients from state mental hospitals to long-term nursing facilities because states were motivated to benefit from the windfall of new federal dollars. The enactment of Medicare (health insurance for those 65 years and over) and Medicaid (medical assistance for low-income people of all ages) in 1965 encouraged the construction of nursing home beds, and the Medicaid programme provided a payment source for patients transferred from state mental hospitals to nursing homes and to general hospitals. Although states were responsible for the full costs of patients in state hospitals, they could now transfer patients to other facilities and have the federal government assume from half to three-quarters of the cost, depending on the state's economic status. This incentive encouraged a massive trans-institutionalisation of long-term patients, primarily elderly patients with dementia who were housed in public mental hospitals for lack of other institutional alternatives. Between 1962 and 1972 the number of patients aged 65 and older in mental hospitals was nearly halved. In 1963 nursing homes cared for nearly 222,000 individuals with mental disorders, of whom 188,000 were 65 or older. Six years later the comparable figures were 427,000 and 368,000. The enactment of Medicaid, in other words, hastened the decline in first admissions of elderly patients into mental hospitals. In 1962 the first admission rate for individuals 65 years of age and older was 163.7 per 100,000; a decade later the comparable figure was 69.2.[28] A study by the General Accounting Office in 1977 noted that Medicaid was 'one of the largest single purchasers of mental health care and the principal Federal programme funding the long-term care of the mentally disabled'. It was also the most significant 'federally sponsored programme affecting de-institutionalisation'.[29] The quality of care in nursing and chronic care facilities (which varied in the extreme) was not an important consideration in the transfer of patients. Indeed, the relocation of elderly patients to extended care facilities was often marked by an increase in mortality. Moreover, many nursing homes provided no psychiatric care. When Bruce C. Vladeck published his study of nursing homes in 1980, he selected as his book title *Unloving Care: The Nursing Home Tragedy.*[30]

To put it another way, intergovernmental relationships – local, state and federal – both shaped and transformed social policy in general and mental health policy in particular.[31] The dramatic increase in nursing home beds from 568,546 in 1963 to 1.4 million beds in 1977 was matched by a comparable increase of non-federal general hospitals with inpatient psychiatric units. In 1963 there were 622 such hospitals with areas for inpatient psychiatric services; only a handful had specialised psychiatric units. Fourteen years later there were 1,056 such hospitals, of which 843 had specialised inpatient psychiatric units.[32] By 1983 general hospitals accounted for nearly two-thirds of the nearly three million inpatient psychiatric episodes. Nevertheless, many of the clients with psychiatric diagnoses who were treated in general hospitals were not necessarily the same as those who would have been patients in state mental hospitals. In 1992 there were 1.7 million discharges from short-stay hospitals. Of this number 53 per cent were for patients with a diagnosis of psychosis, 15 per cent alcohol dependence, and the rest for non-psychiatric depression, anxiety disorders and personality disorders. Length of stays dropped correspondingly. Between 1965 and 1988 the average length of stay in general hospitals was about 12-13 days, as contrasted with inpatient stays of months and even years in state mental hospitals prior to 1965.[33]

During the early stages of de-institutionalisation, many long-term patients in mental hospitals were transferred to different institutions, returned to their families when such families existed and were willing to provide care, or relocated in a variety of community programs and facilities. Other federal programmes hastened the discharge of long-term patients from mental hospitals. In 1956 Congress amended the Social Security Act to enable eligible persons aged 50 and over to receive disability benefits. The Social Security Disability Insurance (ssdi) programme became more inclusive in succeeding years, and ultimately covered the mentally disabled. In 1972 the Social Security Act was further amended to provide coverage for individuals who did not qualify for ssdi. Under the provisions of the Supplemental Security Income for the Aged, the Disabled, and the Blind (ssi), all those whose age or disability precluded them from holding a job became eligible for income support. ssdi and ssi encouraged states to discharge patients from mental hospitals, since federal payments would presumably enable them to live in the community. These individuals received medical coverage under Medicaid; they were also eligible for public housing programmes and food stamps.[34]

A second wave of de-institutionalisation occurred during and after the 1970s. A quite different situation prevailed, however, because of basic demographic trends in the population as a whole and changes in the mental health system. At the end of the Second World War, there was a sharp rise in the number of births, which peaked in the 1960s. Between 1946 and 1960 more than 59 million births were recorded. The disproportionately large size of this age cohort meant that the number of persons at risk from developing severe mental disorders was very high. Morton Kramer, the head of the Biometrics Division at the NIMH, warned that large increases could be expected between 1975 and 1990 'in numbers of persons in high-risk age groups for the use of mental health facilities and correctional institutions.' Moreover, these younger individuals tended to be highly mobile. Whereas 40 per cent of the general population moved between 1975 and 1979, between 62 and 72 per cent of individuals in their twenties changed residences. Like others in their age cohort, the large numbers of young adults with severe and persistent mental disorders also moved frequently both within and between cities and in and out of rural areas.[35]

At the very same time that the cohort born after 1945 was reaching their twenties and thirties, the mental health service system was undergoing profound changes. Before 1970 many persons with severe and persistent mental illnesses were cared for in mental hospitals. If admitted in their youth, they often remained institutionalised for decades, or else were discharged and re-admitted. Hence their care and treatment were centralised within a specific institutional context, and in general they were not visible in the community at large. To be sure, many with severe and chronic mental illnesses were able to reside in the community (particularly if they had caregivers), but in general their presence did not arouse public concern or apprehension.

After 1970 a quite different situation prevailed. By then, mental hospitalisation was already under attack from a variety of quarters. During the 1960s an anti-psychiatry movement had begun to promote the concept that mental illness was a myth that served as a form of social labelling to suppress non-conformist behaviour. A peculiar coalition drawn from the libertarian right and the New Left, associated with such figures as Thomas S. Szasz, R.D. Laing, Erving Goffman, and Thomas J. Scheff, attempted to call into question the very legitimacy of psychiatry and the social control function of mental hospitals.[36] At about the same time, lawyers who had come to maturity during the civil rights struggles of the 1960s transferred their allegiances and began to work to protect the rights and liberties of persons with mental illnesses. Angered by abuses and lack of care, they also shared hostility toward psychiatry. They turned to the legal system to contest involuntary civil commitment, insisted on a right to treatment, and supported the concept of treatment in the least restrictive community alternative.[37] Their attack on mental hospitals led hospital administrators to reduce their resident populations still further in order to meet court-mandated standards of care for those remaining in the hospital. Ironically, per capita expenditures in mental hospitals increased because of the reduced patient population, thus meeting court-ordered mandates. This development, however, did little to improve conditions among the growing number of persons with severe mental illnesses in the community.[38]

Young persons with severe mental disorders who reached maturity at this time were rarely confined for extended periods within mental hospitals. Restless and mobile, they were the first generation to reach adulthood within the community. Although their disorders were not fundamentally different from their predecessors, they behaved in quite different ways. They tended to emulate the behaviour of their age peers, who were often hostile toward convention and authority. Influenced by the critics of psychiatry, young street persons with mental illnesses denied that they were ill and insisted that they were victimised because of their non-conformist behaviour. These young persons exhibited aggressiveness and volatility and were non-compliant. They generally fell into the schizophrenic category (although affective disorders and borderline personalities were also present). Above all, they lacked functional and adaptive skills. As one knowledgeable psychiatrist and his associates noted, these dysfunctional young adults

> seem to be stuck in the transition to adult life, unable to master the tasks of separation and independence. If we examine the nature of their failures, we find them to be based on more or less severe and chronic pathology: thought disorder; affective disorder; personality disorder; and severe deficits in ego functions such as impulse control, reality testing, judgment, modulation of affect, memory, mastery and competence, and integration. In terms of the necessary equipment for community life—the capacity to endure stress, to work consistently toward realistic goals, to relate to other people comfortably over time, to tolerate uncertainty and conflict—these young adults are disabled in a very real and pervasive sense.[39]

Complicating the clinical picture were high rates of drug abuse among these young adults with chronic mental illnesses, which only exacerbated their volatile and non-compliant behaviour. Their mobility and lack of coping skills also resulted in high rates of homelessness. Virtually every community experienced their presence on the streets, in emergency medical facilities, and in correctional institutions.[40] An American Psychiatric Association report on the homeless mentally ill emphasized the tendency of these young persons to drift.

> Apart from their desire to outrun their problems, their symptoms, and their failures, many have great difficulty in achieving closeness and intimacy.
> They drift also in search of autonomy, as a way of denying their dependency, and out of a desire for an isolated life-style. Lack of money often makes them unwelcome, and they may be evicted by family and friends.

And they drift because of a reluctance to become involved in a mental health treatment program or a supportive out-of-home environment [...] [T]hey do not want to see themselves as ill.[41]

The changes in the population with mental disorders and the mental health system had major consequences. In the mental hospital all of the functions of care and treatment were brought together in a single location and unified. That such institutions often failed to meet their obligations was obvious. Yet at a time when other alternatives were lacking, mental hospitals served an indispensable function. Indeed, studies of the patient population suggested a far more variegated portrait of an institution besieged by critics. Morton Kramer and his colleagues at the Biometrics Branch of the NIMH pointed out that longitudinal data revealed declining lengths of stay for particular diagnoses. Between 1940 and 1950, for example, first admissions for schizophrenics increased. Yet the length of stay for such patients had been declining for more than 30 years. In 1948, 56 per cent of all schizophrenics admitted to state hospitals were discharged within 12 months, as compared with only 33 per cent in 1914. In the same period the rise in the number of inpatients with mental diseases of the senium, from 24 to 42 per cent, reflected declining mortality rates (a favourable development that created new problems relating to the care of aged individuals). Such data suggested that the often-repeated generalisations about the 'warehousing' functions of mental hospitals were somewhat inaccurate.[42]

Treatment in the community for clients with multiple needs posed severe challenges, as compared with mental hospital care. In the community (and particularly in large urban areas) clients were widely dispersed, and their successful management depended on bringing together needed services administered by a variety of bureaucracies, each with its own culture, priorities and preferred client populations. Although there were sporadic (and occasionally successful) efforts to integrate these services (psychiatric care and treatment, social services, housing, social support) in meaningful ways, the results in most areas were dismal.

The decentralisation of services and lack of integration made it extraordinarily difficult to deal with individuals with serious disorders in the community, and many became part of the street culture where the use of alcohol and drugs was common. Individuals with a dual diagnosis of a serious mental illness and substance abuse presented such serious problems that many mental health professionals refused to deal with them despite their growing numbers. Moreover, the decline in institutional care created a situation where the 'criminalisation' of persons with mental illnesses became more common. If such individuals were on the streets, they were more likely to engage in acts that attracted the attention of authorities and that ended in arrest and detention. Many persons with serious mental illnesses had encounters with the police, and a significant number were caught up in the criminal justice system rather than the mental health system and incarcerated in prisons. To be sure, collaboration between the two systems was possible, but often the different perspectives, values and cultures of each placed formidable barriers in the way of co-operation.

In the last third of the twentieth century, states pursued a policy of reducing their mental hospital populations by placing barriers in the way of new admissions and only as a last resort. This policy, in conjunction with the vast expansion in the clientele of mental health services and diagnostic categories, shifts in public attitudes and perceptions, changing treatment strategies, and social and economic factors, led to the emergence of a confusing array of organised and unorganised settings for the treatment of persons with mental illnesses. State mental health agencies, which in theory were responsible for administering the mental health system, found themselves faced with declining resources and an increasing inability to influence policy. Multiple sources of funding from a variety of federal programmes administered by independent agencies made it difficult to develop and implement comprehensive, integrated and effective community-based services. Many of the components of community mental health care – income support, housing, social support networks – were designed for other populations (e.g. the poor and the disabled) and often did not fit the needs of persons with severe and cyclic or persistent mental illnesses.

Ironically, the result of de-institutionalisation was fragmentation and disorganisation. Since the 1970s the mental health system has included a bewildering variety of institutions: short-term mental hospitals, state and federal long-term institutions, private psychiatric hospitals, nursing homes, residential care facilities, community mental health centres, outpatient departments of hospitals, community care programmes, community residential institutions for persons with mental disorders with different designations in different states, and client-run and self-help services. This disarray and absence of service integration have led to a situation where many patients with serious mental illnesses were forced to live in homeless shelters, on the streets, and even in prisons.

Conclusion

Although seemingly massive changes have taken place during the latter half of the twentieth century, dissatisfaction with the existing system of mental health services persists. In October, 2002, Michael F. Hogan, chair of the President's New Freedom Commission on Mental Health, sent an Interim Report to the White House. 'America's mental health service delivery system is in shambles,' he wrote in his accompanying letter.

We have found that the system needs dramatic reform because it is incapable of efficiently delivering and financing effective treatments – such

Mental Health Policy in Twentieth-Century America

as medications, psychotherapies, and other services – that have taken decades to develop. Responsibility for these services is scattered among agencies, programs, and levels of government. There are so many programs operating under such different rules that it is often impossible for families and consumers to find the care that they urgently need. The efforts of countless skilled and caring professionals are frustrated by the system's fragmentation. As a result, too many Americans suffer needless disability, and millions of dollars are spent unproductively in a dysfunctional service system that cannot deliver the treatments that work so well.[43]

Can history provide us with a narrative that offers policy guidance? The answer to this ostensibly simple question is extraordinarily complex. Admittedly, history does not provide concrete lessons that spell out precise answers to complex problems. Nevertheless, it offers some broad themes that may provide assistance in policy formulation. At the very least, history suggests that there is a price to be paid for implementing ideology ungrounded in empirical reality, and for making exaggerated rhetorical claims. The ideology of community mental health and the facile assumption that residence in the community would promote adjustment and integration did not take into account the extent of social isolation, exposure to victimisation, inducement to abuse substances, homelessness and criminalisation of persons with mental illnesses. The assumption that CMHCs would assume responsibility for the aftercare and rehabilitation of persons discharged from mental hospitals proved erroneous. The absence of mechanisms of control and accountability permitted CMHCs to focus on new populations of more amenable and attractive clients with less severe problems. Nor does the recent move to managed care for persons with serious mental illnesses offer assurance that the needs of this group will finally be met. Indeed, preliminary evidence suggests that a 'democratisation' of services reduces the intensity of services for patients with more profound disabilities and needs.[44]

When institutional care was the norm, there was a clear recognition that there was a fundamental distinction between its patients and persons experiencing problems of everyday life. The medicalisation of problems of living and the creation of a myriad of psychiatric diagnostic categories far removed from persistent and serious mental illnesses blurred the distinction between the needs of persons with serious disabilities and the population at large with mild disorders, and the former have suffered the consequences of a system that overlooked their needs. Effective community care for those individuals once institutionalised requires a range of functions and services that hospitalisation was intended to provide, from housing and supervision to treatment and rehabilitation.

What is especially notable are the roles played by rhetoric and ideology in the development of mental health policy during the past half century. To dismiss them as simply forms of public posturing is to ignore their consequences.

Rhetoric and ideology shape agendas and debates; they create expectations that in turn mold policies; and they inform the socialisation, training and education of those in professional occupations. The concept of community care and treatment, the belief in prevention, and the corresponding attack on institutional care – all of which played significant policy roles from the 1950s to the present – were not inherently defective. But states, communities and policy advocates lacked the foresight or commitment to finance and to provide required services. Persons with severe and persistent mental illnesses were forced to make their way amidst an unco-ordinated array of programmes, providers and services that happened to be in the community. Many of these individuals, moreover, had to fend on their own, often with unfortunate consequences. At the beginning of the twenty-first century, it is clear that the construction of an integrated and co-ordinated system of mental health care remained an unfulfilled ideal.

Notes

1.   Joanne E. Atay and Ronald W. Manderscheid, *Additions and Resident Patients at End of Year, State and County Mental Hospitals . . . 2001* (Rockville, MD: Center for Mental Health Services, 2003), viii.
2.   Gerald N. Grob, *Mental Illness and American Society, 1875-1940* (Princeton: Princeton University Press, 1983), Chaps. 4, 7.
3.   *Ibid.*
4.   U.S. Bureau of the Census, *Insane and Feeble-Minded in Hospitals and Institutions 1904* (Washington, D.C.: Government Printing Office, 1906), 37; U.S. Bureau of the Census, *Insane and Feeble-Minded in Institutions 1910* (Washington, D.C.: Government Printing Office, 1914), 59; U.S. Bureau of the Census, *Patients in Hospitals for Mental Disease 1923* (Washington, D.C.: Government Printing Office, 1926), 36.
5.   Neil A. Dayton, *New Facts on Mental Disorders: Study of 89,190 Cases* (Springfield, IL: Charles C. Thomas, 1940), 414-38.
6.   American Psychiatric Association, *Report on Patients Over 65 in Public Mental Hospitals* (Washington, D.C.: American Psychiatric Association, 1960).
7.   Morton Kramer, H. Goldstein, R.H. Israel and N.A. Johnson, *A Historical Study of the Disposition of First Admissions to a State Mental Hospital: Experience of Warren State Hospital during the Period 1916-1950* (U.S. Public Health Service *Publication No. 445*: 1955), and the same authors 'Application of Life Table Methodology to the Study of Mental Hospital Populations', in American Psychiatric Association, *Psychiatric Research Report*, v (1956), 49-87.
8.   Thomas W. Salmon, 'Some New Fields in Neurology and Psychiatry', *Journal of Nervous and Mental Disease*, 46 (1917), 90-9. The history of the mental hygiene movement can be followed in Grob, *op. cit.* (note 2), 144-78; Norman Dain, *Clifford W. Beers: Advocate for the Insane* (Pittsburgh: University of Pittsburgh Press, 1980); Margo Horn, *Before It's Too Late: The Child Guidance Movement in the United States, 1922-1945* (Philadelphia: Temple University Press, 1989); and Theresa R. Richard-

son, *The Century of the Child: The Mental Hygiene Movement and Social Policy in the United States and Canada* (Albany: State University of New York Press, 1989).

9.   Lothar B. Kalinowsky and Paul H. Hoch, *Shock Treatments and Other Somatic Procedures in Psychiatry* (New York: Grune & Stratton, 1946), 243.

10.   Raymond G. Fuller, 'A Study of the Administration of State Psychiatric Services', *Mental Hygiene*, 36 (1954), 181-2.

11.   For a typical example, see J.W. Appel and G. Beebe, 'Preventive Psychiatry: An Epidemiologic Approach', *Journal of the American Medical Association*, 131 (1946), 1469-75.

12.   Robert H. Felix, 'Mental Public Health: A Blueprint', presentation at St. Elizabeth's Hospital, April 21, 1945, Felix Papers, National Library of Medicine, Bethesda, Maryland; Felix and R.V. Bowers, 'Mental Hygiene and Socio-Environmental Factors', *Milbank Memorial Fund Quarterly*, 26 (1948), 125-47.

13.   Lawrence J. Friedman, *Menninger: The Family and the Clinic* (New York: Knopf, 1990), 170-80, 194-7; J. Sanbourne Bockoven, *Moral Treatment in Community Mental Health* (New York: Springer Publishing Co., 1972), 114-46.

14.   For a detailed analysis of these developments see Gerald N. Grob, *From Asylum to Community: Mental Health Policy in Modern America* (Princeton: Princeton University Press, 1991).

15.   Morton Kramer, 'Epidemiology, Biostatistics, and Mental Health Planning', in American Psychiatric Association, *Psychiatric Research Report*, xxii (April 1967), 27; Kramer, *Some Implications of Trends in the Usage of Psychiatric Facilities for Community Mental Health Programs and Related Research* (u.s. Public Health Service *Publication 1434:* 1967).

16.   88th Congress, 1st Session, *Mental Health, Hearings before a Subcommittee of the Committee on Interstate and Foreign Commerce House of Representatives . . . 1963* (Washington, d.c.: Government Printing Office, 1963), 100-6.

17.   Rosalyn D. Bass, *CMHC Staffing: Who Minds the Store?* (dhew Publication [adm] 78-686: Washington, d.c., 1978); Paul J. Fink and S.P. Weinstein, 'Whatever Happened to Psychiatry: The Deprofessionalization of Community Mental Health Centers', *American Journal of Psychiatry*, 136 (1979), 406-9.

18.   Maxwell Jones, *The Therapeutic Community: A New Treatment Method in Psychiatry* (New York: Basic Books, 1953); Alfred H. Stanton and Morris S. Schwartz, *The Mental Hospital: A Study of Institutional Participation in Psychiatric Illness and Treatment* (New York: Basic Books, 1954); Milton Greenblatt, Richard H. York, Esther L. Brown and Robert W. Hyde, *From Custodial to Therapeutic Patient Care in Mental Hospitals* (New York: Russell Sage Foundation, 1955); Robert N. Rapoport, *Community as Doctor* (Springfield, il: Charles C. Thomas, 1960).

19.   Council of State Governments, *The Mental Health Programs of the Forty-Eight States: A Report to the Governors' Conference* (Chicago: Council of State Governments, 1950); Milbank Memorial Fund, *The Elements of a Community Mental Health Program* (New York: Milbank Memorial Fund, 1956); Milbank Memorial Fund, *Programs for Community Mental Health* (New York: Milbank Memorial Fund, 1957).

20.   Grob, *op. cit.* (note 14), Chap. 9.

21.   Harold Sampson, D. Ross, B. Engle and F. Livson, 'Feasibility of Community Clinic Treatment for State Mental Hospital Patients', *Archives of Neurology and Psychiatry*, 80 (1958), 71-7. A much longer and more detailed version appeared as *A Study of Suitability for Outpatient Clinic Treatment of State Mental Hospital Admissions* (California Department of Mental Hygiene, *Research Report No. 1*: 1957).

22.   Donald G. Langsley, 'The Community Health Center: Does It Treat Patients?', *Hospital & Community Psychiatry*, 31 (1980), 815-9.

23.   Harris B. Peck, 'A Candid Appraisal of the Community Mental Health Center as a Public Health Agency', *American Journal of Public Health*, 59 (1969), 459-69; Robert Shaw and C. J. Eagle, 'Programmed Failure: The Lincoln Hospital Story', *Community Mental Health Journal*, 7 (1971), 255-63.

24.   Allan V. Horwitz, *Creating Mental Illness* (Chicago: University of Chicago Press, 2002). The publication of DSM-II more than a decade before (actually entitled *Diagnostic and Statistical Manual of Mental Disorders* (2nd ed.: Washington, D.C.: American Psychiatric Association, 1968) in some ways anticipated the radical changes embodied in DSM-III.

25.   David Mechanic, *Mental Health and Social Policy: The Emergence of Managed Care* (4th ed.: Boston: Allyn and Bacon, 1999), 11-4.

26.   This generalisation is based on an examination of the papers of the President's Commission on Mental Health, Record Group 220, Carter Library, Atlanta, Georgia. See also *Report to the President from The President's Commission on Mental Health 1978* (4 vols.: Washington, D.C: Government Printing Office, 1978).

27.   David Mechanic and David A. Rochefort, 'A Policy of Inclusion for the Mentally Ill', *Health Affairs*, 11 (1992), 128-50: 133.

28.   National Institute of Mental Health, *Statistical Note No. 107* (1974), 4; Morton Kramer, *Psychiatric Services and the Changing Institutional Scene, 1950-1985* (DHEW Publication No. [ADM] 77-433: 1977), 80; William Gronfein, 'Incentives and Intentions in Mental Health Policy: A Comparison of the Medicaid and Community Mental Health Programs', *Journal of Health and Social Behavior*, 26 (1985), 192-206; Howard H. Goldman, N. H. Adams and C. Taube, 'Deinstitutionalization: The Data Demythologized', *Hospital & Community Psychiatry*, 34 (1983), 129-34: 133.

29.   General Accounting Office, *Returning the Mentally Disabled to the Community: Government Needs to Do More* (Washington, D.C.: n.p., 1977), 81.

30.   Bruce C. Vladeck, *Unloving Care: The Nursing Home Tragedy* (New York: Basic Books, 1980).

31.   Gerald N. Grob, 'Government and Mental Health Policy: A Structural Analysis', *Milbank Quarterly*, 72 (1994), 471-500.

32.   Charles A. Kiesler and A. E. Sibulkin, *Deinstitutionalization: Myths and Facts About a National Crisis* (Newbury Park, CA: Sage Publications, 1987), 60-1, 115.

33.   *Ibid.*, 66-67; Mechanic, *op. cit.* (note 25), 130; D. Mechanic, D. D. McAlpine and M. Olfson, 'Changing Patterns of Psychiatric Inpatient Care in the United States, 1988-1994', *Archives of General Psychiatry*, 55 (1998), 785-91.

34.   Public Law 92-603, *U.S. Statutes at Large*, 86 (1972): 1329-92; Ann B. Johnson, *Out of Bedlam: The Truth About Deinstitutionalization* (New York: Basic Books, 1990), 96-9.

35.   U.S. Bureau of the Census, *Historical Statistics of the United States: Colonial Times to 1970* (2 vols.: Washington, D.C.: Government Printing Office, 1975), 1, 49; Morton Kramer, *Psychiatric Services and the Changing Institutional Scene, 1950-1985* (DHEW publication [ADM] 77-433: Washington, D.C., 1977), 46; Leona L. Bachrach, 'Young Adult Chronic Patients: An Analytical Review of the Literature', *Hospital & Community Psychiatry*, 33 (1982), 189-97.

36.   Thomas S. Szasz, *The Myth of Mental Illness: Foundations of a Theory of Personal Conduct* (New York: Hoeber-Harper, 1961), and *Law, Liberty, and Psychiatry: An Inquiry Into the Social Uses of Mental Health Practices* (New York: Macmillan, 1963); R.D. Laing, *Sanity, Madness, and the Family* (London: Tavistock, 1964), and *The Politics of Experience and the Bird of Paradise* (New York: Pantheon Books, 1967); Erving Goffman, *Asylums: Essays on the Social Situation of Mental Patients and Other Inmates* (Garden City, N.Y.: Anchor Books, 1961); Thomas J. Scheff, *Being Mentally Ill: A Sociological Theory* (Chicago: Aldine Publishing Co., 1966), and 'Schizophrenia as Ideology', *Schizophrenia Bulletin*, 2 (Fall 1970), 15-19.

37.   See Alan A. Stone, 'Overview: The Right to Treatment: Comments on the Law and Its Impact', *American Journal of Psychiatry*, 132 (1975), 1125-34, and *Mental Health and the Law: A System in Transition* (DHEW Publication No. [ADM] 75-176: 1975); Alexander D. Brooks, *Psychiatry and the Mental Health System* (Boston: Little, Brown, 1974), and the *1980 Supplement* (Boston: Little Brown, 1980); Paul S. Appelbaum, *Almost a Revolution: Mental Health Law and the Limits of Change* (New York: Oxford University Press, 1994).

38.   David Mechanic, 'Judicial Action and Social Change', in Stuart Golann and W. J. Fremouw (eds), *The Right to Treatment for Mental Patients* (New York: Irvington Publishers, 1976), 47-72.

39.   Bert Pepper, H. Ryglewicz and M.C. Kirschner, 'The Uninstitutionalized Generation: A New Breed of Psychiatric Patient', in Pepper and Ryglewicz (eds), *The Young Adult Chronic Patient* (San Francisco: Jossey-Bass, 1982), 5. See also Leona L. Bachrach, 'The Homeless Mentally Ill and Mental Health Services: An Analytical Review of the Literature', in H. Richard Lamb (ed.), *The Homeless Mentally Ill: A Task Force Report of the American Psychiatric Association* (Washington, D.C.: American Psychiatric Association, 1984), 11-53.

40.   Leona L. Bachrach, 'The Concept of Young Adult Chronic Psychiatric Patients: Questions from a Research Perspective', *Hospital & Community Psychiatry*, 35 (1984), 573-80: 574.

41.   H. Richard Lamb, 'Deinstitutionalization and the Homeless Mentally Ill', in Lamb, *op. cit.* (note 39), 65.

42.   Morton Kramer, 'Long Range Studies of Mental Hospital Patients, an Important Area for Research in Chronic Disease', *Milbank Memorial Fund Quarterly*, 31 (1953), 253-64; Kramer et al., *op. cit.* (note 7).

43.   Michael F. Hogan to President George W. Bush, October 29, 2002, *Interim Report of the President's New Freedom Commission on Mental Health*. Available at http://www.mental healthcommissionn.gov/reports/reports.htm (accessed May 16, 2003).

44.   David Mechanic and D.D. McAlpine, 'Mission Unfulfilled: Potholes on the Road to Mental Health Parity', *Health Affairs*, 18 (1999), 7-21.

Gerald N. Grob

CHAPTER 6

Continuities or Ruptures?

Concepts, Institutions and Contexts of Twentieth-Century
German Psychiatry and Mental Health Care

Volker Roelcke

Twentieth-century German psychiatry is conventionally subdivided into three
fairly distinct stages, parallel to German political history. On this basis, the first
decades after 1900 were characterised by the success of academic psychiatrists
(such as Emil Kraepelin or Alois Alzheimer) in the realms of nosology, classification and neuropathology, and the presence of a rationally structured system of
mental health care built on the pillars of university departments and state asylums. The advent of Nazi rule marked the beginning of the second phase, which
lasted from 1933 until 1945. Following this traditional perspective, Nazi mental
health policies were guided by racial ideologies, which were forcefully imposed
on the psychiatric profession. The programmes of eugenic sterilisation and systematic killing of patients ('euthanasia') were mainly supported by lower-rank
psychiatrists working in peripheral asylums, while only a few of the leading
members of the profession were involved. The third stage, beginning after World
War II (and referring to West Germany), was characterised by a slow but more
or less successful 'normalisation' of German psychiatry: an adoption of the programmes and practices of psychiatric care pursued by the international community, such as de-institutionalisation, differentiated use of somatic and psychotherapeutic treatments complemented by community services, and research
particularly in the realms of psychopharmacology and psychiatric genetics.

Such a compartmentalised image certainly reflects important aspects of the
whole century. However, a closer look at the statements of a few significant
psychiatrists throughout the period yields a number of surprises and contradictions to this tripartite periodisation. Thus, for example, both the psychiatric consultant Manfred in der Beek in the late 1950s, and Klaus Dörner, one of the protagonists of the social psychiatry movement since the 1970s (also known as an
historian of psychiatry), pointed to the continuities of reformist programmes in
mental health care since the 1920s, particularly in the treatment of chronic
patients. These continuities bridge the period from the Weimar Republic (exemplified by the asylum director Hermann Simon and his programme of 'activating therapy') through the time of Nazism (exemplified by the programme of

therapy and prevention of Carl Schneider, head of the psychiatric department at Heidelberg University) up to post-war efforts of modernising psychiatric care. This continued in the wake of the 1968 movement and subsequent reform agenda formulated in the Federal Parliament's Inquiry into the State of Psychiatric Care (*Psychiatrie-Enquete des Deutschen Bundestages*, 1975). Dörner emphasized these continuities in spite of his explicit acknowledgment and condemnation of Schneider's pivotal role in the Nazi programme of systematic killing of patients ('euthanasia').[1]

Both these statements and the results of recent research on the history of German eugenics/genetics and 'euthanasia' (see below) suggest that the image of three rather distinct periods may not be adequate to describe the development of twentieth-century German psychiatry. In the following, I shall outline the main issues and trends in the last century by considering three dimensions of psychiatric activity: the professional politics of psychiatrists; the organisation of mental health care; and the realm of psychiatric research. These three dimensions will be followed through the periodisation derived from political history. Throughout, the term 'mental health care' refers to the sum of all activities aimed at treating or caring for individuals considered in their time to be suffering from a psychological disorder, as well as those activities aimed at the prevention of such conditions.

Before 1933: Stabilising Public Order, Creating Scientific Reputation

Politically, this period comprises the late stages of Imperial Germany including World War 1 and the Weimar Republic. Although these changing political contexts were each associated with specific challenges and ramifications for psychiatric care and research, there were strong overarching developments in all three dimensions.

Seen from the perspective of professional politics, German psychiatrists were undertaking strong efforts to create a new identity as a modern medical discipline based on the principles of the natural sciences (in particular, laboratory sciences) and also on statistics and contemporary social sciences. It was their aspiration that their field of work should become recognised as an academic subject equal to all other medical specialties. They also hoped to be able to deliver to state authorities the expertise necessary to help preserve public order, economic efficiency and national strength. This new identity was to substitute for the older image of alienists as a closed group of administrators and rulers of large, isolated asylums, who built their authority on outdated ideas taken from theology, speculative metaphysics or superstition.

In aiming at this new identity, psychiatrists attempted to refashion the structure and location of their institutions, the admission policies for patients, the

recruitment of new members of the profession, the organisation of their training, and finally the modes of producing 'legitimate' knowledge in the form of
plausible and scientifically valid terminology and theories. The beginnings of
such efforts may be traced back to the 1860s. They were exemplified in the establishment by Wilhelm Griesinger of an academic department of psychiatry combined with neurology, together with a new outpatient clinic, at the Charité associated with the University of Berlin. This was followed by initiatives to establish
similar departments of psychiatry (in part also explicitly devoted to 'nervous disorders') at all medical schools, with facilities for teaching students, training
junior staff, and developing research programmes orientated on the natural sciences. Psychiatrists also started to step beyond the borders of their institutions
in order to provide expert interpretations and advice at all levels of public life.
These included law courts, the popular media, the academic world and wider
involvement in social and political matters, such as public order, mental 'overburdening' (*Überbürdung*) by the demands of 'modern life' at school and work,
or sexuality and deviance.[2]

By the first decade of the twentieth century, these long-standing efforts had
led to remarkable results, which were indeed unique in an international comparative perspective. There were academic chairs and university departments of
psychiatry at almost all of the approximately 20 German medical schools;[3]
psychiatry had been integrated into the newly designed curriculum of medical
students; and the long-standing controversies about terminologies and classifi-
cations had been settled after the adoption of the categories created by Emil
Kraepelin and his school. The acknowledged sphere of psychiatric competence
had been extended well beyond the 'traditional' conditions of insanity into the
borderland between healthy and abnormal, including short and transient conditions with fluctuating or vague complaints such as neurasthenia, as well as sexual aberrations.[4] Finally, psychiatric diagnoses (such as hysteria, nervousness
and degeneration) as well as suggestions for interventions had entered the public and political discourse, contributing to the shaping of contemporary interpretations of social life and political agendas.[5] The renaming of the professional association was a symbol for this new self-image and public status. In 1903, the
official name was changed from the Association of German Alienists (*Verein der
deutschen Irrenärzte*) founded in 1864, to the German Association of Psychiatry
(*Deutscher Verein für Psychiatrie*).[6]

An important aspect of the professional strategies of German psychiatrists
consisted of the clear demarcation from and rejection of Freudian psychoanalysis. From the point of view of the established medical disciplines as well as that
of the responsible state authorities, any connection with psychoanalysis might
be understood as a failure of psychiatry to meet the standards of rationality and
method set by the laboratory sciences. These were held in high esteem in late
imperial Germany, and experienced an enormous financial boost from state

Continuities or Ruptures?

agencies. To demonstrate the coming of age of psychiatry in scientific terms, its representatives tried to adopt the conceptual tools, methods and institutional framework of the leading biomedical disciplines of their time. Integrating speculative theories about the origins of dreams or experimentally inaccessible unconscious drives and mechanisms was unacceptable.[7] Only in the mid-1920s, in a period of marked pluralism and moderate public wealth were there signs of a more open attitude amongst some psychiatrists towards theories and practices inspired by psychoanalysis.[8] Significantly, however, the protagonists of such positive evaluations were associated with Austrian and Swiss rather than German institutions.

The leading biomedical disciplines referred to were first neuroanatomy and neuropathology (from the 1860s and 1870s); then physiology (together with experimental psychology); and – from the first decade of the twentieth century – the closely interwoven field of eugenics and genetics. The adoption of the aims and methods of these biomedical disciplines and the natural sciences offered psychiatrists the possibility of gaining the same academic and public prestige as the established medical specialties. These efforts culminated in the joint endeavour of university and asylum psychiatrists to create a German Institute for Psychiatric Research, possibly under the roof of the prestigious Kaiser Wilhelm Society for the Advancement of Sciences (KWS) (*Kaiser-Wilhelm-Gesellschaft zur Förderung der Wissenschaften*). After years of discussions, quarrels and fund-raising activities, the German Research Institute for Psychiatry (*Deutsche Forschungsanstalt für Psychiatrie*, in the following DFA) was founded in Munich in 1917 under the directorship of Emil Kraepelin, independently of the KWS. It was finally integrated into the KWS in 1924.[9] In the mid-1920s, the DFA served in many aspects as the model for the British Institute of Psychiatry established in the late 1920s in association with the Maudsley Hospital in London.[10]

The reverse side of the coin for these professional and scientific aspirations was a specific relationship of psychiatrists to non-medical mental health professions and to psychotherapy – one marked by demarcation and devaluation. Indeed, neither in German university departments of psychiatry nor in the asylums were psychologists, social workers or nurses in a position to share in the processes of decision-making – if they were present at all.[11] The nurses working in the field had no specific training but were rather members of clerical orders or (particularly in the male wards of the asylums) untrained and often recruited from the lower social strata.

Between the 1870s and the beginning of World War I, the most striking aspect of the practice of mental health care was the enormous growth of asylums: e.g. in Prussia from 64 per 100,000 inhabitants in 1875 to 166 in 1905. Whereas the general population increased by 33.4 per cent during these three decades, the number of asylum residents increased by 245 per cent.[12] This growth is usually explained by the convergence of at least four factors: (1) increase in the general population and, in particular, of the urban population coming to the attention of or using the resources of psychiatry; (2) an extension of the sphere of competence of psychiatrists beyond the boundaries of 'traditional' cases of insanity; (3) a more thorough policy of observing, labelling and institutionalising the mentally ill by state authorities; and (4) an increased demand for psychiatric expertise, in particular for legal issues, indicating the increased social status and cultural esteem of psychiatry.

The inpatient care of large-scale asylums was situated mainly in rural areas, but was later supplemented by smaller university hospitals and clinics. The academic departments frequently only dealt with acute 'cases', whereas the asylums were responsible for patients with chronic conditions or those living in rural areas. However, this division of labour was a continuous topic of conflict between the two types of institutions.[13] This division had already been the prevailing answer of the nineteenth century to the 'challenge of madness' (*Irrenfrage*), the contemporary problems perceived to be the result of the increasing numbers of psychiatric patients. And in spite of manifold social, political and cultural changes and upheavals during Germany's twentieth-century history, this institutional and organisational answer turned out to show a remarkable stability. Immediately after the turn of the century, the apparent increase of 'overburdening' syndromes, nervousness and neurasthenia posed an additional challenge to society at large, as well as to the changed psychiatric profession with its enlarged sphere of competence. The reaction was a combined effort of state agencies, the new state-supervised health insurance organisations, and psychiatrists to establish large sanatoria for nervous disorders (*Nervenheilanstalten*), in addition to those for tuberculosis. Frequently, these had hundreds or over a thousand beds and were organised according to the models of asylums. As a 'fringe' phenomenon, a considerable number of small 'nerve clinics' and private hospitals were also established, particularly in large cities, as well as in seaside and mountain resorts; they were administered by doctors alone, or run as single-handed practices.

After World War I, in the democratic Weimar republic, the field of psychiatry experienced a considerable internal differentiation, not least as a result of the marked pluralism that developed in the realm of social, health and educational policies in the emergent welfare state. In urban centres, outpatient services inspired by socialist, psychoanalytic or pedagogic ideals sprang up, often as the result of individual or small-group local initiatives. These had numerous organisational forms and were occasionally supported by social-democratic local authorities, but psychiatrists mostly played a marginal role in them. Such activities were undertaken by psychologists, pedagogues and other non-medical professionals, and were targeted in particular at social maladjustment, sexual problems and other conditions in the borderland between 'normality' and what were considered to be 'proper' mental disorders.

Continuities or Ruptures?

At the level of regions, provinces or states, however, the basic structure of the asylums remained stable, although for a few years, a number of remarkable additional or complementary services were developed and put into practice. These reform approaches included models of early discharge (as developed e.g. in Erlangen/Bavaria); 'activating therapies' (aktivere Therapie) which included physical activities orientated towards everyday life and work, following the programme of Hermann Simon in Gütersloh/Westphalia; and finally, 'social-psychiatric' outpatient services organisationally bound to the asylums (or otherwise mainly independent urban initiatives).[14] In addition, small-scale private hospitals for the wealthy and the single-handed private practices of resident psychiatrists offered services, particularly in larger cities.

From the perspective of psychiatrists of the late nineteenth and early twentieth centuries, there was a triad of both explicit and implicit values associated with these structures of mental health care: (1) stabilizing, increasing or restoring the health of the individual; (2) the prosperity of the national economy; and (3) the (biological) strength of the state.[15] This triad of values was not a specific German feature but rather part of most Western post-enlightenment health policies. However, in the German context from the late nineteenth century, the broader idea of the state was increasingly replaced by the concept of the nation. This implied a presumed common origin and history of the population, social and cultural homogeneity, and the existence of specific national traits, together with the 'otherness' and ultimately inferiority of neighbouring ethnic groups or nations. Accordingly, in mental health care, the goal of improving the strength of the state – or later the nation – became ever more dominant and prioritized over the well-being of the individual.

Both the concept and programme of 'social psychiatry' (Sozialpsychiatrie) as well as the field of psychiatric eugenics and genetics illustrate very well a continuous change in the hierarchical order of the three value orientations identified above. Thus, in the first three decades of the twentieth century, the notion of 'social psychiatry' shifted from a focus on the social origins of the psychiatric disorders of individuals towards an ever stronger preoccupation with the identification and prevention of 'non-social' behaviour to protect the social organism, 'folk-body' (Volkskörper) or race.[16] From the early twentieth century onwards, this development converged with that of eugenics. It also determined the short history of the German version of the mental hygiene movement (psychische Hygiene), which was readily absorbed after 1933 under the roof of racial hygiene. The Deutsche Verein für psychische Hygiene had only been founded in 1925, stimulated by the American Mental Hygiene movement, but from the beginning, it had a certain emphasis on eugenic ideas.[17]

Parallel to this, research into the hereditary origins of mental disorders, beginning in the years after 1900 and inspired by eugenic ideas, experienced a rapid career before and after 1933. In the first decade of the century, Kraepelin and others had formulated the need for a systematic long-term research effort into the hereditary condition of the entire German population. This particularly concerned the modes of genetic transmission for mental disorders, as well as related conditions such as delinquency and sexual aberrations. All these conditions were perceived to be both the expression and the result of an imminent process of degeneration, i.e. a steadily decreasing quality of the genetic pool. To carry out such a far-reaching programme, Kraepelin urged the establishment of a central, state-funded statistical and research institute – a concept that materialized from 1917 in the form of the Department of Genealogy and Demography (*Genealogisch-Demographische Abteilung*, or GDA) of the DFA. Ernst Rüdin, a pupil of Kraepelin, consultant at the psychiatric department in Munich and one of the key figures in the German movement of eugenics and racial hygiene, was appointed head of this new institution, internationally the first in the field of psychiatric genetics. With a new methodology connected to the statistical concept of 'empirical hereditary prognosis' (*empirische Erbprognose*), he had created a paradigm for the field. By 1933/34, Rüdin and his group were internationally perceived as setting the standards in psychiatric genetics. From 1929 until 1934, his department was the main recipient of a considerable five-year grant from the Rockefeller Foundation for a multi-centre research programme aimed at investigating the 'anthropological conditions of the German population'.[18]

In contrast to this increased public spending on eugenically motivated genetic research, resources for mental health care became dramatically scarcer by the end of the 1920s. This in turn induced a restriction of the existing systems of public welfare, with a consequent dismantling of reform schemes such as early discharge or combined outpatient and community services (*offene Fürsorge*). In addition, the increasing social strains caused by high unemployment and poverty reduced the willingness of the population to have dealings with 'abnormal' individuals. For psychiatric institutions, this meant a rise in the average length of stay of patients and, in parallel, an increase in both the absolute and proportional numbers of long-term residents. Because the shortage of funds also affected the financial provision for inpatients, the gap between needs and available resources in psychiatric institutions widened further. The evolving practical problems were a much debated issue at contemporary psychiatric conferences and in publications. Most authors agreed that distinctions had to be made among inpatients on the basis of the prognosis of their condition, and that chronic psychotic and mentally handicapped patients should be housed separately and provision for them kept to a minimum.[19] This concept of differentiated resource allocation – favouring the more healthy (and the economy or the state) at the expense of the weaker patients – lasted well into the Nazi period and turned out to be of deadly consequence.

Continuities or Ruptures?

The Nazi Period (1933-1945): National Strength and Racial Purity

The position of the eugenicist and geneticist Ernst Rüdin in German psychiatry and mental health policy after 1933 is an indicator of the development of this whole field during the Nazi period. Having been appointed director of the whole DFA (in addition to the GDA) in 1931, he succeeded Eugen Fischer as chairman of the German Society of Racial Hygiene in 1934 and was made chairman of the professional association of neurologists and psychiatrists (*Gesellschaft Deutscher Neurologen und Psychiater*) in 1935, as a consequence of intervention by the Reich Ministry of the Interior. In addition, he was the main referee for the field of psychiatry as well as for eugenics and genetics at the German Research Foundation (*Notgemeinschaft Deutscher Wissenschaft/Deutsche Forschungsgemeinschaft*), the main organisation for research funding. He also acted as leading expert advisor for the new regime: from 1933 onwards, he was a member of the expert Committee for Population and Race Policies at the Reich Ministry of the Interior (*Sachverständigenbeirat für Bevölkerungs- und Rassenpolitik*) and chairman of one of the committee's working groups. His advice and guidelines were followed when the new Law for the Prevention of Hereditary Diseased Offspring (*Gesetz zur Verhütung erbkranken Nachwuchses*) was formulated. This law legitimised forced sterilisation of individuals diagnosed as suffering from a number of supposedly hereditary conditions, such as schizophrenia, epilepsy or mental deficiency. It was announced in July 1933, a few months after the Nazi government took over, and put into practice on 1 January 1934. Together with a ministerial officer for public health affairs, Arthur Gütt, and the lawyer and ss-member Falk Ruttke, Rüdin was also author of the official commentary on the implementation of the new law.[20]

Rüdin publicly welcomed the advent of 'the new state' and soon profited in his scientific activities. The number of research positions at the GDA increased sharply after 1933, and until the beginning of the war, Rüdin repeatedly received large additional sums of money from both the Ministry of the Interior and the Chancellory of the Führer for his research into 'creating the scientific foundations for the health and racial policy' of the 'new state'.[21] Although his involvement with the Nazi regime was well known, Rüdin was internationally still regarded as a leading scientist, illustrated by the fact that the Rockefeller Foundation continued the funding of fellowships for promising young scientists from abroad (such as Eliot Slater from the UK) to study at the GDA in Munich well into the late 1930s. He was also invited as a plenary speaker at the Seventh World Congress of Genetics in Edinburgh in 1939.[22]

The case of Rüdin illustrates not only the intricate relationship between psychiatric genetics, eugenics and politics, but also documents that in psychiatry and mental health care, the pluralism of the Weimar period had suddenly changed into a situation dominated by the programmes and practices of eugenics and racial hygiene. This domination may be documented in the dimensions of mental health care (both 'prevention', i.e. sterilization, and selective allocation of therapeutic resources), professional politics and research, which in turn implied the justification or legitimisation of existing and future policies. This change, however, should not be understood in terms of a complete rupture in 1933. Rather, it represented the massive strengthening of eugenicist tendencies that had already been present in the previous decades and, at the same time, the suppression of alternative approaches at the institutional and conceptual levels, paralleled by the systematic exclusion, expulsion and later extermination of Jewish and Socialist doctors.

In the realm of health care, attempts were undertaken to centralise the system of asylums. A standing co-ordinating committee of asylum directors and state officials was set up at the German Communal Council (*Deutscher Gemeindetag*)[23] to evaluate the existing services, in particular psychiatric asylums and homes for the mentally handicapped. It was also meant to formulate strategies for restructuring according to demographic and epidemiological data, and to set goals for diminishing expenditures for those unable to contribute to the national economy. In that context, too, the responsibility for the national statistics of mental disorders was shifted from the professional association of psychiatrists to this central body. Previous debates (which had their origins in the Weimar period) on the rational and effective allocation of scarce resources were continued but now under the premises of the racial state. The result was a further reduction of expenditure on the asylum inmates with a poor prognosis and/or incapable of manual work, whereas more efforts went into new therapeutic approaches for the supposedly more 'valuable' patients. These therapies had been developed in the mid-1930s and included methods such as insulin coma, electroconvulsive therapy, and systematic occupational therapy in the tradition of Hermann Simon, which was also appreciated and practised in the Nazi period. Indeed, protagonists of the later programme of systematic patient killings ('euthanasia'), such as Paul Nitsche and the Heidelberg professor Carl Schneider, were also amongst the most outspoken protagonists of occupational therapy and other reformist approaches.[24]

In the years leading up to the war, the reduction of resources for 'incurable' patients was taken to such an extreme that only the minimum amount of money was available per person to prevent actual starvation. The death of patients weakened by these measures, possibly through an intercurrent infection, was tolerated, although at this stage not systematically intended.[25] Preventive measures following the logic of eugenics were publicly advertised in lectures, exhibitions and the printed media and met with considerable general approval. There was also a continuity in relation to psychotherapy in that it remained of marginal importance for overall mental health care. Professional psychotherapeutic services were restricted to a few urban centres and were completely separated from any psychiatric institutions. One central psychotherapeutic institution continued to exist – the German Institute for Psychological Research and Psychotherapy in Berlin, in the precincts of the former Psychoanalytic Institute, which had been dissolved in 1936. Branches of this institute existed or were founded in Stuttgart, Munich, and a few other cities. They offered an eclectic, explicitly non-psychoanalytic training and (on a small scale) outpatient services. The institute, although marginal in quantitative terms, had a somewhat privileged position due to the fact that its director, Matthias Göring, was a cousin of Hermann Göring, the Reich Minister of Aviation. Psychotherapists from the institute were employed in particular for the treatment and prevention of stress conditions in the Air Force, as well as for applied research in industry aimed at improving the efficacy of work. Finally, they were involved in establishing a specific version of mental hygiene called Psychological Health Guidance (*Seelische Gesundheitsführung*), geared to Nazi health and population policies.[26]

The radicalisation of racially inspired social and health policies during World War II, under severe economic and military constraints, had atrocious consequences in the field of psychiatry. Between 1939 and 1945, a programme of systematic killings ('euthanasia') was implemented to exterminate 'useless' chronic patients who were perceived as a burden, in view both of the needs of war economy and of racial health. Two major strands may be distinguished in this programme. Firstly, the application of various methods and technologies (e.g. gas chambers, overdose of drugs) to patients selected by a centrally distributed catalogue of criteria which varied over time and according to decisions taken by both local personnel and intermediate authorities. Secondly, systematic starvation was intended to kill the weakest out of the asylum population.[27] The resources 'saved' by this programme (in terms of finance, manpower and asylum beds) were to be diverted to intensify the 'active' therapies for those with a good prognosis or made available for wounded soldiers brought back from the war fronts. Altogether, more than 160,000 psychiatric patients and mentally handicapped in the *Reich* fell victim to this specific form of Nazi mental health policies; if the occupied territories are included, the numbers are estimated to be about 250,000-300,000.[28] In this context, psychiatric research was aimed at finding scientifically valid criteria for the differential diagnosis between those valuable for the economy and the race and those not – implying a decision of life or death. Some of these studies, in which members of the elitist DFA were involved, made use of the victims of the 'euthanasia' programme as research subjects.[29]

The Post-World War Two Period: 'Normalisation'

The first few years after the German defeat in May 1945 were marked by the breakdown of the political system, massive material destruction and loss of life due to war, together with the repudiation or loss of norms, values and identification figures which had shaped the public life of the preceding decades. In the public discourse, concepts like 'race', 'nation' or 'German superiority' were suddenly highly controversial and then for some time taboo – although they remained in use in more private circles. The immediate challenges appeared to be the reconstitution of public order, provision of the population with food and elementary health services, and the building up of a reliable administration with the aim to establish a democratic political system. The efforts to meet these challenges soon diverged following the political demarcations between the Eastern, Soviet-occupied zone and the three Western zones governed by the USA, the UK and France. The following account will be restricted to the Western part, from the late 1940s onwards in the political framework of the Federal Republic of Germany.

The policies of de-nazification initiated by the allies and only half-heartedly supported by the German population were designed to keep the new administration and elites free of individuals responsible for Nazi atrocities and to prevent any risks of the future Germany falling back into anti-democratic sentiments. Seen from the contemporary perspective of much of the general population, these policies were a kind of distorted 'justice' of the victors (*Siegerjustiz*). Nevertheless, numerous individuals and social groups within German society felt the necessity to distance themselves from the Nazi past in order to legitimize or at least not to endanger their status in the emerging new state.

The psychiatric profession developed a number of strategies in this context. First, until the mid-1960s, there was a strong tendency to circumvent the topic altogether. Only very few individual psychiatrists felt the need to reflect systematically on the Nazi past of their profession and the atrocities experienced by the victims, to share the new insights with the public, or to draw conclusions for the further organisation and practice of psychiatric care.[30] The dominating reluctance of psychiatrists to comment on the past resonated with the ambiguous policies of both local and regional authorities in politically 'cleansing' their professional staff, since these professionals were needed for the urgent rebuilding of institutions and services. There were, of course, considerable regional differences in such policies, dependent in part on guidelines of the military governments and on the political views and priorities of individual officers.[31] In general, however, it may be stated that the responsible public authorities prioritised the functioning of their respective institutions over the investigation of individual responsibilities. Such ambiguous attitudes met with the similarly ambivalent legal prosecutions of doctors involved in the systematic patient killings or other Nazi atrocities. Almost all the trials related to these issues concentrated on individual culpability but marginalised or neglected the structural preconditions that had enabled the specific psychiatric practices of the period. And in many if not most of these trials, all available information to exonerate the defendants was taken into consideration, including testimonies of colleagues of rather

Continuities or Ruptures?

dubious value – with the result that only very few of the accused were finally sentenced, and most of these were released after some time.[32]

On the part of the psychiatric profession itself, there was – similarly – set priority on protecting the public image of the group, as opposed to any thorough inquiry into individual and group responsibility. Almost no contradiction came from colleagues when past activities of members of the profession, even as active experts within the 'euthanasia' organisation, were re-interpreted as 'subversive', allegedly aimed at reducing the number of selected victims for the killing programme to an absolute minimum.[33] Representatives of the profession created an image of the past according to which the systematic killings were a phenomenon almost completely restricted to the sphere of the asylums, with mainly lower-rank psychiatrists actively involved and university psychiatry almost unaffected. Regarding mental health policies and psychiatric research, it was argued that the priorities followed here had nothing to do with the standards and rationalities of 'proper psychiatry' but were rather part of irrational and perverse ideologies followed by the Nazi leadership and imposed on the profession. Only after 1945 – so they formulated – was it possible for psychiatrists to return to pre-Nazi traditions in practice and research.[34] This image of the past, together with the half-hearted policies of regional authorities and courts, legitimized continuities at the level of the psychiatric establishment regarding both therapeutic and research programmes. It also implied a dissociation of the majority of the profession from the atrocities of the Nazi period.

The necessity to demonstrate distance from the Nazi past, combined with the wish of younger psychiatrists for alternative approaches to mental disorders, also led to a remarkable resurgence of long-existing approaches framed as 'anthropological psychiatry', which had been completely marginalised since the early 1930s. These approaches were inspired by phenomenological philosophy in the tradition of Husserl and by specific Swiss developments from psychoanalysis, merged with the philosophy of Heidegger (*Daseinsanalyse*). From the late 1940s to the 1960s, they resulted in elaborate and very idealistic debates about appropriate terminologies, theories and attitudes for understanding and interacting with the mentally disordered patient. Perhaps not accidentally, the sphere of politics and the social context of the life of psychiatric patients – either in the community or in institutions – were almost completely absent in these debates. Similarly, they had little or no effect on the everyday practice of mental health care. These 'anthropological' concepts allowed extensive deliberations on the subjectivity of the patient which did not – at least at first glance – rely on the theories and terminologies of psychoanalysis.

These debates, however, paved the way for more thorough and lasting changes, on both the conceptual and the practical level. There was a shift from theories of mental disease based on somatic models towards those acknowledging the impact of psychological and social factors. This was accompanied by a dramatic increase in awareness of the completely inadequate living conditions of psychiatric patients, both in institutions and in the community. The shift on the conceptual level was also a reaction to practical challenges. In the post-World War II period, together with health insurance agencies and courts, psychiatrists were confronted with many individuals who presented with a wide range of mental symptoms, apparently connected with their exposure to the battlefield, imprisonment or even torture. Psychiatric experts often had difficulty in accommodating the presented clinical pictures within existing disease categories and were thus looking for alternatives. The concept of 'dystrophy' was a first attempt to account for these 'atypical' psychiatric conditions.[35] It implied long-term effects of malnourishment and starvation on the brain and concomitant psychological dysfunctioning, and thus opened up discussions about the impact of 'external' (although still somatic) factors, in contrast to the previous hegemony of the notion of 'constitution'. This concept of 'dystrophy' was readily accepted in court cases dealing with claims for pensions or compensations and thus contributed to a less stigmatized position for the affected individuals.[36] A further step was the acknowledgment of states of 'illness without disease' (*Kranksein ohne Krankheit*), which presupposed that a real disease is somatic in nature, but that there are serious conditions of psychological suffering without such a somatic correlate.[37] With this state of affairs, in the second half of the 1950s, German psychiatry had reached a conceptual openness which had existed in the early years of the Weimar Republic, when the experiences with war trauma had resulted in similar debates and related programmes for practical help. In the mid-1920s, however, both economic and professional considerations had led to a decision of the Reich Insurance Office (*Reichsversicherungsamt*) not to accept a causal connection between war trauma and neurosis anymore.[38]

From the mid-1960s onwards, awareness of the suffering of those persecuted during the Holocaust as well as of the poor condition of mental health care led to the formation of a new movement of social psychiatry.[39] One significant feature of this movement was the opening up of the psychiatric profession to the expertise of psychologists, nurses and social workers, together with the willingness to integrate these professions in decision-taking processes and political interventions.[40] Important steps in this development were the formation in 1970 of the 'Mannheim circle' – an open forum of debate for all health care professions – and in 1971, the foundation of the German Society for Social Psychiatry (*Deutsche Gesellschaft für soziale Psychiatrie*) as well as the *Aktion Psychisch Kranke*, a lobby of psychiatric patients in which patient representatives and mental health professionals joined forces.[41] These events have, of course, to be seen in the wider context of the students' movement of 1968 and the post-68 emergence of social movements that brought the problems of socially marginal groups to the centre of the political agenda.[42] Whereas the protagonists of the former initiatives (e.g. M. Bauer, K. Dörner, A. Finzen, M. Richartz) came mainly from

Continuities or Ruptures?

young residents at university departments or from asylums, a further, partly related initiative was brought forward by a small group of psychiatrists in leading academic positions (C. Kulenkampff, H. Häfner, K. Kisker).

These protagonists managed to persuade a Member of the Federal Parliament (Walter Picard, of the Christian Democratic Union/CDU) to propose an official inquiry into the state of mental health care. In June 1971, Parliament agreed to set up an expert committee for such a systematic investigation. A preliminary report, published in 1973, stated that 'a great number of psychiatric patients and mentally disabled staying in psychiatric institutions have to live in extremely poor conditions, indeed in part intolerable for human beings'.[43] The final report, in 1975, to a large degree confirmed this diagnosis and formulated a number of principles and recommendations: (1) community care; (2) comprehensive care adapted to the needs of psychiatric patients and the mentally handicapped; (3) co-ordinating all mental health care services according to the established needs of those concerned; (4) equality of psychiatric patients with somatic patients.[44] These recommendations implied that there should be a redirection of institutionalised care towards smaller psychiatric units in general hospitals, community-based day or night facilities, or 'sheltered homes' where small groups of patients could live in the community, supported by psychiatric social workers and nurses.

Thus, from the 1970s, for the first time in twentieth-century German psychiatry and mental health care, the monopoly and isolation of the psychiatric profession were substantially broken up. Large-scale asylums were no longer considered the adequate answer to the problems of individuals with mental disorders. At the same time, the expertise of non-medical professions was integrated into therapeutic concepts and practices, as well as to a certain degree into academic psychiatric research. The developments triggered by these events in the late 1960s and early 1970s are still ongoing, in a gradual process of de-centralisation and establishing community care. This process has taken place at a fairly moderate tempo, compared with some other Western countries, and certainly more slowly than the early protagonists of these programmes had hoped for. From 1971 to 1990, the number of psychiatric units in general hospitals increased from 21 to 90, with an average of 70–90 beds (compared to often more than 1,000 or even 2,000 beds in the former asylums). The former asylums (now also called *Krankenhaus*, 'hospital') themselves decreased remarkably in size (towards a target of ca. 600 beds) and were converted into 'psychiatric centres', with integrated small departments of internal medicine and neurology and affiliated community services.[45] The establishment of complementary community services with opportunities for sheltered housing or work, however, is even today far behind the original plans of the 1970s and also below the standards of some neighbouring countries (in particular the Netherlands, Switzerland and Scandinavia). Similarly, the goal of introducing specific training in psychiatric nursing has been propagated vehemently since the 1960s, but even in the early 1990s, a considerable proportion of the nursing staff – in particular in the asylums/psychiatric centres – did not have such training.

Another long-lasting phenomenon which reached from the beginning of the twentieth century to well beyond the political ruptures of 1933 and 1945 was the almost complete dissociation of psychiatry and mental health care from psychoanalysis and related forms of psychotherapy. Due to the persistent resistance of psychiatrists to the establishment of psychotherapeutic units or programmes in psychiatric institutions and at the same time political pressures to introduce psychotherapeutic facilities both in the academic field and in health care, a completely separate institutionalisation occurred of a combined field of 'psychosomatic medicine and psychotherapy'. This was at the level of medical schools, in the form of sanatoria and rehabilitation hospitals, and finally through private psychotherapeutic practitioners. The first academic programme in this field was established in 1949-50 at the University of Heidelberg, with a number of others following in the early 1950s. From the 1970s, this specific subject was integrated into the medical curriculum, and appropriate departments were set up at all German medical schools. At the same time, after the cost-efficiency of systematic psychotherapy for certain groups of patients had been documented in a controlled, long-term study in 1965,[46] analytical psychotherapy was introduced into the general health insurance in 1967 and was thus (on medical recommendation) accessible to more than 80 per cent of the population. It was only in the early 1990s – in the context of a major restructuring of postgraduate medical training – that psychiatrists and psychological psychotherapists agreed to establish a common certified training in 'psychotherapeutic medicine', including methods from several psychotherapeutic schools. Other non-medical professionals, such as social workers, were only allowed to practise psychotherapy in exceptional cases. This also implied the establishment of new professional associations, integrating different disciplinary and theoretical backgrounds (psychiatry and psychology; psychoanalysis and behavioural therapy), and in many cases the absorption of the former departments of psychosomatic medicine and psychotherapy in existing psychiatric hospitals.[47]

A final point is the impact of the introduction of new drugs such as neuroleptics and anti-depressants on mental health care from the 1950s onwards. No reliable data are available as to the consequences on the overall numbers of patients in psychiatric institutions, or the average duration of inpatient care, but the effects are likely to have been similar to those in the neighbouring countries. The influence of the available drug treatments on the newly emerging 'culture of psychiatric pharmacotherapy' was illustrated at the 99th annual conference of the German Psychiatric Association in 1970, where the general theme was the 'state of the art' of contemporary psychiatry. Rudolf Degkwitz, Professor of Psychiatry at the University of Freiburg, spoke on 'modern psychopharmacology'. From a systematic survey of 689 publications on the effect of the new drugs since their introduction in the mid-1950s, he found that only a very small minority of these publications had really taken into consideration the elementary standards of clinical trials, and that their results were thus most dubious. In particular, side-effects had not really been studied in a systematic way. However, this had been made almost impossible since an expert memorandum commissioned by the *Deutsche Forschungsgemeinschaft*, the main body for research funding, stated that to stop neuroleptic treatment in order to look into persistent, non-reversible side-effects was not ethically acceptable.[48] Thus, the plausibility of the positive effects of this treatment was such that – in spite of the absence of methodically sound evidence – it was considered to be against good therapeutic practice to withhold such treatment for a limited time for research purposes.

Conclusion

The main features in the development of twentieth-century German psychiatry described above clearly document considerable continuities overarching the political breaks of 1933 and 1945 but also point to a number of important discontinuities.

The continuities include the persistence of institutional structures of inpatient services predominantly in large-scale mental hospitals which was only questioned in the wake of the social movements of the late 1960s and early 1970s. Parallel to these institutional structures, there were equally persistent initiatives to complement or reform the available inpatient services by programmes to activate patients and re-integrate them into the community through early discharge and outpatient services connected to institutional care. Although these attempts met with considerable resonance at the level of psychiatric discourse and were in some cases also used as models for similar programmes abroad (in particular Simon's *aktivere Therapie*), they remained local phenomena that did not have a lasting effect on the general structure of mental health care. However, this also changed in the last third of the century, in connection with broader social and cultural developments. A third dimension of continuity is apparent in the long-standing devaluation and subordination of non-medical personnel (such as psychologists, social workers and psychiatric nurses) in mental health care settings. The integration of these professional groups into decision-taking processes also began only in the late 1960s, and even today is only realized to a lesser degree than in neighbouring countries such as Switzerland or the Netherlands. A further form of continuity can be seen in the strong orientation of the majority of the psychiatric profession towards the natural sciences and a concomitant antagonism to psychodynamic approaches. This feature resulted in the establishment of an independent medical specialty

– 'psychosomatic medicine and psychotherapy' – in the post-World War II period. As a result, psychotherapy did not develop as a branch of psychiatry, but separately in the context of psychosomatic medicine.

Discontinuities may be found at the level of psychiatric practitioners as well as that of therapeutic practice and research programmes. One consequence of the Nazi takeover was the forced migration of a considerable number of practitioners in the field of mental health care. It also led to a re-configuration of psychiatric practice and research according to the principles of eugenics and genetics. However, these principles had certainly been present and to a certain extent effective before, in particular during the last years of the Weimar republic and in the context of the economic crisis of the late 1920s and early 1930s. This re-configuration cannot therefore be adequately interpreted as a 'break' but rather as an increasingly rapid narrowing down of political and scientific concepts to those favoured by the eugenic/racial hygiene movement and the new state. Indeed, it might be argued that medicine and politics used each other as mutual resources.[49]

The end of World War II may be seen even less as a break cutting through the whole realm of psychiatry and mental health care. Marked changes occurred mainly at the material level, with extensive destruction of buildings and other infrastructure, as well as on the general political level, with the breakdown of the Nazi regime and transition to a democratic society. These changes had, of course, repercussions for health care in general, and psychiatry in particular. However, although there was a limited degree of discontinuity at the level of personnel as a consequence of jurisdiction (e.g. P. Nitsche), suicide (M. de Crinis, C. Schneider) or retirement (E. Rüdin), the great majority of psychiatric professionals as well as nurses and administrative staff active during the Nazi period continued working. Continuities predominate also at the level of institutional structures, therapeutic concepts, and in the relationships between psychiatrists and non-psychiatric professions in the field of mental health care. A marked break in 1945 may be identified only in psychiatric research, where eugenically inspired genetic programmes disappeared almost completely until the mid-1980s.

In view of this complex history, the persistence of the image of three distinct periods of twentieth-century German psychiatry is in need of explanation. One hypothesis might be that this conventional periodisation is considerably influenced by the self-perception and outward representation by post-World War II German psychiatric professionals. This consisted of the reshaping of their professional identity and politics, which needed a clear demarcation between 'proper' German psychiatric traditions and events that were the result of political pressure in the Nazi period. A full exploration of this hypothesis, however, would not only require a reconstruction of twentieth-century German psychiatry but would also need a complementary analysis of the debates, strategies and contexts of those psychiatrists (and historians of psychiatry) who formulated this 'discontinuity' interpretation of history. Such a comprehensive analysis will be a task for further research.

Notes

1.   See M. in der Beek, *Praktische Psychiatrie* (Berlin: De Gruyter, 1957); K. Dörner, 'Carl Schneider: Genialer Therapeut, moderner ökologischer Systemtheoretiker und Euthanasiemörder', *Psychiatrische Praxis*, 12 (1986), 112-14.

2.   See V. Roelcke, 'Die Entwicklung der Psychiatrie zwischen 1880 und 1932: Theoriebildung, Institutionen, Interaktionen mit zeitgenössischer Wissenschafts- und Sozialpolitik', in R. vom Bruch and B. Kaderas (eds), *Wissenschaften und Wissenschaftspolitik: Bestandsaufnahmen zu Formationen, Brüchen und Kontinuitäten im Deutschland des 20. Jahrhunderts* (Stuttgart: Franz Steiner, 2002), 109-24; E. Engstrom, *Clinical Psychiatry in Imperial Germany. A History of Psychiatric Practice* (Ithaca/London: Cornell University Press, 2003).

3.   See Engstrom, *ibid.*

4.   See the contributions by D. Kaufmann, H.-P. Schmiedebach, and V. Roelcke, in M. Gijswijt-Hofstra and R. Porter (eds), *Cultures of Neurasthenia from Beard to the First World War* (Amsterdam: Rodopi, 2001).

5.   See V. Roelcke, 'Biologizing social facts. An early 20th century debate on Kraepelin's concepts of culture, neurasthenia, and degeneration', *Culture, Medicine, and Psychiatry*, 21 (1997), 383-403; V. Roelcke, *Krankheit und Kulturkritik. Psychiatrische Gesellschaftsdiagnosen im bürgerlichen Zeitalter, 1790-1914* (Frankfurt am Main: Campus, 1999), chaps. 5-6; J. Radkau, *Das Zeitalter der Nervosität* (München: Hanser, 1998).

6.   See [Report on] 'Jahresversammlung des Deutschen Vereins für Psychiatrie', *Allgemeine Zeitschrift für Psychiatrie*, 60 (1903), 905-78: 906.

7.   A. Hoche, 'Über den Wert der Psychoanalyse', *Archiv für Psychiatrie und Nervenkrankheiten*, 51 (1913), 1055-79; O. Bumke, *Die Psychoanalyse. Eine Kritik* (Berlin: Springer, 1931).

8.   L. Binswanger, *Einführung in die Probleme der Allgemeinen Psychologie* (Berlin: Springer, 1922); Paul Schilder, *Seele und Leben. Grundsätzliches zur Psychologie der Schizophrenie und Paraphrenie, zur Psychoanalyse und zur Psychologie* (Berlin: Springer, 1923).

9.   See M.M. Weber, '"Ein Forschungsinstitut für Psychiatrie": Die Entwicklung der Deutschen Forschungsanstalt für Psychiatrie München 1918-1945', *Sudhoffs Archiv*, 75 (1991), 74-89.

10.   R. Hayward, 'Making Psychiatry British: The Maudsley and the Munich Model', in V. Roelcke and P. Weindling (eds), *Inspiration – Co-operation – Migration: American-British-German Relations in Psychiatry, c. 1870-1945* (in preparation).

11.   This may be illustrated by the example of Eugen Kahn: V. Roelcke, 'Cultures of Psychiatry in Munich and Yale, ca. 1930: The case of Eugen Kahn', in V. Roelcke and P. Weindling (eds), *op. cit.* (note 10).

12. D. Blasius, *Der verwaltete Wahnsinn. Eine Sozialgeschichte des Irrenhauses* (Frankfurt am Main: S. Fischer, 1980), 84. Parallel but not as extensive increases have been found for the European neighbours. In the Netherlands, e.g. there were 52 asylum inmates per 100,000 inhabitants by 1860, compared to 144 per 100,000 in 1900. *Ibidem*, quoting D. Schermers, 'Die niederländische Irrenanstaltspflege in den Jahren 1875-1900', *Zeitschrift für die gesamte Neurologie und Psychiatrie*, 3 (1910), 284-306.

13. See Engstrom, *op. cit.* (note 2).

14. See H.-L. Siemen, '*Menschen blieben auf der Strecke ...*'. *Psychiatrie zwischen Reform und Nationalsozialismus* (Gütersloh: van Hoddis, 1987); B. Walter, *Psychiatrie und Gesellschaft in der Moderne. Geisteskrankenfürsorge in der Provinz Westfalen zwischen Kaiserreich und NS-Regime* (Paderborn: Schöningh, 1996). See H. Simon, *Aktivere Krankenbehandlung in der Irrenanstalt* (Berlin 1929, repr. Gütersloh 1969, and Bonn: Psychiatrie Verlag, 1986).

15. See e.g. E. Kraepelin, *Die psychiatrischen Aufgaben des Staates* (Jena: Fischer, 1900); E. Kraepelin, 'Hundert Jahre Psychiatrie', *Zeitschrift für die gesamte Neurologie und Psychiatrie*, 38 (1918), 189-275. Also K. Fürstner, *Wie ist die Fürsorge für Gemütskranke von Aerzten und Laien zu fördern?* (Berlin: Karger, 1900); F. Jolly, 'Rede zur Eröffnung der Jahresversammlung des Vereins der deutschen Irrenärzte etc.', *Allgemeine Zeitschrift für Psychiatrie*, 34 (1901), 694-707. See also Engstrom, *op. cit.* (note 2), passim.

16. H.-P. Schmiedebach and S. Priebe, 'Social psychiatry and open psychiatric care in late 19th and early 20th century Germany', in E. Engstrom and V. Roelcke (eds), *Psychiatrie im 19. Jahrhundert. Forschungen zu Institutionen, Praktiken und Kontroversen im deutschsprachigen Raum* (Basel: Schwabe, 2003), 263-81. See also H.-P. Schmiedebach and S. Priebe, 'Social Psychiatry in Germany in the Twentieth Century: Ideas and Models', *Medical History*, 48 (2004), 449-72.

17. See P. Weindling, *Health, Race, and German Politics between National Unification and Nazism, 1870-1945* (Cambridge: Cambridge University Press, 1989). And Walter, *op. cit.* (note 14).

18. See V. Roelcke, 'Programm und Praxis der psychiatrischen Genetik an der Deutschen Forschungsanstalt für Psychiatrie unter Ernst Rüdin', *Medizinhistorisches Journal*, 37 (2002), 21-55. For a contemporary evaluation from abroad, see A. Lewis, 'Inheritance of Mental Disorders', in Ch. P. Blacker (ed.), *The Chances of Morbid Inheritance* (London: H. K. Lewis, 1934), 86-133: 87.

19. See e.g. E. Friedlander, 'Kann die Versorgung der Geisteskranken billiger gestaltet werden und wie?', *Psychiatrisch-Neurologische Wochenschrift*, 24 (1932), 373-81. See Siemen, *op. cit.* (note 14), 102-5.

20. *Gesetz zur Verhütung erbkranken Nachwuchses*, bearbeitet und erläutert von Arthur Gütt, Ernst Rüdin, Falk Ruttke (Munich: Lehmanns, 1934).

21. For the full archival source, see Roelcke, 'Progamm', *op. cit.* (note 18), 43-4.

22. See *ibid.*, 45, note 69.

23. The German Communal Council had been founded in December 1933 following an order of the new regime to centralize all communal administrative authorities throughout the Reich, including e.g. the *Deutscher Städtetag*, the *Reichsstädtebund*,

the *Deutscher Landgemeindetag*, and the *Verband der Preussischen Provinzen*, and to create one authoritative institution for interaction with state and party instances. See H. Faulstich, *Hungersterben in der Psychiatrie 1914-1949* (Freiburg: Lambertus, 1998), 109-10.

24. C. Schneider, *Behandlung und Verhütung der Geisteskrankheiten* (Berlin: Springer, 1939). On Schneider, see V. Roelcke, G. Hohendorf, M. Rotzoll, 'Psychiatric research and "euthanasia". The case of the psychiatric department at the University of Heidelberg, 1941-1945', *History of Psychiatry*, 5 (1994), 517-32.

25. See Faulstich, *op. cit.* (note 23), esp. 109-28.

26. G. Cocks, *Psychotherapy in the Third Reich. The Göring Institute* (New York/ Oxford, Oxford University Press, 1985). For the specific form of Nazi mental hygiene, see V. Roelcke, '"Zivilisationsschäden am Menschen" und ihre Bekämpfung: Das Projekt einer seelischen "Gesundheitsführung" im Nationalsozialismus', *Medizinhistorisches Journal*, 31 (1996), 3-48.

27. Faulstich, *op. cit.* (note 23).

28. H. Faulstich, 'Die Zahl der "Euthanasie"-Opfer', in A. Frewer, C. Eickhoff (eds), *'Euthanasie' und die aktuelle Sterbehilfe-Debatte. Die historischen Hintergründe medizinischer Ethik* (Frankfurt am Main: Campus, 2000), 218-34.

29. See V. Roelcke, 'Psychiatrische Wissenschaft im Kontext nationalsozialistischer Politik und "Euthanasie". Zur Rolle von Ernst Ruedin und der Deutschen Forschungsanstalt für Psychiatrie', in D. Kaufmann (ed.), *Die Kaiser-Wilhelm-Gesellschaft im Nationalsozialismus. Bestandsaufnahme und Perspektiven der Forschung* (Göttingen: Wallstein, 2000), 112-50.

30. Psychiatrists who did confront themselves with the past were e.g. W. Leibbrand (ed.), *Um die Menschenrechte der Geisteskranken* (Nürnberg: Die Egge, 1946). G. Schmidt, *Selektion in der Heilanstalt 1939-1945* (completed in 1946) (Stuttgart: Evangelisches Verlagswerk, 1965); A. von Platen-Hallermund, *Die Tötung Geisteskranker in Deutschland* (Frankfurt: Verlag der Frankfurter Hefte, 1948).

31. See the chapter by Franz-Werner Kersting in this volume.

32. See D. de Mildt, *In the Name of the People: Perpetrators of Genocide in the Reflection of their Post-War Prosecution in West Germany. The 'Euthanasia' and 'Aktion Reinhard' Trial Cases* (The Hague: Nijhoff, 1996).

33. See e.g. the cases of Kurt Pohlisch and Friedrich Panse who, after a short intermission, were allowed to take up their positions again: Pohlisch as Chair of the Department of Psychiatry at the University of Bonn, Panse as consultant who was later (in 1955) appointed Professor of Psychiatry in Düsseldorf. U. Heyll, 'Friedrich Panse und die psychiatrische Erbforschung', in M.G. Esch, K. Griese et al. (eds), *Die Medizinische Akademie Düsseldorf im Nationalsozialismus* (Essen: Klartext, 1997), 318-40.

34. H. Ehrhardt, *Euthanasie und Vernichtung 'lebensunwerten Lebens'* (Stuttgart: Enke, 1965).

35. See e.g. H.-H. Rauschelbach, 'Zur Klinik der Spätfolge nach Hungerdystrophie', *Fortschritte der Psychiatrie, Neurologie und ihrer Grenzgebiete*, 22 (1954), 214-26.

36. *Anhaltspunkte für die ärztliche Gutachtertätigkeit im Versorgungswesen.* Guidelines edited by the Federal Ministry of Work and Social Affairs: in edition of 1952:

p. 45, ed. of 1954: p. 78; ed. of 1958: p. 120-122; see S. Goltermann, 'Psychisches Leid und herrschende Lehre. Der Wissenschaftswandel in der westdeutschen Psychiatrie der Nachkriegszeit', in B. Weisbrod (ed.), *Akademische Vergangenheitspolitik. Beiträge zur Wissenschaftskultur der Nachkriegszeit* (Göttingen: Wallstein, 2002), 263-80.

37.   See e.g. H. Mueller-Suur, 'Abgrenzung neurotischer Erkrankungen gegenüber der Norm', in V.E. Frankl and V.E. von Gebsattel (eds), *Handbuch für Neurosenlehre und Psychotherapie*, vol. 1 (München/ Berlin: Urban & Schwarzenberg, 1959), 250-62; Goltermann, *op. cit.* (note 36), 273.

38.   See G.A. Eghigian, 'The German Welfare State as a Discourse of Trauma', in M. Micale and P. Lerner (eds), *Traumatic Pasts. History, Psychiatry, and Trauma in the Modern Age, 1870-1930* (Cambridge: Cambridge University Press, 2001), 92-114.

39.   F.-W. Kersting (ed.), *Psychiatriereform als Gesellschaftsreform. Die Hypothek des Nationalsozialismus und der Aufbruch der sechziger Jahre* (Paderborn: Schöningh, 2003).

40.   On the history of psychiatric nursing in Germany, see D. Falkenstein, '*Ein guter Wärter ist das vorzüglichst Heilmittel...': Zur Entwicklung der Irrenpflege vom Durchgangs- zum Ausbildungsberuf* (Frankfurt am Main: Mabuse, 2000).

41.   See M. Bauer, 'Reform als soziale Bewegung: Der "Mannheimer Kreis" und die Gründung der "Deutschen Gesellschaft für Soziale Psychiatrie"', in Kersting (ed.), *op. cit.* (note 39), 155-63.

42.   F.-W. Kersting, 'Psychiatriereform und '68', *Westfälische Forschungen*, 48 (1998), 283-95.

43.   Quoted in Bundesminister für Jugend, Familie, Frauen und Gesundheit (ed.), *Empfehlungen der Expertenkommission der Bundesregierung zur Reform der Versorgung im psychiatrischen und psychotherapeutisch/ psychosomatischen Bereich* (Bonn: Bundesminister für Jugend, Familie, Frauen und Gesundheit, 11 November 1988), 3.

44.   *Bericht über die Lage der Psychiatrie in der Bundesrepublik Deutschland.* Deutscher Bundestag, Drucksache 7/4200 + 4201 (Bonn, 1975).

45.   On these developments, see M. Bauer and R. Engfer, 'Entwicklung und Bewährung psychiatrischer Versorgung in der Bundesrepublik Deutschland', in A. Thom and E. Wulff (eds), *Psychiatrie im Wandel. Erfahrungen und Perspektiven in Ost und West* (Bonn: Psychiatrie-Verlag, 1990), 413-429.

46.   A. Dührssen and E. Jorswieck, 'Eine empirisch-statistische Untersuchung zur Leistungsfähigkeit psychoanalytischer Behandlung', *Nervenarzt*, 36 (1965), 166-9.

47.   For an overview, see V. Roelcke, 'Psychotherapy between Medicine, Psychoanalysis and Politics: Concepts, Practices, and Institutions in Germany, c. 1945-1992', *Medical History*, 48 (2004), 473-92.

48.   R. Degkwitz, 'Zur Bilanz der modernen Psychopharmakologie', in H.E. Ehrhardt (ed.), *Perspektiven der heutigen Psychiatrie* (Frankfurt am Main: Gerhards, 1972), 364-71.

49. See on this interpretation M. Ash, 'Wissenschaft und Politik als Ressourcen für einander', in vom Bruch and Kaderas (eds), *op. cit.* (note 2), 32-49.

CHAPTER 7

Care and Control in a Communist State

The Place of Politics in East German Psychiatry

Greg Eghigian[1]

The Politics of Psychiatry in the Twentieth Century

No sooner had the Berlin Wall come down in 1989 than questions began to be asked about the role psychiatry, clinical psychology and psychotherapy had played in East Germany's authoritarian regime. Since its founding in 1949, the German Democratic Republic (GDR) and its governing communist party (the *Sozialistische Einheitspartei Deutschlands* or SED) had been among the USSR's most stalwart allies. With the reunification of Germany, western German policy-makers, eastern German reformers and international observers, well aware of the Soviet practice of committing dissidents to psychiatric institutions, wondered aloud whether the same kind of systematic abuse of psychiatry had taken place in the GDR as well.

In the years that followed, journalists uncovered horrible living conditions in some facilities, most infamously in the psychiatric hospital and prison at Waldheim.[2] Former East German clinicians told of being restricted in their use of psychotherapies and how fears of denunciation prompted a climate of distrust among psychiatrists and between psychiatrists and patients.[3] Federal and state commissions were convened to investigate these and other individual accusations. In the end, the evidence has indicated that party officials, security forces and some psychiatric professionals were willing to use the mental health system as a policing tool for rounding up and warehousing those deemed social undesirables, such as alcoholics, prostitutes and delinquents. Nevertheless, there is no evidence indicating that political opponents were systematically committed to psychiatric facilities as in the Soviet Union, and the best estimate is that at most around one to two per cent of all East German psychiatrists and psychotherapists ever broke the confidence of their patients by providing privileged information to State Security.[4]

The lines of questioning opened up by these investigations raise a host of substantive and methodological questions for the history of twentieth-century psychiatry. Was there something essentially 'communist' about East German (and by extension, post-war Eastern European) psychiatry? Do politically authoritarian regimes necessarily translate into totalitarian psychiatric regimens? What have political ideologies had to do with the form and content of psychiatric ideas and services? Marked by mass eugenic sterilisation, the deliberate killing of 'incurables', and the rise of patient advocacy and anti-psychiatry movements, twentieth-century psychiatry – and particularly twentieth-century German psychiatry – has proven to be deeply entangled in the ideological conflicts and party politics of its time, for good and ill. But what exactly was the nature of these entanglements?

To say that modern psychiatry is political is, of course, hardly novel. Already in the 1960s and 1970s, observers such as Klaus Doerner, Michel Foucault, George Rosen, Andrew Scull and Thomas Szasz attempted to outline and explain the social control functions of psychiatry in the modern age.[5] Yet while the spectre of the twentieth century hovers more or less ominously in the background of these studies, their authors were more interested in tracing the origins rather than directly exploring the social dynamics of the peculiar relationship between contemporary politics and psychiatry. More recently, historians in the United States, Great Britain, and the Netherlands have remedied this oversight by investigating the growing prominence of the psychological sciences (psychiatry, psychology, psychotherapy) in a variety of public endeavours over the last century.[6] This new generation of scholars tends not to find the function of the psychological sciences in their serving as a tool for social control but rather stresses the compatibility of psychiatry and psychology with the modern liberal project of promoting more autonomous, intelligent, happy and enterprising citizens.

As plausible as the contention might seem that there is an inherent connection between liberalism and the psychological sciences, it is one that requires an international or comparative perspective to confirm it. Few, if any, of the histories mentioned however, consider that contemporaneous fascist and communist societies might have undergone similar changes – a fact that would call into question the thesis of a psychological liberalism. Take the example of National Socialist Germany. Evidence indicates that authorities, scholars, clinicians and the general public in the years 1933-1945 found cause to expand the public role of the psychological sciences as part of Nazi party efforts to fundamentally transform society. Psychology, for instance, was professionalised for the first time as an independent discipline, while psychotherapy was used to help ailing members of the party and military, and psychiatric institutions and personnel employed in the mass sterilisation and genocide of undesirables.[7] Though both the party and the state were driven by an all-encompassing, essentialising racial eugenics, policies toward a wide range of deviants – including the mentally ill, alcoholics, juvenile delinquents, homosexuals and violent criminals – did not simply aim at identifying, segregating and exterminating those deemed abnormal. Rather, even during the war, administrators at all levels were keen on distinguishing between those individuals who could and those who could not be 'rehabilitated'. As a result, authorities remained surprisingly curious about the life histories, psychological abilities and family environments of patients, prisoners and detainees, and enlisted the aid of clinicians to help arrive at a prognosis and plan for treatment.[8]

Recent social histories of the Soviet Union tell a similar story there. Studies have shown that there was an enormous everyday preoccupation with the narrative reconstruction of life histories and technologies of self-perfection immediately after the revolution and throughout the Stalinist years.[9] This grass-roots development served as both cause and effect in the concerted efforts of communist party officials, scientists and clinicians to understand and exploit the inner workings of individuals in order to realise the utopian ambition of creating a revolutionary 'new man'.[10] Many, therefore, believed that communist ideological ambitions and psychiatric knowledge were compatible (though, as I will show, this compatibility was not always apparent to everyone, nor was it always welcome).

Thus, we can see a trend, cutting across national and ideological boundaries, that constitutes one of the defining features of psychiatric and psychotherapeutic practice in the twentieth century. In liberal, fascist and communist societies alike, psychiatry and psychotherapy took on a prominent role in the management of (ab)normality. In particular, psychiatric professionals, political authorities and the general public came to see psychiatry's work of classifying, assessing and attempting to reintegrate human beings into everyday life as a vital part of efforts to reform and reinvent society. Categorising the conduct of psychiatrists and psychotherapists in totalitarian regimes as examples of 'collaboration', 'resistance' and 'acquiescence', as has most often been the case up to now, not only fails to acknowledge this basic trans-national development. It overlooks how psychiatric systems have changed over time and how other non-political, often unintentional, factors have helped shape modern psychiatric care.

Psychiatry in the Early GDR

What role did communism and the communist party play in the structure and substance of East German psychiatry? To begin with, it needs to be pointed out that if Soviet-style communism proved to be generally receptive to psychiatric knowledge and professionals over the course of the twentieth century, this receptiveness was not uniform. At any given point in time, there were, in fact, influential communist party functionaries who were more or less antagonistic toward psychiatry and its practitioners. This was especially the case in the early GDR. The founding leaders of the SED – many, like party chief Walter Ulbricht, having spent the war in exile in the Soviet Union – returned to Germany dismissive of both the native intelligentsia (*Bildungsbürgertum*) and conventional academic knowledge. Party officials were particularly dismissive of human sciences such as sociology, criminology and forensic psychology, rejecting them as 'bourgeois' endeavours inadequate for understanding anti-social behaviour in a socialist society. Crime and delinquency, instead, were to be seen as expressions of class struggle, driven not by 'personal' motivations but rather by political 'enemies of worker and peasant power'.[11] As a result, psychopathological and psychological explanations of deviant behaviour, which previously played an important role in German criminal justice and social services, were marginalised in party debates throughout the 1950s.

This suspicion of 'bourgeois' forms of knowledge was accompanied by a corresponding distrust of psychiatrists. Under National Socialism, psychiatric personnel had helped murder some 200,000 psychiatric patients as part of the state's eugenic agenda, a legacy not easily forgotten. In fact, officials found that for years after 1945, family members in East Germany remained reticent about placing their loved ones in the hands of institutional psychiatry due to the latter's recent history. Moreover, while some facility directors, clinicians and nurses were dismissed as part of de-Nazification immediately after the war, a critical shortage of qualified staff quickly compelled authorities to retain numerous personnel with Nazi connections.[12] One government estimate in 1947 indicated that 48 per cent of all psychiatrists and neurologists in the Soviet-Occupied Zone had been members of the Nazi Party. By June of that year, however, only around 15 per cent had joined the communist party.[13] Taking into consideration the fact that physicians were also among those groups of professionals most prone to fleeing to the West over the course of the 1940s and 1950s, it is hardly surprising that many in the SED remained highly suspicious about the political loyalty and reliability of East German psychiatrists well into the early 1960s.

During the first decade of the GDR, psychiatric care itself, like the rest of East German society at this time, was stamped by two other factors: Soviet occupation and shortages. Upon reaching the outskirts of Berlin, Soviet troops plundered every major psychiatric facility surrounding the German capital. Fear among staff prompted a considerable number of personnel to commit suicide as the Red Army approached. Upon entering individual hospital grounds, Soviet soldiers routinely raped both nurses and female patients. After this, troops occupied large portions of facilities, using them to house soldiers and commandeering food, beds, mattresses and blankets.[14] Sources indicate that the mortality rate among patients during the first month of occupation was around 20 per cent, though improving considerably thereafter.[15] Nonetheless, daily rations for patients in these early months after the war were meagre, consisting mostly of bread and potatoes.[16]

Facilities were generally undercrowded up until around 1950, housing only about one-fifth of the patient population of 1936.[17] All told, immediately after the war, there were only around 6,000 registered psychiatric patients in the Soviet-Occupied Zone. This was due, in part, to the public perception of German psychiatric hospitals as killing facilities. But more than anything else, the small number of patients in the early years of occupation had more to do with patients and staff fleeing the Red Army. Reports at the time also indicate that the Soviet authorities, during at least the first year of occupation, were eager to release patients since this made more resources available for troops.

It was only in the late 1940s and early 1950s that conditions began to 'normalise' in East German psychiatric hospitals. The turn of the decade witnessed a massive transfer of patient populations from Eastern Europe (many being mentally ill German prisoners of war) and West Germany into East German facilities, as part of the general process of repatriating German citizens.[18] At the same time, the Red Army gradually withdrew its troops from psychiatric hospitals, making it possible for authorities to increase the number of psychiatric beds to 15,000 by the end of 1948. By 1955, the GDR could boast of having 15.2 psychiatric beds per 10,000 residents. This began what would be a virtually unbroken period of increasing overcrowding in psychiatric hospitals and clinics. The number of psychiatric beds eventually rose to a high of 19.8 per 10,000 residents in 1975, only finally decreasing to 16.4 beds in the late 1980s.[19] The problem of overcrowding was only exacerbated by the 'brain drain' that plagued East Germany before the building of the Berlin Wall in 1961 as professionals, particularly those in health and social services, fled to the West in the years before the border was restrictively policed.

Ironically, the general result of all these profound changes was to reinforce continuities in German psychiatry. The general lack of funds and personnel coupled with the retention of Nazi-era clinicians had the effect of assuring that neurology and the natural sciences – both of which had played dominant roles in German institutional psychiatry since the second half of the nineteenth century[20] – continued to provide the guiding paradigms in East German mental health care. Even the new commitment to Marxist-Leninist dogma contributed to this trend. Efforts were made at this time to Sovietise psychiatry and psychology as sciences. Soviet psychological literature and practices were held up as models for research and treatment. The sole psychiatric and psychotherapeutic journal in the GDR, *Psychiatrie, Neurologie, und medizinische Psychologie*, was founded in 1949, and it institutionalised the practice of citing and translating prominent Soviet scholarship in the field. Still, while there was an attempt to 'Pavlovise' East German psychiatry and psychology, it never really succeeded; indeed, it aimed at little more than turning the two disciplines into more formally natural, instead of human, sciences.[21] More than anything else, the Sovietisation campaign reinforced a biological approach to psychiatric disorders, a renunciation of psychological testing, and a reliance on conventional forms of work therapy in the tradition of Simon's active therapy and Makarenko's collective work regimen.[22] It also had the effect of forcing psychoanalysis underground, the discipline being officially renounced for not being materialistic enough.[23]

Psychiatry and Reform, 1960-1975

Around 1960, however, the reserve with which communist party officials greeted psychiatry and clinical psychology began to wane quickly. Changes in party doctrine and mental health care during the 1960s and into the early 1970s led to the articulation of new ideals of normality and rehabilitation. For the first time, the SED explicitly endorsed the expansion of psychiatric and psychological work, as psychiatrists and psychologists were asked to play prominent roles in a variety of social reform projects.

Party politics had much to do with this. Beginning around the start of the decade, the SED embarked on a comprehensive reform of the country's economic, legal, health care and educational systems as part of de-Stalinisation. Under 'The New Economic System' (1963-1969), 'scientific-ness', technical innovation and expert know-how were all hailed as the keys to realising the new goals of socialism, and a new generation of psychiatrists, psychologists, social workers and social scientists was recruited to advance the cause.[24] In addition, the building of the Berlin Wall in 1961, surprisingly enough, also encouraged reformist thinking inside the communist party. Ideologues could no longer blame everything on Western influences, compelling party officials to look 'inward' (both domestically and subjectively) to explain deviant thinking and behaviour, and thereby leading them for the first time to entertain more psychological and psychopathological explanations of social conduct.

Therapeutic, intellectual and structural changes within psychiatry contributed something as well to this reformist atmosphere. The successful introduction of neuroleptic drugs into psychiatric facilities beginning in the mid-1950s, the emergence of anti-psychiatry and alternative psychiatry movements in Western Europe and West Germany, and the end of the mass emigration of East German physicians gave clinicians their first opportunity since the war to imagine reforming and planning long-term institutional care.[25] Borrowing heavily from the ideas of West German advocates of what became known as social psychiatry, groups of East German psychiatrists in 1963 (in the so-called Rodewischer Theses) and again in 1974 (in the Brandenburger Theses) laid out principles and an agenda for creating a psychiatric health care system more responsive to the individual rehabilitative needs of the mentally ill. Among other things, these included a greater appreciation for the social causes of mental illness and more emphasis on outpatient and transitional care.[26]

The emergence of a psycho-social and non-custodial approach to mental health care in East Germany inspired a broader reconsideration of social policies in areas such as juvenile delinquency, alcohol and drug abuse, and compulsory psychiatric commitment.[27] In 1966, for instance, a government commission was set up to examine those factors believed responsible for some of the most common forms of anti-social behaviour. After consulting with law enforcement, health officials, and social services, the commission recommended that priority be given to better accommodating and medically treating the mentally ill and alcoholics, as well as finding ways to better extend assistance to dysfunctional families.[28]

On one level, this reformist turn in party, administrative and clinical approaches toward the mentally ill, delinquents and anti-socials reflected a change in international standards and practices. Since the mid-1950s, international mental health care had begun to distance itself from depth psychology and the essentialism of earlier psychiatric eugenics to embrace more environmental approaches to personality, stressing communication, learning, interpersonal relations, family therapy and education.[29] This was the very same time when states were becoming more engaged in revisiting such social issues as sexual liberation, juvenile delinquency and alternatives to incarceration.[30] Thus, one must acknowledge the presence here of a trans-national trend, whereby political, scientific, and clinical institutions met one another deep in civil society, in the realm of social and interpersonal relations and problems, to reciprocally develop a new view of social intervention.

At the same time, this social-therapeutic vision, placed in the context of the height of the Cold War, opened up new lines of connection and tension between the social control and the helping functions of psychiatric and social services. De-Stalinisation provoked a great deal of anxiety within the SED, and the focus on preventive mental health care reflected this. The participation of young people in the unrest of 1953, the large numbers of them who fled to the West in the 1950s, and their receptiveness to American popular culture led officials to see the young as one of the principal risks to national security.[31] State and party apprehension, therefore, was very much at the heart of the campaign to identify, isolate and rehabilitate so-called at-risk (gefährdete) youth.[32]

As criminal justice and health policy in the GDR were being renegotiated in the 1960s and early 1970s, those involved in providing inpatient psychiatric services found themselves called upon to respond to two, often mutually exclusive, sets of demands: on the one hand, an internationally recognised appeal by practitioners and patients to open up facilities both literally and figuratively; on the other, the insistence of police and prosecutors that psychiatric facilities assume responsibility for properly isolating dangerous deviants from the population at large.[33] In attempting to address both sets of concerns, East German psychiatric care was beset by the kinds of contradictions that characterised so much of East German institutional life.

A telling example involves the law governing involuntary psychiatric commitment. Up until 1968, the forcible hospitalisation of an individual in an East

German psychiatric facility was regulated by a Prussian police ordinance from 1931 (itself little changed since its original form dating back to 1794). While voluntary hospitalisation was certainly possible and psychiatrists could play a role in advising courts about the mental status of institutionalised individuals, the ordinance made compulsory commitment a matter for police and judges to decide based primarily on public security concerns. A directive of the Ministry of Health in 1959 attempted to give health administrators and district doctors more say in the process, but this proved ineffective. Throughout the 1960s, psychiatrists, health and social service administrators, and justice and police officials discussed reforming the existing law, with an eye toward reorienting it around medical certification and prognosis. The new psychiatric commitment law of 11 June 1968 did just that. It not only made a medically certified diagnosis a prerequisite for hospitalising individuals, it also mandated that individuals be informed of the reasons for their commitment, they be given access to the courts to petition for their release, and a time limit of six weeks be placed on most forms of institutionalisation.[34]

In practice, however, things worked quite differently. To be sure, evidence indicates that the number of compulsory commitments decreased during the 1970s. Even after passage of the law, however, the General Prosecutor's Office in Berlin continued to press psychiatric facilities to house habitual criminals and delinquents who were deemed a danger to the community but who showed few, if any, signs of mental illness – a practice that proved to be widespread in the GDR.[35] The Ministry of Health and a number of health care professionals decried the practice of using hospitals and clinics for such purposes as medically and legally irresponsible, while a host of studies conducted by East German researchers in the years 1974-1986 consistently showed that the psychiatric commitment law was routinely being misapplied and abused. Administrative forms often provided no clinical diagnosis. Alcoholics were frequently committed without there being any acute medical emergency. And, most glaringly, the law was being used to confine various socially marginalised individuals – including the elderly, 'a-socials', the so-called 'work shy', repeat offenders and prostitutes – in psychiatric facilities.[36] The most infamous example of this came in the summer of 1973. In preparation for the Tenth World Festival of Youth and Students meeting in East Berlin, hundreds of East Germans – most not meeting the criteria for involuntary hospitalisation – were apprehended and committed to psychiatric facilities throughout the GDR in order to remove from the streets anyone 'who might damage our image'.[37] At least one director of a psychiatric hospital believed the project worked well enough to draw up plans for a more permanent system for registering and institutionalising delinquents and 'a-socials'.[38]

Psychiatry in the Wake of Détente

By the mid-1970s, then, psychiatric services in the GDR were being challenged on three different fronts: calls for the progressive reform of psychiatric care, an insistence by criminal justice officials that facilities assume more security responsibilities, and all coupled with a shortage of available beds. Added to this was yet another pronounced shift in party canon and state policies. In 1971, Erich Honecker became head of the SED and state (positions he held until 1989). Under his leadership, East Germany embarked on a new economic modernisation campaign that included opening up international relations and cultural exchange with the West. This brought with it not only a greater exposure to foreign influences but also, at the same time, an increasing invasiveness of state security during the last decade and a half of the GDR. As geographical and discursive boundaries opened up – and particularly after Mikhail Gorbachev's introduction of *glasnost* in 1985 – the head of the Ministry for State Security (the Stasi), Erich Mielke, held fast to his image of the agency as a shield against a new wave of foreign and domestic threats to socialist society. Over the course of the 1960s and 1970s, the Stasi underwent unprecedented growth in its size and reach, the number of its personnel rising from 20,000 in 1961 to 81,500 in 1982.[39]

In looking at how psychiatrists and health care officials responded to this highly politicised environment, one which pitted advocates of incarceration against proponents of decarceration, it is worth noting that all sides agreed on the need for a neater division of their labour. In the process, the seeming incompatibility of security and therapeutic approaches to anti-social, criminal and otherwise conspicuous behaviour promoted a demand for finer differentiation between criminals and the mentally ill according to their potential 'dangerousness' and reformability. This only served to augment the increasingly prominent role being played by psychiatrists and psychologists in the criminal justice system and in social policy in general.

This all resulted in some clinicians and researchers becoming more directly involved in the surveillance and social control of ostensibly 'normal' East German citizens.[40] But these practitioners appear to have been in the minority. What far more psychiatric professionals contributed to was the minting of a rehabilitative ideal that enjoyed wide currency in administrative, legal, party political, policy-making, scientific and clinical circles. This rehabilitative ideal – in general, conceptualising the actions of criminals and delinquents as expressions of pathologies, stressing treatment instead of punishment, advocating greater de-institutionalisation and outpatient care – assumed an ever greater prominence during the Honecker years. So much so, that by the late 1970s and 1980s, social care (*Fürsorge*) as such had become associated with the methods and approaches of the human sciences. *They* represented the 'soft line' in contrast to the 'hard line' of ideologues, police and state security. Psychology, psychiatry, psychotherapy, social work, sociology, pedagogy, social policy, criminal justice, youth assistance: all became wrapped up in one another, and at a time when East German intellectual life was more open than ever to international influences.[41]

Thus, psychiatry during the last decade or so of the GDR arguably had its greatest social impact in advocating and disseminating novel ideas and values. The thaw in foreign relations between West and East Germany beginning in the early 1970s, for instance, bolstered advocates of mental health care reform in the GDR. By the early 1980s, Western influences were in clear evidence. For the first time, journals and monographs extensively cited West German and American alongside the conventional Russian studies. Psycho-diagnostic tools and tests such as the MMPI, long repudiated in East Germany, were introduced into clinical and pedagogical training and work.[42] And it became acceptable to explicitly invoke the ideas of such prominent figures as Erik Erikson, Hans Eysenck, Maxwell Jones and Carl Rogers.[43]

The demand for Western ideas and research was in large measure a manifestation of the growing interest in transitional and outpatient care. Psychotherapy and community mental health came to enjoy greater profiles than ever before. While there had always been figures in East Germany, such as Kurt Höck, who insisted on the commensurability of talk therapies and socialism, party functionaries and pedagogues had generally harboured reservations about individual psychotherapy. Instead, in keeping with the socialist ethos of collectivism and productivity, work, occupational and group therapies remained the most widely practised forms of psychotherapy well into the 1980s.[44] With official acceptance of community- and client-based rehabilitation projects, however, the climate was conducive to experimentation and to testing the boundaries of acceptability. Under these conditions, more individualised forms of psychotherapy began to gain a foothold. Marriage and Sexual Counseling Centres, first set up in the mid-1960s, were expanded, marketing counseling services for singles as well as couples.[45] At the same time, clinicians sympathetic to psychoanalysis found ways to insinuate depth-psychological methods into everyday practice under the guise of so-called 'dynamic group psychotherapy' in the 1970s and 'dynamic individual psychotherapy' in the 1980s.[46]

Thus, even before Gorbachev's reforms, East German psychiatry and psychotherapy were undergoing a phase of 'openness'. Receptiveness to international influences and standards was evident in the growing number of international conferences attended and hosted by East German clinicians and researchers.[47] At the same time, professional discussions about the challenges and problems facing mental health care in the GDR became franker. Two of the leading figures behind the social psychiatry reform movement, for instance, attempted to establish a code of professional ethics for psychiatry that made explicit reference to the World Psychiatric Association's 'Declaration of Hawaii' of 1977, which had condemned the abuse of psychiatry in the Soviet Union.[48]

Care and Control in a Communist State

And although newspapers and magazines avoided mentioning such things in public, clinicians used conferences and academic journals to discuss such matters as alcohol and drug abuse, depression, and East Germany's disturbingly high suicide rate (the third highest in the world by the late 1980s).[49]

Despite the greater openness and the avowed commitment to psychotherapy and community mental health, however, social psychiatry and an 'open-door policy' were rarely put into practice in the GDR. The reformist ambitions first set out in the Rodewischer and Brandenburger Theses were never realised for a variety of reasons: lack of adequate funding, a shortage of personnel, and the persistent distrust of police and criminal justice officials toward deviants of all kinds. Some de-institutionalisation was evident, to be sure. The number of long-term patients, for instance, was reduced between 1976 and 1985 from 14.7 to 12.5 beds per 10,000 residents. In addition, the number of discharged patients (per 10,000 residents) rose from 30.5 in 1975 to 36 in 1987, while the length of stay in stationary care sank from an average of 200 days annually to 155 days over this same period of time.[50] But with few separate facilities for mentally disabled and elderly patients, the system remained highly centralised, dominated by closed, large and often dilapidated hospitals occupied mainly by patients with chronic and degenerative disorders.[51] At the same time, biological explanations and psycho-tropic drugs continued to dominate the landscape of mental health care right up until the fall of the Berlin Wall in 1989. Moreover, to make matters worse, the criminally mentally ill were largely integrated into the general population of psychiatric hospitals and clinics, with sometimes disastrous consequences.[52] Clinicians, social workers and administrators did bring these discrepancies to the attention of government and party officials throughout the 1980s, but to no avail. A literally bankrupt state that had been running huge deficits since the late 1970s simply did not have the resources for – and, in some circles, the interest in – innovation.

Conclusions

The historical evidence indicates that it would be overly simplistic to say that communist ideology and party politics determined the form and substance of psychiatry in the GDR. That said, without question, politics and ideology did play a formative role in the development of East German psychiatry. At different moments and in different contexts, various political interests had a direct bearing on psychiatric work. These intersections of political and psychiatric ideas, values, purposes and institutions might usefully be organised into two types of encounters.

On the one hand, there were *sites of apparent incompatibility and tension* between the political and the psychiatric. These were instances where party or state interests, situated largely *outside the psychiatric community*, attempted or succeeded in dictating what psychiatrists, researchers and patients could do. In these instances, post-war Marxism-Leninism and Stalinist as well as post-Stalinist statecraft had very direct effects on mental health care in the GDR. One of the most glaring examples, we have seen, was the attempt of the criminal justice system to force mental hospitals to assume more security responsibilities in the last two decades of the regime. To this could be added the Soviet occupation of psychiatric hospitals in the late-1940s, the attempted 'Sovietisation' of research in the 1950s, the party's influence on career advancement, the ban on psychoanalysis, and the fiscal retrenchment of the 1970s and 1980s. In most of these cases, large numbers of psychiatrists perceived and opposed the intervention of political authorities as invasive and counter-productive.

On the other hand, there were also *sites of accepted compatibility and agreement* between the political and psychiatric communities. Here political influences came not only *from outside, but also from within, organised psychiatry.* In these instances, psychiatry, psychology and psychotherapy reciprocated, providing political authorities and policy-makers with the language and tools to psychopathologise deviants, criminals, and delinquents and offering a progressive vision of social concern and care. Not all political authorities – nor all psychiatrists, for that matter – shared an affinity for this new rehabilitative ideal inspired by social psychiatry. Police and state security often complained that such 'soft' approaches to deviance only promoted more aberrant behaviour in the population. But legislators, courts and social policy-makers, by and large, embraced at least the ideals behind reform psychiatry.

The convergence of the seemingly incommensurable impulses of mental health care reform (informed by social psychiatry) and control over deviant behaviour (informed by state security) had two effects. It provided more than a kind of counter-discourse to the positions of hard-liners. The psychopathologisation of anti-social conduct, the 'discovery' of the dysfunctional family, and the return of the concept of 'personality' in the 1960s and 1970s all also made it possible to conceive of a more invasive approach to social intervention in the name of treating those 'at risk'. In a state like the GDR, whose governing ideology was Marxism-Leninism and whose ostensible raison d'etre was looking after the comprehensive welfare of its citizens (*Fürsorgestaat*), 'caring for' its citizens meant something quite peculiar.[53] It meant ensuring that the individual did not get 'off track' in his or her linear development toward becoming a proper socialist citizen. Social control could now be extended beyond simply modifying conspicuous behaviour. It now, in good conscience, could involve monitoring and enforcing life histories, with the intention of preventing potentially destructive and self-destructive attitudes and conduct. In the end, East Germany did come to blur distinctions between care and control, mental illness and crime, but just as often without as with the support of the psychiatric community and driven just as much by fiscal and administrative exigency as by any ideological commitment.

Care and Control in a Communist State

Notes

1.   An earlier, much shorter version of this essay was published as 'Was There a Communist Psychiatry? Politics and East German Psychiatric Care', *Harvard Review of Psychiatry*, 10 (2002), 346-68. Copyright 2002, from 'Was There a Communist Psychiatry? Politics and East German Psychiatric Care' by Greg Eghigian (Reproduced by permission of Taylor & Francis, Inc.).

2.   E. Klee, *Irrsinn Ost – Irrsinn West: Psychiatrie in Deutschland* (Frankfurt: Fischer, 1993).

3.   H.-J.Maaz, *Behind the Wall: The Inner Life of Communist Germany* (New York and London: Norton, 1995); A. Simon, *Versuch mir und anderen die ostdeutsche Moral zu erklären* (Gießen: Psychosozial, 1995); F.R. Groß, *Jenseits des Limes: 40 Jahre Psychiater in der DDR* (Bonn: Psychiatrie, 1996).

4.   S. Süß, *Politisch mißbraucht? Psychiatrie und Staatssicherheit in der DDR* (Berlin: Ch. Links, 1999).

5.   M. Foucault, *Histoire de la Folie à l'âge classique* (Paris: Plon, 1961) ; T. Szasz, *The Myth of Mental Illness: Foundations of a Theory of Personal Conduct* (New York: Harper and Row, 1961); G. Rosen, *Madness in Society: Chapters in the Historical Sociology of Mental Illness* (Chicago: University of Chicago Press, 1968); K. Dörner, *Bürger und Irre: Zur Sozialgeschichte und Wissenschschaftssoziologie der Psychiatrie* (Frankfurt a.M.: Europäische Verlagsanstalt, 1969); A. Scull, *Museums of Madness: The Social Organization of Insanity in Nineteenth-Century England* (London: Allen Lane, 1979).

6.   E. Lunbeck, *The Psychiatric Persuasion: Knowledge, Gender, and Power in Modern America* (Princeton: Princeton University Press, 1994); E. Herman, *The Romance of American Psychology: Political Culture in the Age of Experts* (Berkeley and Los Angeles: University of California Press, 1995); N. Rose, *Inventing Our Selves: Psychology, Power, and Personhood* (New York and Cambridge: Cambridge University Press, 1996); E.S. Moskowitz, *In Therapy We Trust: America's Obsession with Self-Fulfillment* (Baltimore: Johns Hopkins University Press, 2001); J. Jansz and P. van Drunen (eds), *A Social History of Psychology* (Oxford and Cambridge: Blackwell, 2003).

7.   H.-W. Schmuhl, *Rassenhygiene, Nationalsozialismus, Euthanasie: Von der Verhütung zur Vernichtung 'lebensunwerten Lebens'* (Göttingen: Vandenhoeck & Ruprecht, 1987); U. Geuter, *The Professionalization of Psychology in Nazi Germany* (Cambridge and New York: Cambridge University Press, 1992); M. Burleigh, *Death and Deliverance: 'Euthanasia' in Germany, 1900-1945* (Cambridge and New York: Cambridge University Press, 1995); G. Cocks, *Psychotherapy in the Third Reich: The Göring Institute* (New Brunswick and London: Transaction, 1997).

8.   I discuss this in 'The Psychological Curiosity of Totalitarianisms: The Promise and Limits of Rehabilitation in Nazi and East Germany' (unpublished paper), American Historical Association Conference, Seattle, WA, January 2005. See also H. Oosterhuis, 'Medicine, Male Bonding, and Homosexuality in Nazi Germany', *Journal of Contemporary History*, 32 (1997), 187-205.

9.   S. Kotkin, *Magnetic Mountain: Stalinism as Civilization* (Berkeley: University of California Press, 1995); O. Kharkhordin, *The Collective and the Individual in Russia: A Study of Practices* (Berkeley: University of California Press, 1999); A. Krylova,

'"Healers of Wounded Souls": The Crisis of Private Life in Soviet Literature, 1944-1946', *Journal of Modern History*, 73 (2001), 307-31; *idem*, 'The Tenacious Liberal Subject in Soviet Studies', *Kritika*, 1 (2001), 119-46; I. Sirotkina, *Diagnosing Literary Genius: A Cultural History of Psychiatry in Russia, 1880-1930* (Baltimore: Johns Hopkins University Press, 2002).

10.   R. Bauer, *The New Man in Soviet Psychology* (Cambridge: Harvard University Press, 1968); A. Kozulin, *Psychology in Utopia* (Cambridge: MIT Press, 1984); M. Thielen, *Sowjetische Psychologie und Marxismus: Geschichte und Kritik* (Frankfurt and New York: Campus, 1984); D. Joravsky, *Russian Psychology* (Oxford: Blackwell, 1989); M.A. Miller, *Freud and the Bolsheviks: Psychoanalysis in Imperial Russia and the Soviet Union* (New Haven and London: Yale University Press, 1998).

11.   B. Gertig and R. Schädlich, *Lehrbuch für Kriminalisten: Die allgemeinen Verfahren und Arbeitsmethoden der Kriminalistik* (Berlin: Verlag für Fachliteratur der Volkspolizei, 1955), 3.

12.   See the article by Franz-Werner Kersting in this volume.

13.   Bundesarchiv (hereafter, BArch), DQ 1/1901, Zusammenstellung der Psychiater und Neurologen, 19 June 1947, p. 457.

14.   Brandenburgisches Landeshauptarchiv (hereafter, BLHA), Rep 211/656a, Vermerk über Ereignisse in Görden, 31 May 1945. A. Thom, 'Die Nachkriegslage der Psychiatrie in Sachsen 1945-1948', *Sozialpsychiatrische Informationen*, 24 (1994), 8-12.

15.   L.M. Köhler, *Entwicklungsprobleme im Fachgebiet Neurologie/Psychiatrie im Land Brandenburg in der Zeit vom Mai 1945 bis 1952* (Diss. Dr. med. Karl-Marx-Universität, 1986).

16.   On the poor nutritional conditions in German psychiatric facilities throughout the first half of the twentieth century, see H. Faulstich, *Hungersterben in der Psychiatrie, 1914-1949* (Freiburg: Lambertus, 1998).

17.   Landesarchiv Berlin, C Rep 118/178, Magistrat Gross-Berlin, Abteilung Gesundheitswesen an Hauptjugendamt, 29 April 1948.

18.   BLHA, Rep 221/940, Peschke an Ministerium für Arbeit und Sozialwesen, 29 December 1949.

19.   It should be noted that the number of psychiatric beds differed wildly from region to region in East Germany, ranging from 4 to 30 thirty per 10,000 residents. See K. Weise and M. Uhle, 'Entwicklungsformen und derzeitige Wirkungsbedingungen der Psychiatrie in der Deutschen Demokratischen Republik', in A. Thom and E. Wulff (eds), *Psychiatrie im Wandel: Erfahrungen und Perspektiven in Ost und West* (Bonn: Psychiatrie, 1990), 440-61: 441-42.

20.   E.J. Engstrom, *Clinical Psychiatry in Imperial Germany: A History of Psychiatric Practice* (Ithaca and London: Cornell University Press, 2003).

21.   A. Mette, 'Bericht über die Arbeitstagung der Staatlichen Pawlow-Kommission der Deutschen Demokratischen Republik vom 15.-17. 1. 1954 in Leipzig', *Psychiatrie, Neurologie, und medizinische Psychologie*, 6 (1954), 173-80; Stefan Busse, '"Von der Sowjetwissenschaft lernen": Pawlowismus und Psychologie', *Psychologie und Geschichte*, 8 (1998), 150-73.

22.   Hermann Nobbe, 'Über eine Erweiterung der Aufgaben der Landesheilanstalten', *Psychiatrie, Neurologie, und medizinische Psychologie*, 3 (1951), 25-8; D. Müller-

Hegemann, 'Die Bedeutung der Arbeitstherapie in der Gegenwart', *Psychiatrie, Neurologie, und medizinische Psychologie,* 4 (1952), 97-101; L. Sprung and H. Sprung, 'Geschichte der Psychodiagnostik in der Deutschen Demokratischen Republik – Ausbildung, Weiterbildung, Forschung, Praxis', *Psychologie und Geschichte,* 7 (1995), 115-40.

23.   H. Bernhardt and R. Lockot, *Mit ohne Freud: Zur Geschichte der Psychoanalyse in Ostdeutschland* (Giessen: Psychosozial, 2000).

24.   J. Roesler, 'Die Wirtschaftsreform der DDR in den sechziger Jahren: Einstieg, Entwicklungsprobleme, und Abbruch', *Zeitschrift für Geschichtswissenschaft,* 38 (1990), 979-1003; Jeffrey Kopstein, 'Ulbricht Embattled: The Quest for Socialist Modernity in the Light of New Sources', *Europe-Asia Studies,* 46 (1994), 597-615; M.G. Ash, 'Wissenschaft, Politik, und Modernität in der DDR: Ansätze zu einer Neubetrachtung', in K. Weisemann, P. Kröner, and R. Toellner (eds), *Wissenschaft und Politik: Genetik und Humangenetik in der DDR 1949-1989* (Münster: LIT, 1997), 1-25; Ulrike Schuster, *Mut zum eigenen Denken? DDR-Studenten und Freie Deutsche Jugend, 1961-1965* (Berlin: Metropol, 1999).

25.   U. Hoffmann-Richter, H. Haselbeck, and R. Engfer (eds), *Sozialpsychiatrie vor der Enquête* (Bonn: Psychiatrie, 1997); A.-S. Ernst, 'Von der bürgerlichen zur sozialistischen Profession? Ärzte in der DDR, 1945-1961', in R. Bessel and R. Jessen (eds), *Die Grenzen der Diktatur: Staat und Gesellschaft in der DDR* (Göttingen: Vandenhoeck & Ruprecht, 1996), 25-48; A. Thom and E. Wulff, 'Vergleichende Betrachtungen: Gemeinsamkeiten, Divergenzen, und erkennbare Perspektiven struktureller Wandlungen der psychiatrischen Versorgungssysteme', in Thom and Wulff (eds), *op. cit.* (note 19), 587-602.

26.   'Empfehlungen des internationalen Symposions über psychiatrische Rehabilitation vom 23. bis 25. Mai 1963 in Rodewisch i. V.', in H.F. Späte, A. Thom, and K. Weise (eds), *Theorie, Geschichte, und aktuelle Tendenzen in der Psychiatrie* (Jena: G. Fischer, 1982), 166-70; S. Schirmer, K. Müller, H.F. Späte, 'Brandenburger Thesen zur Therapeutischen Gemeinschaft', *Psychiatrie, Neurologie, und medizinische Psychologie,* 28 (1976), 21-5; A. Thom, 'Auf dem Wege zu einer Psychiatrie der sozialistischen Gesellschaft', *Psychiatrie, Neurologie, und medizinische Psychologie,* 26 (1974), 578-87.

27.   D. Müller-Hegemann, 'Psychohygiene und Psychotherapie in ihrer Stellung zum Fragenkomplex "Sozialismus, wissenschaftlich-technische Revolution und Medizin"', *Psychiatrie, Neurologie, und medizinische Psychologie,* 20 (1968), 153-55.

28.   BArch, DQ1/6033, Bericht über die Ergebnisse der Arbeit der Kommission mit Schlußfolgerungen zur Erziehung und Kontrolle Asozialer und kriminell Gefährdeter, 1967.

29.   See G.R. Vandenbos, N.A. Cummings, and P.H. Deleon, 'A Century of Psychotherapy: Economic and Environmental Influences', in D.K. Freedheim (ed.), *History of Psychotherapy* (Washington: APA, 1992), 65-102; G.N. Grob, *The Mad Among Us* (New York and Toronto: Free Press, 1994), 249-78; P. Cushman, *Constructing the Self, Constructing America: A Cultural History of Psychotherapy* (Boston: Addison-Wesley, 1995), 210-78; E. Shorter, *A History of Psychiatry* (New York: Wiley & Sons, 1997), 229-38, 272-87; M. Gijswijt-Hofstra and R. Porter (eds), *Cultures of Psychiatry*

and Mental Health Care in Postwar Britain and the Netherlands (Amsterdam and Atlanta: Rodopi, 1998).

30.   A. Marwick, *The Sixties: Cultural Revolution in Britain, France, Italy, and the United States, c. 1958-1974* (Oxford and New York: Oxford University Press, 1998).

31.   D. Wierling, 'Die Jugend als innerer Feind: Konflikte in der Erziehungsdiktatur der sechziger Jahre', in H. Kaelble, J. Kocka, and H. Zwahr (eds), *Sozialgeschichte der DDR* (Stuttgart: Klett-Cotta, 1994), 404-25; P. Skyba, *Vom Hoffnungsträger zum Sicherheitsrisiko: Jugend in der DDR und Jugendpolitik der SED 1949-1961* (Cologne: Böhlau, 2000).

32.   V. Zimmermann, *'Den neuen Menschen schaffen': Die Umerziehung von schwererziehbaren und straffälligen Jugendlichen in der DDR, 1945-1990* (Cologne: Böhlau, 2004).

33.   This very issue was at the heart of a lively disagreement between the General Prosecutor's Office and the Ministry of Health in the years 1974-1975. See the records in BArch, DP 3/1194.

34.   K.-R. Otto, 'Das Recht als Instrument zur Förderung der sozialen Integration', in Thom and Wulff (eds), *op. cit.* (note 19), 150-65.

35.   BArch, DP1/VA 2459, Heinz Bleuler to Dr. Wünsche, Ministerium der Justiz, Hauptabteilung 1, 5 November 1968.

36.   C. Gold and R. Gold, *Zur Problematik der befristeten ärztlichen Einweisung durch Anordnung bei Alkoholismus: Ein kritischer Beitrag zur Anwendung des Gesetzes über die Einweisung in stationäre Einrichtunge für psychisch Kranke vom 11. Juni 1968* (Diss. Dr. med: Akademie für Ärztliche Fortbildung der DDR, 1980); G. Weißheit, *Erfahrungen der Bezirksnervenklinik Brandenburg mit der Einweisung von Patienten nach §6 des Gesetzes über die Einweisung in stationäre Einrichtungen für psychisch Kranke vom 11. 6. 1968* (Diss. Dr. med., Akademie für Ärztliche Fortbildung der DDR, 1986). Individuals aged 60 and over represented a disproportionately large number of commitments. This was due to the fact that the law was being used as a way to temporarily house elderly individuals awaiting an opening in a nursing home.

37.   Süß, *op. cit.* (note 4), 523-34.

38.   BLHA, Rep. 601, Nr. 2653, Dr. Barylla, Entwurf an alle Kreispsychiater, poliklinisch tätige Nervenärzte und psychiatrische Fürsorgerinnen bzw. Fürsorger, 1 November 1973.

39.   J. Gieselke, *Mielke-Konzern: Die Geschichte der Stasi, 1945-1990* (Stuttgart and Munich: Deutsche Verlags-Anstalt, 2001), 72-3.

40.   K. Behnke and J. Fuchs (eds), *Zersetzung der Seele: Psychologie und Psychiatrie im Dienste der Stasi* (Hamburg: Rotbuch, 1995).

41.   For more on how this rehabilitative ideal took shape in the 1960s and 1970s, see G. Eghigian, 'The Psychologization of the Socialist Self: East German Forensic Psychology and its Deviants, 1945-1975', *German History*, 22 (2004), 181-205.

42.   Sprung and Sprung, *op. cit.* (note 22).

43.   See, for instance, H. Eichhorn, 'Zum Konzept der Therapeutischen Gemeinschaft', *Psychiatrie, Neurologie, und medizinische Psychologie*, 35 (1983), 449-59.

44.   P. Sommer, 'Kurt Höck und die psychotherapeutische Abteilung am "Haus der Gesundheit" in Berlin: Institutionelle und zeitgeschichtliche Aspekte der

Entwicklung der Gruppenpsychotherapie in der DDR', *Gruppenpsychotherapie und Gruppendynamik*, 33 (1997), 130-47.

45.   For an interesting example of the marketing of these centers in women's magazines, see BArch, DQ 1/13733, I. Starke, 'Beratungsstellen helfen – Wenn Ehen in Gefahr sind', *Für Dich*, 20 (August 1979), no page numbers included.

46.   C. Leuenberger, 'Socialist Psychotherapy and Its Dissidents', *Journal of the History of the Behavioral Sciences*, 37 (2001), 261-73.

47.   The first of what would be periodic meetings of the International Psychotherapy Symposium of Socialist Countries was held in 1973, and the city of Leipzig was chosen to host the 22nd World Congress for Psychology in 1980.

48.   H.F. Späte and A. Thom, 'Ethische Prinzipien und moralische Normen des psychiatrischen Handelns in der sozialistischen Gesellschaft', *Psychiatrie, Neurologie, und medizinische Psychologie*, 36 (1984), 385-93. On the Declaration of Hawaii, see H. Rome, 'Psychiatry as Ideology', *Psychiatric Annals*, 7 (1977), 4-7.

49.   'Bericht über die Tagung der Medizinischen Gesellschaft der Bezirke Cottbus-Frankfurt/Oder...', *Psychiatrie, Neurologie, und medizinische Psychologie*, 29 (1977), 502-4; E. Lange (ed.), *Depression: Ergebnisse des Symposiums der Sektion Psychiatrie der Gesellschaft für Psychiatrie und Neurologie der DDR vom 29./30. Oktober 1986 in Neubrandenburg* (Leipzig: S. Hirzel, 1988); H. von Keyserlingk, V. Kielstein and J. Rogge (eds), *Diagnostik und Therapie Suchtkranker: Ergebnisse der 1. Arbeitstagung der Arbeitsgruppe 'Suchtkrankheiten' der Sektion Psychiatrie der Gesellschaft für Psychiatrie und Neurologie der DDR, Wustrow, 27.-30. Oktober 1987* (Berlin: Volk und Gesundheit, 1988); Süß, *op. cit.* (note 4), 86-95.

50.   See Weise and Uhle, 'Entwicklungsformen', in Thom and Wulff (eds), *op. cit.* (note 19), 440-61: 443.

51.   M. Uhle, 'Zur Betreuung chronisch Kranker in der DDR: Erkenntnisse, Ansprüche, Realitäten und Perspektiven', in Thom and Wulff (eds), *op. cit.* (note 19), 237-53; Groß, *op. cit.* (note 3), 202. According to Uhle, chronic patients took up some two-thirds of all psychiatric beds in the GDR by 1985.

52.   Klee, *op. cit.* (note 2), 35-71. K.-P. Dahle, *Zur Versorgung forensisch-psychiatrischer Patienten in den neuen Bundesländern: Bestandaufnahme und Empfehlungen* (Baden-Baden: Nomos, 1995), 12-20. Prisons in East Germany offered little by way of mental health care for inmates, a fact of which the party and government were well aware. See M. Ochernal, *Die Aufgaben der Psychiatrie im Strafvollzug der DDR* (Diss. Dr. sc. med.: Humboldt-Universität Berlin, 1971).

53.   K. Jarausch, 'Care and Coercion: The GDR as Welfare Dictatorship', in Konrad H. Jarausch (ed.), *Dictatorship as Experience: Towards a Socio-Cultural History of the GDR* (New York and Oxford: Berghahn, 1999), 47-69.

CHAPTER 8

Between the National Socialist 'Euthanasia Programme' and Reform

Asylum Psychiatry in West Germany, 1940-1975

Franz-Werner Kersting[*]

Martin Schrenk's Speech for 'Restitution'

We have to catch up with regard to asylum psychiatry – just like all other countries... President *Kennedy* has expressed this insight, and it would be desirable for other governments also to identify with his message. But psychiatry in Germany faces yet other *special, historically determined 'remains'*. One of the medical problems of psychiatry is to discuss the question of *'restitution'*... Restitution is possible and necessary [in psychiatry as well]: First with regard to the surviving victims, then – as a substitute so to speak – with regard to the ill and those in need of care now living in our society, those who were not at all affected by Hitler's euthanasia, but should be regarded as representatives of the victims. – How much more humane the existence of those who are ill and placed in our care could be today if we had had no '1933-1945' has to remain open... *Kennedy's* message is very serious, and his nation does not have to bear the burden of this legacy. What would the message of a *German* president or chancellor look like? Today it is still missing.[1]

These clear and sensitive sentences were spoken by the psychiatrist Martin Schrenk. He voiced his – up to now unknown – appeal during the 16th Advanced Education Week (*Fortbildungswoche*) of the Westphalian State Hospital in Gütersloh, held in the beginning of October 1963. Martin Schrenk, born in 1922, was almost 41 years old at that time and employed at the Baden State Psychiatric Hospital in Emmendingen.[2] He belonged to the generation marked by Hitler Youth, war and reconstruction, who were predominantly born between 1920 and 1930. In 1945, this generation was faced, both materially and mentally, with a world in ruins. *Die skeptische Generation* (The Sceptical Generation) – the title of a book published in 1957 by the well-known German sociologist Helmut Schelsky[3] – became the synonym for the internal and external image of this youth, caught between National Socialism and democracy.[4]

During the war, after he had been wounded as a young soldier, Schrenk had begun his medical studies at the University of Heidelberg, where he belonged to the close circle of students around Viktor von Weizsäcker, who supervised his graduation in 1949.[5] As we know today, during the time when Weizsäcker temporarily held the chair in neurology at the University of Breslau (from 1941 to the end of the war), brains and spinal marrow from murdered girls and boys were sent from the Upper Silesian 'children's euthanasia' ward Loben/Lubliniec to the Neurological Institute in Breslau led by him, where they were examined by Hans-Joachim Scherer.[6] On the other hand, Schrenk's academic teacher was one of the few people who attempted the first critical discussions of the National Socialist 'euthanasia' policy soon after the war. In Weizsäcker's case, this was his 1947/48 treatise '"Euthanasia" and human experiments'. It appeared in the annual 'Psyche' by the Heidelberg publishing house Lambert Schneider, co-published by Alexander Mitscherlich.[7] At that time, Schneider also published the first ground-breaking documentation by Mitscherlich and Fred Mielke about the Nuremberg Doctors Trial.[8]

Before his time as an assistant doctor at the Weizsäcker clinic in Heidelberg from 1951-1955, Schrenk had spent a year as a visiting doctor with Max Müller in Bern, a time he retroactively described as his true 'apprenticeship in the psychiatry of the present'.[9] From 1961 to 1965, he worked at the State Hospital Emmendingen. Then, he also turned to international psychiatric history.[10] As a further point in his life, he worked from 1972 as professor of psychotherapy and psychosomatic medicine at the University Hospital of the Saarland in Homburg/Saar and was founding director of the corresponding institute. Martin Schrenk died in 1995.

The foreign example he quoted was John F. Kennedy's famous 'Special Message to the Congress on Mental Illness and Mental Retardation' of 5 February 1963, where the President declared his support for a large national investment and reform programme in aid of the mentally ill and mentally handicapped.[11] In Germany, several years were to pass before Social Democrat Willy Brandt was the first Chancellor to mention explicitly the 'physically or mentally handicapped' in his equally memorable government statement of 28 October 1969.[12]

Brandt's call for more solidarity with these fellow human beings was part of his well-known dictum 'Dare More Democracy!'. It corresponded with the beginning of the health and socio-political reform movement that coincided almost exactly with the Federal Republic's 'Social Democratic Decade'. Then, both the ideology and structure of the mental health care system started to change fundamentally, influenced by the atmosphere of the latter half of the 1960s and the work of the 1971-75 Psychiatry Commission (*Psychiatrie-Enquete*) of the German Parliament (*Bundestag*).

Problem Definition

Martin Schrenk's appeal can serve as a guideline for a socio-historical approach to the West German reform impulses towards a more modern and humane view and treatment of the mentally ill and handicapped.[13] First of all, the significance which the burden of the Nazi campaign of extermination against psychiatric patients had for the reform process of German post-war psychiatry will be considered. Fundamental reform ideas were articulated well before the Commission began work. From the 1950s, many individual initiatives to improve the living and working conditions in mental hospitals had already breathed the spirit of change.

However, the situation of West German psychiatry was not really made public before the social changes of the late 1960s and early 1970s. In its narrower sense, the reform discourse was partly obscured by broad cultural expressions, particularly with regard to the 'anti-psychiatry' movement. This latter featured prominently in both film and literature and in various circles of the 'leftist scene'. The Socialist Patients Collective Heidelberg (*Sozialistisches Patientenkollektiv Heidelberg/SPK*) became especially well-known.

These questions will be explored mainly with regard to the regional example of Westphalia/North Rhine-Westphalia, though many *structural* conditions point beyond this region, bordering on the Netherlands. After the Second World War, this state maintained a particular Prussian tradition: the 'provincial associations' (*Provinzialverbände*). These were autonomous regional and communal administrative organisations with a wide range of duties, among them the care for the mentally ill. In the territory of North Rhine-Westphalia, they were re-founded in 1946 and were named *Landschaftsverband Rheinland/LVR* and *Landschaftsverband Westfalen-Lippe/LWL* from 1953.[14] Thus, the LWL took over responsibility for the seven large regional asylums (*Provinzial-Heilanstalten*) in Dortmund-Aplerbeck, Eickelborn, Gütersloh, Lengerich, Marsberg, Warstein and Münster from its predecessor. Up to the end of 1960, they were called 'State Asylums and Hospitals' (*Landesheil- und Krankenanstalten*), then 'Westphalian State Hospitals' (*Westfälische Landeskrankenhäuser*), and today they are known as the 'Westphalian Psychiatric Clinics' (*Westfälische Psychiatrie-Kliniken*).

National Socialist Crimes against the Mentally Ill

Until 1945,[15] throughout the Reich (including the annexed territories) altogether about 400,000 men and women were robbed of their fertility through forced sterilisation according to the 'Law for the Prevention of Hereditarily Diseased Offspring' (*Gesetz zur Verhütung erbkranken Nachwuchses*) motivated by ideas of racial hygiene. Nearly 3,300 patients from the Westphalian provincial asylums were part of these frightening 'statistics of mutilation'.[16] Many victims, predominantly women, died as a result of the severe operations. Up to the end of the war, more than 200,000 people in the territory of the Reich fell victim to the advancing radicalisation of National Socialist health and race policies, when these took the form of the murder of patients – the 'euthanasia' crimes.[17]

Among these were the acts of transfer and murder directed specifically against *Jewish* patients in 1940, the subsequent registration, transfer and murder by gas, '*Action T4*' during 1940/41, and the parallel extermination of handicapped children and youths. The scenes of the Westphalian 'children's euthanasia', Niedermarsberg and Dortmund-Aplerbeck, lay within the region itself, while the T4 transports of 1941 ended for most of the 2,800 'selected' Westphalian patients in the Hessian annihilation asylum of Hadamar. In 1943, a second large wave of transfers followed, totaling about 2,850 asylum inmates from Westphalia. These transports mainly ended in asylums in the south of Germany.

Officially, the renewed mass transfers were justified with reference to the increasing danger of air raids – as 'disaster control measures'.[18] In fact, a main motivation for them was to make room in the asylums for military hospitals of the *Wehrmacht* and to evacuate urban hospitals and clinics for the physically ill. For instance, in 1943, the Eickelborn asylum was used as alternative site for the State Clinic for Women in Bochum. It also harboured a huge military hospital. Together with the destruction of asylum buildings caused by the war, these extensive cross-occupancies contributed to a general catastrophic deterioration of conditions in German psychiatric institutes. Many patients were forced to live in cramped conditions, to share beds, or to make do with straw sacks on the ground. Medical care and social attention were nearly impossible, as military conscription had severely reduced available manpower. In Westphalian asylums, a ward doctor would eventually be responsible for up to 800 patients.

Sanitary conditions also steadily deteriorated. Furthermore, patients increasingly suffered from serious malnourishment and from skin diseases. The malnourishment was the result of a general development which had set in even before the war. Based on racial hygiene and cost-benefit calculations relating to the armaments policy, the standard of basic care devoted to the mentally ill was first cut back and then increasingly reduced strictly according to the ability to undertake work considered 'vital to the war effort'. Throughout the Reich, very many patients in the asylums died of starvation (as had already happened during the First World War), especially since malnutrition combined with overdosing medication was now used in some hospitals as a more indirect way of killing, in conformity with the 'euthanasia' policy.[19] In total 'with about 96,000 victims, more mentally ill died from lack of care, malnourishment and murder by medication than were murdered during Action T4'![20]

Post-war in Asylum Psychiatry

In Westphalia as well, care for the mentally ill experienced a kind of 'post-war' (*Nachkrieg*)[21] and remained for a long time in the shadow of the 'ruined conditions at the end of the war'.[22] In spite of the political transformation from 8 May 1945, everyday life in the mental hospitals was clouded by the continuing disastrous conditions. Often, the situation became even worse. So the 'Hunger Years' (*Hungerjahre*) of the 'Collapsed Society' (*Zusammenbruchgesellschaft*) began, primarily affecting asylum patients, with a resulting death rate often far exceeding the rates of the preceding National Socialist era![23] Compared with other regions and hospitals, however, overall developments in the Westphalian provincial hospitals were less dramatic.[24] In October 1945, Werner Hartwich, director of the mental hospital at Gütersloh, described all his patients as undernourished and demanded for them the same increase in calorie intake as was granted to the physically ill in general hospitals.[25] Moreover, many patients not only had to suffer from hunger but were freezing, as the 'fuel allocation' in both winters between 1945 and 1947 was totally insufficient.[26] According to an eyewitness account, in Lengerich, patients froze to death in their beds.[27]

The extensive cross-allocation of space in mental hospitals for military hospitals, municipal surrogate hospitals and other non-psychiatric institutions also continued. British occupational forces continued to use some military hospitals of the *Wehrmacht*, while other emptied buildings were immediately used again as new emergency accommodation. For instance, the state hospitals in Dortmund-Aplerbeck and Warstein now housed Russian and Polish 'displaced persons', while Eickelborn – parts of the *Wehrmacht* hospital cleared only at the beginning of 1947 – had to accommodate the administrative, educational and care units of the municipal school for the deaf from Soest, as well as an old people's home 'for fugitives from the east and evacuated persons in need of care'. Both facilities remained there well into the 1950s. The last departments of the Bochum State Clinic for Women, still accommodated there, were finally withdrawn from Eickelborn in 1949.[28]

Next to delays in reconstructing destroyed buildings and the use of wards for treating specific war and post-war casualties, the continuing cross-occupancies were responsible for the fact that even at the end of 1954, the LWL was unable to use 28 of its sanatorium buildings for their defined purpose![29] Therefore, the acute overcrowding of the available wards and dormitories often continued. Simultaneously, the swift ending or at least reduction of these material wants was impossible during the 'time of debris' (*Trümmerzeit*). With regard to laundry, clothing and other essential items, the Westphalian mental hospitals still lived 'on the barest subsistence level' during the first post-war years.[30] Floors, walls, ceilings and technical installations were usually in a desolate condition. Moreover, many patients still had to use open toilets built directly into the dormitories. As the dormitories were tightly packed with (bunk) beds, it was impossible to provide small bedside lockers for the patients.

This dismal state of affairs was criticized by a national commission inspecting the state hospital in Aplerbeck at the beginning of 1950 on behalf of the North Rhine-Westphalian Ministry of Social Welfare. That nearly 15 years had passed since the last inspection in June 1935 also indicates the long neglect of minimal standards regarding the care for the mentally ill. The renovation and modernisation efforts that the commission demanded regarding Aplerbeck were also required for all other mental hospitals – and not only in Westphalia. However, the patients' diet at least was described as 'good and sufficient'.[31]

Confronting the National Socialist Past

The disastrous legacies of National Socialism resulted in a persistent moral discrediting of asylum psychiatry. Therefore, the re-activation of outpatient care (*Außenfürsorge*), after years of neglect, met with considerable resistance. In 1952, Wilhelm Schneider, director of the state hospital in Gütersloh, reported:

> Outpatient care had been stopped during the war and had to be re-constructed slowly and carefully, because, due to the National Socialist methods (forced sterilization, euthanasia), all measures connected with psychiatry were met with deep mistrust.[32]

This mistrust was especially deep-rooted with regard to the victims directly affected by these 'methods' and their families. Many of them had tried to prevent the risk to life and limb during the 'Third Reich', through courageous resistance.[33] Their mistrust was additionally fuelled by the bitter experience that many accountable Nazi criminals and accomplices were either not brought to justice, or only inadequately. In Hagen, for instance, a father tried to encourage the criminal investigation of his son's 'euthanasia' death. In the summer of 1941, Josef G. had been transferred from the asylum in Warstein to Hadamar, where he 'suddenly deceased'.[34] His father repeatedly wrote petitions to the legal authorities in 1947, but received no satisfactory response. He therefore wrote to the senior public prosecutor at the district court in Frankfurt/Main: 'I hope to expect [after all], that the offenders will be arrested without exception, in the interest of humanity and above all [...so that] the mentally ill [can] once again entrust themselves confidently to the asylums'.[35]

The judicial investigation of National Socialist crimes against the mentally ill in Westphalia also remained far behind expectations.[36] As a result, many distinctive features of the provincial policy confirm the well-known image of appalling continuities with regard to personnel and the general tabooing of their own

National Socialist legacy.[37] The continued full-time employment of the Aplerbeck 'children's euthanasia' doctor, Theodor Niebel, belongs in this context. After the war, Niebel, a rank-and-file member of the Nazi party since 1937, evaded the de-nazification regulations and remained in office until retiring normally in 1968, all the while benefiting from promotional advantages gained for participating in the murder of children. However, research also indicates some disciplinary measures and criminal prosecutions against responsible parties (mainly in the form of the Westphalian 'Euthanasia' Trial),[38] as well as some early self-critical reflection on the burden of the National Socialist past with regard to politics, medical care and society.

In Westphalia, Rudolf Amelunxen (born in 1888), administrative expert and member of the *Zentrum*, the Catholic party from before 1933, was the main voice in this regard. The British military government appointed him to be Senior Executive (*Oberpräsident*) of the province of Westphalia in 1945 and then the first Prime Minister of North Rhine-Westphalia, in 1946. With courageous public initiatives and speeches, Amelunxen strongly promoted a serious discussion of the 'German cataclysm' (historian Friedrich Meinecke) – especially in front of young people from the 'sceptical generation' and with specific reference to the National Socialist mass murder of the mentally ill.[39]

For Amelunxen, a return to peace and social democracy was unthinkable without serious, self-critical reflection on the National Socialist destruction of both values. Even then, he imagined a 'culture of peace', not merely understood as the absence of violence – military or otherwise – but also as social respect and enforcement of human, citizen and minority rights – including the rights of the mentally ill. The specific challenge to West German society regarding the transformation from the 'cult of war' to a 'culture of peace' was to confront the National Socialist past as a single whole.[40]

However, like other remarkable efforts of the immediate post-war era,[41] for the time being, Amelunxen's initiatives simply ran aground, due to the general atmosphere of social *Stille* (philosopher Hermann Lübbe) and the widespread wish to put an end to the criminal prosecution and exclusion from office of former Nazi activists which were commonly encountered during the transition to the 1950s.[42]

Early Reform and '*Vergangenheitsbewältigung*' ('Confronting the Past')

During the late 1950s and the early 1960s, the indifference and callousness regarding National Socialism displayed by the majority of West German society finally started to concern a small group of psychiatrists from the 'sceptical generation'.[43] Their impulse coincided with a period when the National Socialist past 'returned to haunt'[44] the Federal Republic, becoming an object of public debate.

The Ulm *Einsatzgruppen* (operational groups, killing units) Trial in 1958 and a wave of anti-Semitic acts culminating during the winter of 1959/60 were major causes of this development. The trial made it obvious that those responsible for a whole range of crimes had not been prosecuted and that these remained un-atoned for. At the start of the 1960s, the Eichmann Trial in Jerusalem was followed by the spectacular Auschwitz Trial in Frankfurt. At the same time, from 1959, the scandal surrounding the physician Werner Heyde (using the alias 'Dr. Fritz Sawade') who had continued his professional career in camouflage but was also deliberately covered up for, shed a glaring light on continuities from the 'Third Reich' to the Federal Republic.[45] Heyde was one of the main perpetrators responsible for the National Socialist murder of the mentally ill. Finally, the first reprint of documentation of the Nuremberg Doctors' Trial by Alexander Mitscherlich and Fred Mielke appeared in 1960.[46]

It is still hardly known that the psychiatrists mentioned above also helped to bring about the 'return' of the Nazi past into public debate. Among them, in addition to Martin Schrenk, were the Westphalian asylum doctor Manfred in der Beeck (born in 1920), the Heidelberg psychiatrists Walter von Baeyer (born in 1904), Heinz Häfner and Karl Peter Kisker (both born in 1926), and the director of the University of Tübingen Psychiatric Clinic, Walter Schulte (born in 1910). They can be regarded as 'harbingers' of the West German 'culture of peace', for they started to put into practice what Rudolf Amelunxen had already demanded in 1946. These reform-minded doctors combined reflection on their profession's National Socialist history and the corresponding public mistrust with criticism of the continuing inhumane state of affairs in psychiatric medicine. Earlier than others, they admitted that, in international comparison, blatant lack of reform in West German psychiatry was not least a product of the devastations that the National Socialist regime wreaked on the care of the mentally ill. They considered the West German body politic, medical profession and society morally indebted to their mentally ill and handicapped citizens – and demanded the modernisation of psychiatry.

This combination of confronting the past and advancing reform was additionally promoted by a comparative view of developments in psychiatry abroad, mainly in the Western world. It was considered important to re-establish connections to the profession's international scientific community, to overcome the post-war isolation of German psychiatry, and to regain trust and reputation. This view was also driven by the experiences that individual doctors gained abroad and the progressive programmes developed by the World Health Organisation.

With his book 'Practical Psychiatry' (*Praktische Psychiatrie*),[47] Manfred in der Beeck, then working at the mental hospital in Münster, pointed in a similar direction in 1957, even before Martin Schrenk. This book was based on and continued the work of Hermann Simon, director of the Gütersloh State Hospital, who had earned international renown during the 1920s with his concept of treating patients in a more active manner by work therapy ('*aktivere Krankenbehand-lung*').[48] In der Beeck aimed to provide a 'summary of the questions and problems raised by Simon with regard to the future development of psychiatry'.[49] He was also influenced by visits to psychiatric institutions in France, England, Italy and the Netherlands. The 'silence' in Germany with regard to its National Socialist past filled him with discomfort. While Schrenk was especially influenced by Weizsäcker's study '"Euthanasia" and human experiments', In der Beeck owed much to his mentor, the psychiatrist Gerhard Schmidt.

In 1947, In der Beeck had started to work with Schmidt at the Lübeck Medical Centre. For a time, this hospital also treated the psychiatric disorders of Jewish 'Exodus' refugees. In der Beeck saw this work as a chance for some 'restitution', while only a short time before Schmidt had written an impressive report on the 'euthanasia' actions at the mental hospital Egelfing-Haar near Munich during his provisional directorship of this institution. Though Schmidt's study 'Selection at the Asylum 1939-45' from 1945/46 is now regarded as one of the early classics in 'euthanasia' research, a publisher could only be found for it after almost 20 years.[50]

In 1957, In der Beeck called for a modern 'individual psychiatry' which would be able to transform traditional mental asylums into proper hospitals accepted by society at large. Looking back at the years before 1933, he concluded that Germany had long been one of the 'fast ships [...] in modern psychiatric therapy':

Then [1933] came the years in which those mentally and spiritually damaged were merely administrated, then sterilised, and finally gassed, despite the organic methods of treatment which were coming to light at that very time. We still have to atone for a considerable burden of guilt for what happened to our patients in the asylums during that time! It is intolerable that those who are mentally suffering should continue to be viewed and treated as second-class humans and fourth-class patients.[51]

In the case of Heidelberg professor Walter von Baeyer and his two assistant medical directors, Häfner and Kisker, their commitment to reform, based on their reflection on the Nazi years, was doubtless strengthened by their intense involvement with the 'Psychiatry of the Persecuted'. This was the title of a major innovative and internationally acclaimed study on 'Psychopathological experiences and assessments of victims of National Socialist persecution and comparable extreme stress', which the three published in 1964.[52] Schrenk reviewed this book for the *Frankfurter Allgemeine Zeitung*.[53] The study also promoted Walter von Baeyer's appointment to the post of Vice President of the World Psychiatric Association (1966-1971).[54]

Like his colleague Walter Schulte in Tübingen, Baeyer also participated in the contemporary joint series of lectures on the National Socialist past held at

West German universities. Both spoke about the Nazi crimes in psychiatry.[55] Their lectures were not designed to be apologetic, but rather marked by the intention to document, examine and reflect. The criticism with regard to their profession also did not leave out the connection between the Nazi murder of the mentally ill and the striking mistrust and obstruction of reform that West German psychiatry faced during the post-war years.

'Reform before Reform'

The psychiatrists mentioned above were in the forefront of those representatives of their profession who, from the 1950s, anticipated the basic ideas and demands of the later 'Psychiatry Commission' programme.

The Heidelberg psychiatrists, for instance, were setting up model transitional homes, day and night clinics, post-care patient 'clubs', and advanced socio-psychiatric training courses for nursing staff.[56] In 1965, Häfner, Baeyer and Kisker published a memorandum entitled 'Urgent reforms in the Federal Republic's psychiatric medical care: On the necessity to construct socio-psychiatric institutions (psychiatric community centres)'. However, this was only published in a small and rather obscure psychiatric journal.[57]

In the daily routine of mental hospitals,[58] the reform proposals at first concentrated on the consolidation of the care situation and then on a partial 'internal modernisation' of the therapeutic infrastructure. The Westphalian State Hospital in Gütersloh, headed by Walter Schulte, offered a relatively progressive example. Schulte and his successor, Walter Theodor Winkler, together with their colleagues, encouraged both structural and social measures: old dormitories were reduced in size, patients' toilets were enclosed, patients were provided with their own lockers, they were paid for their work and involved in producing a hospital newspaper. During the 1950s, the first radio and TV sets also appeared in the wards.

The introduction of modern forms of occupational and group therapy, replacing the older work therapies, and the 'therapeutic [ward] communities', based on English models, signified a paradigm change away from the traditional, scientific, hierarchical view of the patient as an 'object' or 'case' and towards his/her perception and recognition as 'an individual character' with specific needs.

These were first beginnings of a 'treatment partnership'[59] between medical personnel and patients. With the introduction of therapeutic group discussions, the former strict separation between the sexes was partially overcome for the first time. Nevertheless, these new approaches in therapy were accompanied by the continued use of traditional somatic methods of treatment, e.g. electroshocks.

Use of the new psychiatric drugs chlorpromazine and reserpine, introduced in 1952, also remained ambivalent: they changed the internal climate of the state hospitals considerably – by reducing the wards for the chronically restless, less-ening the usual restrictions, producing the principle of the 'open door', and shortening the average length of stay.[60] In contrast, however, due to the some-times excessive use of psychiatric drugs, in many wards 'the problem,' as Walter Schulte said, 'no longer was the unrest, but rather this quite disturbing silence of stiffness, paralysis and dullness'.[61] Here, the traditional habits of the asylums proved again to be a barrier against a broader development of available new approaches in therapy.

An important feature of this partial modernisation was the increasing intern-al differentiation (not only in Westphalia)[62] of asylum care with the introduction of specialised wards. Certainly, the chronically ill were still treated in the same institution as those who were less afflicted. But alongside traditional differentia-tions between 'calm' and 'restless' individuals, patients began to be increasingly separated according to age or symptoms, e.g. neurological or psychiatric. Fi-nally, since the 1950s the difficult and underprivileged situation of the person-nel of mental hospitals was debated.[63] The first reform measures were imple-mented with the 'Nursing Law' (*Krankenpflegegesetz*) in 1957.[64]

At a very early stage, hospital directors like Schulte and Winkler in Gütersloh or Stefan Wieser in Bremen were aware that progressive *internal* measures had to be followed with a corresponding *external* orientation. No amount of radical reforms could begin to take root as long as society at large failed to show more understanding and responsibility for the mentally ill. Accordingly, as early as the mid-1960s, they began to use modern public relations methods like radio talks and television broadcasts to advocate more transparency, tolerance and trust between psychiatrists and the general public.[65]

In 1966, the 'German Welfare Day' Conference (*Deutscher Fürsorgetag*) was organised with the theme 'Society's Responsibility for the Mentally Ill'.[66] The principal spokesmen at this event were from the 'Action Committee for Im-proving the Help for the Mentally Ill', founded in 1959.[67] Several remarkable local initiatives that occurred in the former GDR at the same time show that many reform ideas were 'in the air' around the turn of the 1960s.[68]

1968 – A Turning Point in the History of Psychiatry

All pioneers of reform had in common that they were not able to communicate with a wider public. In the FRG, the 'leap' from limited internal to socially ac-cepted modernisation of psychiatric care only succeeded as a result of the upheav-als happening between the late 1960s and early 1970s. The peak of this develop-ment was not only marked by the anti-authoritarian protests of the 'Extra-parliamentary Opposition' (APO) and the students in 1967/68, but also by Willy Brandt's government proclamation in October 1969. The combination of psychiatric reform and the '68 Movement' highlights the 'cultural-revolutionary' and far-reaching effects that this time of upheaval had on the whole of society. This transformation also triggered other comparable social awakenings and movements: the women's liberation movement, the ecology movement, educational reform, and military and police reform. But the rapid spread of a new political and ideological consciousness also led to a polarisation and radicalisation of the political atmosphere and associated personal grievances. This change in the social climate was not only the medium but also, to a certain extent, the 'price' of the widespread internal drive towards democratising the Federal Republic.[69]

Psychiatry as an institution and a profession, its political and social environment and the anti-authoritarian protest movement now entered a dynamic inter-relationship. The basic events which fuelled this development and the ensuing results occurred during a brief period between 1970 and 1971. They were:

(1) The first debates at the German Doctors' Day (*Deutscher Ärztetag*) and the German Society for Psychiatry & Psychiatric Treatment (*Deutsche Gesellschaft für Psychiatrie und Nervenheilkunde*) with regard to improving psychiatric care.

(2) The 'Action for the Mentally Ill' (*Aktion psychisch Kranke*), founded on the initiative of professionals in psychiatry and politics, to realize the interests of patients at a political level.

(3) The 'Mannheim Circle' established by nurses, care workers, social workers, occupational therapists, doctors, psychologists and sociologists working in psychiatric clinics or closely related institutions. This gave rise to the German Society for Social Psychiatry (DGSP) with its publication *Sozialpsychiatrische Informationen*.[70]

(4) The 'Gütersloh Further Training Week', which coined 'the [later] often quoted expression of the "miserable and degrading circumstances" in large psychiatric hospitals'.[71]

(5) A conference held at the 'Protestant Academy' in Loccum entitled 'The Mentally Ill and the Society', at which 130 representatives from psychiatry, politics and the general public passed a reform-orientated resolution to be sent to the Parliamentary Committee for Youth, Family & Health.[72]

(6) Two public hearings held by the above Committee.

(7) Finally, an appeal from the German *Bundestag* to the relevant Ministry, primarily initiated by CDU (Christian Democratic Union) member of parliament Walter Picard (1923-2000), calling for a 'committee of experts to be appointed to report on the state of psychiatry in the Federal Republic' – the Psychiatry Commission headed by psychiatrist Caspar Kulenkampff (1921-2002).[73]

This Commission published an interim report in 1973,[74] followed by a final report in 1975,[75] which was only discussed in the Bundestag four years later, however. Parallel to the work of the Commission, regional psychiatry plans were devised and passed at the state level.

The expert report radically questioned the traditional structures of care. Several characteristics were described as in need of reform, primarily the size of mental hospitals and their remote geographical position, considered to be counter-productive to the need for a care system closely connected to the communities, their vast catchment areas, the over-long stay of inpatients, the overcrowded dormitories, the quantity and quality of personnel recruitment, and finally the unacceptable accommodation of many patients.

In the eyes of the experts, a large proportion of psychiatrically disturbed old people, the majority of the mentally handicapped, alcohol addicts and the chronically ill (not in need of urgent hospitalisation) were no longer in need of psychiatric inpatient care and were therefore not being treated according to their needs.[76]

The 'Socialisation' of Psychiatry

How is the dynamic inter-relationship between psychiatry reform and the '68 Movement' to be explained? Three perspectives can be subsumed under the heuristic working concept of 'socialisation of psychiatry' (*Vergesellschaftung der Psychiatrie*). This term helps to explain the genesis, formation and aims of the reform movement. It does not imply that psychiatry immediately discarded its traditional position on the fringes of society. It might therefore be suitable to use the term 'socialisation of psychiatry' as a complementary concept to the better-known 'de-institutionalisation'.

First: In the context of the anti-authoritarian criticism of society and its traditions – aimed against 'the institutions' – and a more highly developed sensitivity about social issues, as well as human and civil rights (especially of fringe groups),[77] psychiatry had become a breeding-ground for social and political issues. It had become a topic of public interest, beyond the narrow confines of the mental hospitals.[78] A good indicator of this was the public response to Frank Fischer's 1969 publication *Madhouses: The Sick Accuse*. This 'historian and scholar of German literature and language' had 'studied' the everyday life at mental asylums as a psychiatric 'amateur', primarily by working for several months as an 'auxiliary nurse-attendant' at various institutions. First interim results of his investigations had already been published in the weekly *Die Zeit* in 1967.[79]

Mental illness now became increasingly regarded as a social problem. A widespread criticism of psychiatry and society that regarded itself as anti-repressive and emancipative popularised the concept of the American sociologists Everett Hughes and Erving Goffman, describing mental hospitals as 'total institutions'. It was no accident that around 1970 Goffman's book *Asylums. Essays on the Social Situation of Mental Patients and Other Inmates*, originally published in 1961, appeared in a German translation.[80] About the same time, Michel Foucault's

1961 classic *Folie et déraison. Histoire de la folie à l'âge classique* was also published in German.[81]

Foucault's thesis of the 'great confinement'[82] of the mad appeared to 'de-mystify' the history of psychiatry. Until then, it had been chiefly depicted as a history of medical and humanitarian progress under the banner of 'bourgeois' enlightenment and reason. Foucault's perspective and his reception laid the foundations for a revisionist socio-historical approach with a place in the broad context of politics, administration, economics and society.

The first generation of critical revisionist histories of psychiatry started with Klaus Dörner's study 'Citizens and Madmen', published in 1969.[83] Dörner, a doctor and sociologist, described his work both with regard to 'time' and 'contents' as 'a product [...] of the anti-authoritarian student movement' and as providing a helpful impulse to the 'psychiatry movement in Germany and Italy'.[84] His book was indeed translated into several languages including Italian. Conversely, in 1971, the German publishing house Suhrkamp put out the translation of a volume edited by radical Italian psychiatry reformer Franco Basaglia, entitled *Die negierte Institution oder Die Gemeinschaft der Ausgeschlossenen.*[85]

Anti-Psychiatry

This leads directly to the second point: The '68 movement was not least a *media* event, where the flourishing press, but also television and radio, played a major role, for instance by drawing attention to the protagonists involved in psychiatry abroad, thus promoting them as role models. This particular phenomenon in the very heterogeneous 'socialisation of psychiatry' introduced one of the more radical variations of the reform movement, 'anti-psychiatry', to the interested general public.[86]

Among the proponents of the international anti-psychiatric debate of the 1960s and 1970s were – next to Basaglia, Goffman and, in part, Foucault – the English psychiatrists Ronald Laing and David Cooper and their American colleague Thomas Szasz. Put briefly and neglecting different positions in detail, they refused to label psychic dysfunctions as disease, but rather defined them as a consequence of social processes of rejection and discriminating exclusion from the alleged 'normal' and 'healthy' majority of society. To them, the old hierarchically structured mental hospitals were similar to prisons for ensuring social control, stigmatisation and legal incapacitation – with the doctors to a certain extent seen as 'agents' of this system. Along the same lines, Tilman Fischer recently took the following quotation as the title of his study dealing with the position of Heinar Kipphardt's novel *März* ('March')[87] in the context of the anti-psychiatry debate: '*Gesund ist, wer andere zermalmt*' (He is healthy, who crushes others).[88]

The Socialist Patients Collective Heidelberg (SPK)

A specifically West German case of the cultural effects of anti-psychiatry was the 'Socialist Patients Collective in Heidelberg' (SPK).[89] This short-lived and highly controversial organisation emerged in February 1970 around the psychiatrist Wolfgang Huber and comprised about 500 patients when it closed down in the summer of 1971. By then, it had become widely known. The collective developed out of Huber's outpatient department at the psychiatric clinic of the University of Heidelberg. He wanted to strengthen the rights of the patients and to dismantle the old hierarchy in the relations between doctor and client. After conflicts with the management and Huber's official dismissal, his department developed into an independent entity, in rooms outside the clinic. For a short time, SPK members and sympathizers squatted in the staff rooms and offices of the clinic and university board. It was temporarily tolerated as an institution of the university, but in late autumn of 1970, the university administration and the State Department for Education and Cultural Affairs finally revoked this authorization. From then on, the collective had to reckon with being shut down – possibly even by force.

In April 1971, the situation escalated after a female SPK patient committed suicide. Then, in June, when unknown parties shot at a policeman in the small town of Wiesenbach near Heidelberg, flats and houses of SPK members were searched in the hunt for suspected members of the left-wing terrorist group 'Red Army Faction' (*Rote Armee Fraktion/RAF*). Huber and other members of the SPK were arrested. Trials followed and sentences were imposed for participation in a criminal association, the manufacture of explosive materials, and the forgery of documents. Altogether, more than a dozen young SPK members joined the 'armed struggle' of the RAF, among them Margrit Schiller (born in 1948). Already influenced by the student movement of the late 1960s, she had separated herself from her conservative parental home, bourgeois way of living, close ties to the church, and traditional sexual ethics. Her real left politicisation and radicalisation, however, only started after she joined the SPK. Schiller has vividly described these experiences in her autobiography:

> There was a Marx working group, a Hegel working group, a working group on anti-psychiatry and one on the New Left analysis of society. I registered immediately for one-on-one discussions, called 'single agitation' in the SPK. During the sessions, I had an immense need to initially speak about me, my biography, my insecurities, my fears and my search for something different. At first, I went to the SPK several times a week exclusively for this reason. There, I realized that my loneliness and sadness and the many problems I had with myself were not my personal and inescapable fate... I started to become curious about history and politics. In

Between the National Socialist 'Euthanasia Programme' and Reform the SPK, there were books about the Nazi crimes during the Second World War. I read them and could hardly sleep at night, struck with horror... After a few weeks, I felt at home in the SPK. I participated in several working groups, wrote leaflets with others, reproduced them on the small machine, felt well and worked with the others as energetically as I could. On the old record player, time and again we listened to the song '*Macht kaputt, was euch kaputtmacht*' [rough English equivalent: 'Break what breaks you'] by the group *Ton, Steine, Scherben* and sang along as loud as we could, because at that time the text expressed exactly how we felt. There was always something going on. Small or larger groups of people heatedly discussed the latest events, the situation in the world, books or personal questions. Protest actions or demonstrations were prepared.[90]

Margrit Schiller's memories illustrate the typical contemporary interaction of youthful 'consumerism' and 'hedonism' with left 'politicisation',[91] and then turn towards the SPK's response to anti-psychiatry. It modified and radicalised the ideas of anti-psychiatry; its motto read: 'Turn illness into a weapon!' This slogan was also used as the title for a widespread agitation text, with an introduction by Jean-Paul Sartre.[92] Illness was explained as a human reaction to the sickening capitalist society; the patients themselves, as self-aware 'revolutionary subjects', should now smash this system. In other words, 'the recognition of the social backgrounds of illness' should be 'transformed into revolutionary action' – even leading to 'invoking the sacrificial death for the revolution: "To come to life in this way, it must be put at stake."'[93]

This Marx-orientated anti-psychiatric concept and interpretation of the relationship between illness and society therefore constituted an important medium of left sub- and counter-cultural radicalisation. For that reason, anti-psychiatry constituted one of the driving forces of the broad militant left discourse about 'repression' and 'anti-repression' during the 1970s. But it simultaneously helped to facilitate the contemporary social and political climate in the FRG which, towards the end of the 1960s, gave rise to the reform movement modernising and humanizing the treatment of the mentally ill and handicapped.

Finally, the National Socialist past played a central role alongside anti-psychiatry in the specifically West German SPK conflict. Members of the SPK had gone so far as to compare themselves to the victims of the Nazi 'euthanasia' and genocide policies. Once again, according to their perceptions of their inner and the outer world, a sick 'fascist' or 'fascist-like' society was on the verge of 'shutting away' or even 'liquidating' patients and undesirables.[94] Their medical 'opponents' at the Heidelberg psychiatric clinic were compared to National Socialist 'euthanasia' experts.[95]

These accusations must have hit the Heidelberg psychiatrists Baeyer, Häfner and Kisker particularly hard. For precisely these three had provided the first important impulses during the 1950s and 1960s for reforming psychiatry and, in doing so, had reflected critically on their profession's National Socialist past. Understandably, these psychiatrists suffered personal emotional wounds during the s p k conflict.[96] As a result, their original liberal position was replaced by a defensive attitude, dismissing everything that was regarded as 'Sixties' and 'left-wing'. They shared this shock with many others of the older 'sceptical' postwar generation.[97] This development was once again significant for the social climate in which the conflict with the juvenile leftist radicalism occurred.

Psychiatry and 'Democratisation'

'Socialisation of psychiatry' can explain a third basic aspect of the interactions between psychiatric reform and '1968'. This points beyond the early phases of the reform movement to the practical everyday concerns of psychiatric reform. Overcoming the old system of mental hospitals and developing a new culture of therapeutic and rehabilitative care required opening up psychiatry to the public at large, by introducing outpatient, part-time inpatient, and other complementary services, increasing the number of independent psychiatrists and neurologists, and creating self-help groups for patients and their families. This demanded a social atmosphere relying more on a spirit of citizenship than on obedience, thus dismantling the old hierarchies and reducing the reciprocal fears between psychiatry and the outside world. The late 1960s promoted such tendencies of democratisation and liberalisation.

These trends affected the mental hospitals via a younger generation of incoming practitioners. The traditional rigid, directorial attitudes and the superior status of doctors gave way, though increasingly not without conflicts, to a style of work which was more democratic, friendly and team-spirited. In part, this was because additional new groups of professionals (like psychologists and social workers) had to be integrated. At the same time, new social structures and a change in the social climate were indispensable if patient care was to become more open, individual and democratic.

Conclusions

The focus on the 'take-off' period of the West German psychiatric reform movement and the analysis of several, basically positive, long-term trends should not obscure the specific limits, drawbacks and 'costs' accompanying the reform process. The 'price' that the politicisation and ideological radicalisation of the social climate around 1968 claimed with regard to the West German culture of discussion and conflict during the 1970s – up to the trail of blood left behind by RAF

Between the National Socialist 'Euthanasia Programme' and Reform terrorism – has been described. In the context of this topic, however, the question of the social 'costs' has to be primarily asked with regard to the situation of the mentally ill and handicapped. Many chronically ill patients remained 'on the edges of psychiatry reform' because, in the course of scaling down and modernising large state hospitals during the 1970s and 1980s, they were merely transferred to ill-equipped or understaffed nursing homes.[98]

In this regard, the 'de-institutionalisation' of psychiatry sometimes degenerated to a simple 'trans-institutionalisation'[99] of welfare problem groups and responsibilities. This 'dark area' of the German psychiatry reform still has to be illuminated more systematically. Further research on the many delays and temporal differences in the regional and local implementation of the Psychiatry Commission's programme is also necessary. Such a discerning historical examination of the reform process may also promote a sensitivity for continuing deficits and possible new threats to an equal treatment of the mentally and the physically ill.

Notes

*   I would like to thank Christoph Tiemann/Münster and Roy Kift/Castrop-Rauxel for translating the text into English and Hugh Freeman/London for his final editorial comments and corrections.

1.   M. Schrenk, 'Ärztliche und organisatorische Fragen der "Anstalts"-Psychiatrie', in *Referate der Gütersloher Fortbildungswoche 1963* (Gütersloh: Selbstverlag der Psychiatrie-Klinik, 1963), 13-20. See also the reprint in: M. Schrenk, *Schriften 1949-1989*, 3 vols ([Homburg/Saar]: Selbstverlag, [1989]), vol. 1, 224-31.

2.   For Schrenk's biography see: P. Achilles, 'Laudatio. Im Namen der Mitarbeiter des Instituts', in Universität des Saarlandes (ed.), *Umwelt – Inwelt – Mitwelt. Jubiläumssymposion zum 65. Geburtstag von Prof. Dr. Martin Schrenk und zum 15jährigen Bestehen des Instituts für klinische Psychotherapie* (Saarbrücken: Universität, 1988), 7-20. For the psychiatric history of Emmendingen, see: G. Richter (ed.), *Die Fahrt ins Graue(n). Die Heil- und Pflegeanstalt Emmendingen 1933-1945 und danach* (Emmendingen: Zentrum für Psychiatrie, 2002).

3.   H. Schelsky, *Die skeptische Generation. Eine Soziologie der deutschen Jugend* (Düsseldorf/Köln: Diederichs, 1957).

4.   F.-W. Kersting, 'Helmut Schelskys "Skeptische Generation" von 1957. Zur Publikations- und Wirkungsgeschichte eines Standardwerkes', *Vierteljahrshefte für Zeitgeschichte*, 50 (2002), 465-95.

5.   M. Schrenk, *Anthropologische Krankengeschichte aus der Tuberkuloseklinik*, medical dissertation (Heidelberg: [no publisher], 1949); also printed in: Schrenk, *Schriften, op. cit.* (note 1), vol. 1, 1-73.

6.   See especially: U. Benzenhöfer, 'Viktor von Weizsäcker und Breslau', *Jahrbuch der Schlesischen Friedrich-Wilhelms-Universität zu Breslau*, 36/37 (1995/96), 454-66: 463-66; C. Penselin, *'Bemerkungen zu den Vorwürfen, Viktor von Weizsäcker sei in die nationalsozialistische Vernichtungspolitik verstrickt gewesen'* in U. Benzenhöfer (ed.),

Anthropologische Medizin und Sozialmedizin im Werk Viktor von Weizsäckers (Frankfurt am Main: Peter Lang, 1994), 123-37. The question of whether Weizsäcker knew about or was even involved in these occurrences is here doubted or denied, but is still not finally answered.

7.   V. v. Weizsäcker, '"Euthanasie" und Menschenversuche', *Psyche. Ein Jahrbuch für Tiefenpsychologie und Menschenkunde in Forschung und Praxis*, 1 (1947-48), 68-102.

8.   A. Mitscherlich and F. Mielke (eds), *Das Diktat der Menschenverachtung. Eine Dokumentation* (Heidelberg: Lambert Schneider, 1947). Later followed: *idem* (eds), *Wissenschaft ohne Menschlichkeit. Medizinische und eugenische Irrwege unter Diktatur, Bürokratie und Krieg. Mit e. Vorw. der Arbeitsgemeinschaft der Westdeutschen Ärztekammern* (Heidelberg: Lambert Schneider, 1949); several later paperback editions entitled: *Medizin ohne Menschlichkeit. Dokumente des Nürnberger Ärzteprozesses* (Frankfurt/M.: Fischer, 1960ff.). Last but not least, see: Alice Platen-Hallermund, *Die Tötung Geisteskranker in Deutschland. Aus der deutschen Ärztekommission beim amerikanischen Militärgericht* (Frankfurt am Main: Verlag der Frankfurter Hefte, 1948; Reprint Bonn: Psychiatrieverlag, 1993).

9.   M. Schrenk, *Über den Umgang mit Geisteskranken. Die Entwicklung der psychiatrischen Therapie vom "moralischen Regime" in England und Frankreich zu den "psychischen Curmethoden" in Deutschland* (Berlin: Springer-Verlag, 1973), VI (foreword).

10.   *Ibid.*

11.   The 'Special Message' is printed in: *Public Papers of the Presidents of the United States: John F. Kennedy. Containing the Public Messages, Speeches, and Statements of the President*, January 1 to November 22, 1963 (Washington, DC : United States Government Printing Office, 1964), 126-37.

12.   See for the full text of the speech: K. v. Beyme (ed.), *Die großen Regierungserklärungen der deutschen Bundeskanzler von Adenauer bis Schmidt* (München: Carl Hanser, 1979), 251-81. See for the broader context: W. Brandt, *Berliner Ausgabe*, vol. 7: *Mehr Demokratie wagen. Innen- und Gesellschaftspolitik 1966-1974*, adapted by Wolther von Kieseritzky (Bonn: Dietz, 2001).

13.   In stark contrast to the broad research on the history of National Socialist psychiatry, historical research on German psychiatry *after* 1945 is still in its beginnings.

14.   A. Weißer (ed.), *Staat und Selbstverwaltung. Quellen zur Entstehung der nordrhein-westfälischen Landschaftsverbandsordnung* (Paderborn: Schöningh, 2003); K. Teppe (ed.), *Selbstverwaltungsprinzip und Herrschaftsordnung. Bilanz und Perspektiven landschaftlicher Selbstverwaltung in Westfalen* (Münster: Aschendorff, 1987).

15.   For the following, see especially: B. Walter, *Psychiatrie und Gesellschaft in der Moderne. Geisteskrankenfürsorge in der Provinz Westfalen zwischen Kaiserreich und NS-Regime* (Paderborn: Schöningh, 1996); F.-W. Kersting, *Anstaltsärzte zwischen Kaiserreich und Bundesrepublik. Das Beispiel Westfalen* (Paderborn: Schöningh, 1996); *idem* and H.-W. Schmuhl (eds), *Quellen zur Geschichte der Anstaltspsychiatrie in Westfalen*, vol. 2: *1914 – 1955* (Paderborn: Schöningh, 2004); K. Teppe, *Massenmord auf dem Dienstweg. Hitlers 'Euthanasie'-Erlass und seine Durchführung in den Westfälischen Provinzialheilanstalten* (Münster: LWL, 1989). The latest study on the overall develop-

ment is: W. Süß, *Der 'Volkskörper' im Krieg. Gesundheitspolitik, Gesundheitsverhältnisse und Krankenmord im nationalsozialistischen Deutschland 1939-1945* (München: Oldenbourg, 2003).

16. Teppe, *op. cit.* (note 15), 11.

17. This does not include the territories annexed or occupied by Hitler's Germany. See H. Faulstich, 'Die Zahl der "Euthanasie"-Opfer', in A. Frewer and C. Eickhoff (eds), *'Euthanasie' und aktuelle Sterbehilfe-Debatte. Die historischen Hintergründe medizinischer Ethik* (Frankfurt am Main: Campus, 2000), 218-32.

18. Walter, *op. cit.* (note 15), 756ff.

19. This is not really true with regard to Westphalia.

20. H. Faulstich, 'Die Anstaltspsychiatrie unter den Bedingungen der "Zusammenbruchgesellschaft"', in F.-W. Kersting (ed.), *Psychiatriereform als Gesellschaftsreform. Die Hypothek des Nationalsozialismus und der Aufbruch der sechziger Jahre* (Paderborn: Schöningh, 2003), 21-30: 21.

21. See on the use of the term and its perspective in: K. Naumann, 'Einleitung', in *idem* (ed.), *Nachkrieg in Deutschland* (Hamburg: Hamburger Edition, 2001), 9-26.

22. Faulstich, *op. cit.* (note 20), 23.

23. H. Faulstich, *Hungersterben in der Psychiatrie 1914-1949. Mit einer Topographie der NS-Psychiatrie* (Freiburg/Br.: Lambertus, 1998), 661ff.

24. *Ibid.*, 706f.

25. *Hartwich an Kreisernährungsamt Wiedenbrück*, 20 October 1945, in Kersting and Schmuhl (eds), *op. cit.* (note 15), document no. 191.

26. *Protokoll der Konferenz der westfälischen Anstaltsdirektoren*, 2 July 1946, in *ibid.*, document no. 176.

27. Kersting, *op. cit.* (note 15), 360.

28. With regard to this post-war development see Lanschaftsverband Westfalen-Lippe/LWL (ed.), *Landesheilanstalt Eickelborn 1883-1958* ([Münster]: LWL, 1958), 10-11.

29. See the administrative draft *Wie viel Betten braucht der Landschaftsverband Westfalen-Lippe für die Geisteskrankenfürsorge?*, 6 December 1954, in: Kersting and Schmuhl (eds), *op. cit.* (note 15), document no. 179. An initial examination of this source can be found in: Sabine Hanrath, *Zwischen 'Euthanasie' und Psychiatriereform. Anstaltspsychiatrie in Westfalen und Brandenburg: Ein deutsch-deutscher Vergleich (1945-1964)* (Paderborn: Schöningh, 2002), 276ff.

30. *Referat Wernzes zur wirtschaftlichen Lage der Landesheilanstalten*, 20 July 1950, in Kersting and Schmuhl (eds), *op. cit.* (note 15), document no. 177.

31. *Bericht der Besuchskommission an den nordrhein-westfälischen Sozialminister*, 15 January 1950, in *ibid.*, document no. 194.

32. *Schneider an Provinzial-Verwaltung*, 22 February 1952, in *ibid.*, document no. 182.

33. *Ibid.*, documents no. 118ff. and 157ff.

34. *Josef G. an den Präsidenten des Oberlandesgerichts Hamm*, 16 January 1947, in: *ibid.*, document no. 203.

35. *Josef G. an den Oberstaatsanwalt beim Landgericht Frankfurt am Main*, 16 June 1947, in: *ibid.*, document no. 204.

36. See, more extensively: Kersting, *op. cit.* (note 15), 339ff.

37.   See the latest study: E. Klee, *Das Personenlexikon zum Dritten Reich. Wer war was vor und nach 1945* (Frankfurt/M.: S. Fischer, 2003).

38.   See K. Teppe, 'Bewältigung von Vergangenheit? Der westfälische "Euthanasie"-Prozess', in F.-W. Kersting, K. Teppe, B. Walter (eds), *Nach Hadamar. Zum Verhältnis von Psychiatrie und Gesellschaft im 20. Jahrhundert* (Paderborn: Schöningh, 1993), 202-52.

39.   See especially his speech '*Barrikaden der Freiheit*', 6 November 1946, in *Wege zum Volksstaat. Ansprachen des Ministerpräsidenten Dr. Amelunxen* (Düsseldorf: Merkur-Verlag, 1947), 53-64. Partial reprint in: Kersting and Schmuhl (eds), *op. cit.* (note 15), document no. 197.

40.   F.-W. Kersting, 'Die "junge Generation" zwischen Kriegs- und Friedenskultur', in Th. Kühne (ed.), *Von der Kriegskultur zur Friedenskultur? Zum Mentalitätswandel in Deutschland seit 1945* (Hamburg: LIT, 2000), 64-77; F.-W. Kersting, 'Vor Ernst Klee. Die NS-Medizinverbrechen als Reformimpuls', in *idem, op. cit.* (note 20), 63-80.

41.   See note 8.

42.   See especially N. Frei, *Vergangenheitspolitik. Die Anfänge der Bundesrepublik und die NS-Vergangenheit* (München: C.H. Beck, 1997).

43.   For the following see, more extensively: Kersting, *op. cit.* (note 40).

44.   Expression based on: D. Siegfried, 'Zwischen Aufarbeitung und Schlußstrich. Der Umgang mit der NS-Vergangenheit in den beiden deutschen Staaten 1958 bis 1969', in A. Schildt, D. Siegfried, Karl Christian Lammers (eds), *Dynamische Zeiten. Die 6oer Jahre in den beiden deutschen Gesellschaften* (Hamburg: Christians, 2000), 77-113: 78.

45.   K.-D. Godau-Schüttke, *Die Heyde/Sawade-Affäre. Wie Juristen und Mediziner den NS-Euthanasieprofessor Heyde nach 1945 deckten und straflos blieben* (Baden-Baden: Nomos, 1998). T. Freimüller, 'Mediziner: Operation Volkskörper', in N. Frei, *Hitlers Eliten nach 1945. In Zusammenarbeit mit T. Freimüller* et al. (München: dtv, 2003), 13-68: 53ff.

46.   See note 8.

47.   M. in der Beeck, *Praktische Psychiatrie* (Berlin: De Gruyter, 1957).

48.   H. Simon, *Aktivere Krankenbehandlung in der Irrenanstalt* (Berlin: de Gruyter, 1929; reprint: Gütersloh: Westfälisches Landeskrankenhaus, 1969, and Bonn: Psychiatrie-Verlag, 1986). Simon's activities are nowadays regarded more critically by modern research, cf. B. Walter, 'Hermann Simon – Psychiatriereformer, Sozialdarwinist, Nationalsozialist?', *Der Nervenarzt*, 73 (2002), no. 11, 1047-54.

49.   In der Beeck, *op. cit.* (note 47), 11.

50.   G. Schmidt, *Selektion in der Heilanstalt 1939-1945*. Geleitwort von Karl Jaspers (Stuttgart: Ev. Verlagswerk, 1965).

51.   All quotations In der Beeck, *op. cit.* (note 47), 109-11.

52.   W. Ritter von Baeyer, H. Häfner, K.P. Kisker, *Psychiatrie der Verfolgten. Psychopathologische und gutachtliche Erfahrungen an Opfern der nationalsozialistischen Verfolgung und vergleichbarer Extrembelastungen* (Berlin: Springer, 1964).

53.   M. Schrenk, 'Folgen des Terrors', *Frankfurter Allgemeine Zeitung*, 12 December 1964.

54.   Ch. Pross, *Wiedergutmachung. Der Kleinkrieg gegen die Opfer* (Frankfurt/M.: Athenäum, 1988), 155.

55.   W. Schulte, '"Euthanasie" und Sterilisation', in A. Flitner (ed.), *Deutsches Geistesleben und Nationalsozialismus. Eine Vortragsreihe der Universität Tübingen mit einem Nachwort von Hermann Diem* (Stuttgart: Rainer Wunderlich Verlag, 1965), 73-89; W. v. Baeyer, 'Die Bestätigung der NS-Ideologie in der Medizin unter besonderer Berücksichtigung der Euthanasie', in *Universitätstage 1966. Veröffentlichung der Freien Universität Berlin. Nationalsozialismus und die deutsche Universität* (Berlin: De Gruyter, 1966), 63-75.

56.   H. Häfner, 'Die Inquisition der psychisch Kranken geht ihrem Ende entgegen. Die Geschichte der Psychiatrie-Enquete und Psychiatriereform in Deutschland', in Kersting (ed.), *op. cit.* (note 20), 113-40: 127f.

57.   H. Häfner, W.R. v. Baeyer, K. P. Kisker, 'Dringliche Reformen in der psychiatrischen Krankenversorgung der Bundesrepublik. Über die Notwendigkeit des Aufbaus sozialpsychiatrischer Einrichtungen (psychiatrischer Gemeindezentren)', *helfen und heilen. Diagnose und Therapie in der Rehabilitation*, no. 4 (1965), 118-25.

58.   The following overview is based on: Kersting and Schmuhl (eds), *op. cit.* (note 15), 1ff. (introduction) and documents no. 175ff.; Hanrath, *op. cit.* (note 29), 275ff., 302ff.

59.   Term coined by: H. Häfner, *Das Rätsel Schizophrenie. Eine Krankheit wird entschlüsselt* (München: Beck, 2001), 10.

60.   W.Th. Winkler, 'Fortschritte der psychiatrischen Therapie in den letzten 50 Jahren', in Landschaftsverband Westfalen-Lippe (ed.), *Wandlungen der Psychiatrie in fünfzig Jahren. Entwicklungen im Bereich des Landschaftsverbandes Westfalen-Lippe. Herausgegeben aus Anlass des fünfzigjährigen Bestehens des Westfälischen Landeskrankenhauses Gütersloh* (Dortmund: Ardey, 1969), 9-47: 25ff.

61.   W. Schulte, *Klinik der 'Anstalts'-Psychiatrie* (Stuttgart: Thieme, 1962), 113.

62.   G. Engelbracht, *Von der Nervenklinik zum Zentralkrankenhaus Bremen-Ost. Die Geschichte der Bremer Psychiatrie 1945-1977* (Bremen: Edition Temmen, 2004).

63.   See especially the comment of the 'head nurse' ('*Oberpflegerin*') of the state hospital Gütersloh, Eva von Gadow: *Gedanken über die Ausbildung von Irrenpflegepersonal* (1953), in Kersting and Schmuhl (eds), *op. cit.* (note 15), document no. 196.

64.   Hanrath, *op. cit.* (note 29), 285ff.

65.   V. Jakob, '"Wartesaal *mit* Hoffnung". Psychiatrie und Reform im Spiegel zeitgenössischer Filme aus Gütersloh, Bremen und Eickelborn (1963/1967). Versuch einer Bewertung', in Kersting (ed.), *op. cit.* (note 20), 141-48. With regard to the public relations of Bremen hospital director Stefan Wieser see also: St. Wieser, *Isolation. Vom schwierigen Menschen zum hoffnungslosen Fall. Die soziale Karriere des psychisch Kranken*, ed. and introduced by Wolfgang Kirchesch (Reinbek: Rowohlt, 1973). Engelbracht, *op. cit.* (note 62).

66.   H. Reschke (ed.), *Die Verantwortung der Gesellschaft für ihre psychisch Kranken* (Frankfurt/M.: Eigenverlag des Deutschen Vereins für öffentliche und private Fürsorge, 1967).

67.   Hanrath, *op. cit.* (note 29), 327ff.

68.   J. Schulz, 'Die Rodewischer Thesen von 1963 – ein Versuch zur Reform der DDR-Psychiatrie', in Kersting (ed.), *op. cit.* (note 20), 87-100: 97ff. Also: *Von den Rodewischer Thesen zum Gemeindepsychiatrischen Verbund – Erinnerung und Ausblick* [Schwerpunktthema], *Symptom. Leipziger Beiträge zu Psychiatrie & Verrücktheit*, no. 5, 2000, 1ff.; K.-D. Waldmann, '30 Jahre offene Psychiatrie – ein Erfahrungsbericht', *Sozialpsychiatrische Informationen*, 28 (1998), 24-27.

69.   This summary is based on: F.-W. Kersting, 'Entzauberung des Mythos? Aus-gangsbedingungen und Tendenzen einer gesellschaftsgeschichtlichen Standortbe-stimmung der westdeutschen "68er"-Bewegung', *Westfälische Forschungen* 48 (1998), 1-19. Many comparable perspectives and results now in: J. Calließ (ed.), *Die Reform-zeit des Erfolgsmodells BRD. Die Nachgeborenen erforschen die Jahre, die ihre Eltern und Lehrer geprägt haben* (Rehburg-Loccum: Evangelische Akademie Loccum, 2004).

70.   M. Bauer, 'Reform als soziale Bewegung: Der "Mannheimer Kreis" und die Gründung der "Deutschen Gesellschaft für Soziale Psychiatrie"', in Kersting (ed.), *op. cit.* (note 20), 155-63.

71.   K. Dörner, 'Einführung', in *idem* (ed.), *Jetzt wird's ernst – die Psychiatrie-Reform beginnt! Wie setzen wir die "Empfehlungen der Experten-Kommission der Bundesregie-rung zur Reform der psychiatrischen Versorgung" in die Praxis um? 41. Gütersloher Fort-bildungswoche 1989* (Gütersloh: Jakob von Hoddis, 1990), 7-10: 7.

72.   H. Lauter and J.-E. Meyer (eds), *Der psychisch Kranke und die Gesellschaft. Tagung der Evangelischen Akademie Loccum, Oktober 1970* (Stuttgart: Thieme, 1971).

73.   H. Häfner, 'Caspar Kulenkampff (1922-2002)', *Der Nervenarzt* 73 (2002), 1105-06.

74.   *Sachverständigen-Kommission zur Erarbeitung der Enquete über die Lage der Psy-chiatrie in der BRD, Zwischenbericht* (Bonn: Bundestag, 1973; Bundestagsdrucksache 7/1124).

75.   *Enquete-Bericht über die Lage der Psychiatrie in der Bundesrepublik – Zur politi-schen und psychotherapeutisch/psychosomatischen Versorgung in der Bevölkerung*, 2 vols (Bonn: Bundestag, 1975; Bundestagsdrucksache 7/4200 and 7/4201).

76.   *Ibid.*, here especially the summary, vol. 1, 6ff. For the history of the Psychiatry Commission now also see: Aktion Psychisch Kranke (ed.), *25 Jahre Psychiatrie-Enquete*, 2 vols (Bonn: Psychiatrie-Verlag, 2001).

77.   W. Rudloff, 'Sozialstaat, Randgruppen und bundesrepublikanische Gesell-schaft. Umbrüche und Entwicklungen in den sechziger und frühen siebziger Jah-ren', in Kersting (ed.), *op. cit.* (note 20), 181-219: 204ff.

78.   C. Kulenkampff, 'Erkenntnisinteresse und Pragmatismus. Erinnerungen an die Zeit von 1945 bis 1970', in K. Dörner (ed.), *Fortschritte der Psychiatrie im Umgang mit Menschen. Wert und Verwertung des Menschen im 20. Jahrhundert, 36. Gütersloher Fortbildungswoche* (Rehburg-Loccum: Psychiatrie-Verlag, 1985) 127-38: 137.

79.   F. Fischer, *Irrenhäuser. Kranke klagen an* (München: Kurt Desch, 1969), insb. 10f. (Vorwort). *Die Zeit* is also mentioned here.

80.   E. Goffman, *Asyle. Über die Situation psychiatrischer Patienten und anderer Insas-sen* (Frankfurt/M.: Suhrkamp, 1972).

81.   M. Foucault, *Wahnsinn und Gesellschaft* (Frankfurt/Main: Suhrkamp, 1969).

82.   *Ibid.*, 68ff.

83. K. Dörner, *Bürger und Irre. Zur Sozialgeschichte und Wissenschaftssoziologie der Psychiatrie* (Frankfurt/M.: Europäische Verlagsanstalt, 1969; Pocketbook, new edition Frankfurt/M.: Europäische Verlagsanstalt, 1984)

84. *Ibid.* (Dörner's preface in the 1984 edition).

85. F. Basaglia, *Die negierte Institution oder Die Gemeinschaft der Ausgeschlossenen. Ein Experiment der psychiatrischen Klinik in Görz* (Frankfurt/M.: Suhrkamp, 1971; since 1973 also available as paperback in the 'edition suhrkamp': Frankfurt/M.; ital. original: 1968).

86. T. Fischer, *'Gesund ist, wer andere zermalmt'. Heinar Kipphardts 'März' im Kontext der Antipsychiatrie-Debatte* (Bielefeld: Aisthesis-Verlag, 1999), especially 97ff. Häfner, *op. cit.* (note 59), 71f.

87. H. Kipphardt, *März. Roman* (München: Bertelsmann/'AutorenEdition', 1976). Before he wrote the novel, Kipphardt produced the TV movie 'Leben des schizophrenen Dichters Alexander März' (first broadcast on the channel ZDF: 23 June 1975).

88. See note 86.

89. Along with my own research, the following is based on: C. Brink, 'Radikale Psychiatriekritik in der Bundesrepublik. Zum Sozialistischen Patientenkollektiv in Heidelberg', in Kersting (ed.), *op. cit.* (note 20), 165-79; *Idem*, '(Anti-)Psychiatrie und Politik. Über das Sozialistische Patientenkollektiv Heidelberg', in R. Faber and E. Stölting (eds), *Die Phantasie an die Macht? 1968 – Versuch einer Bilanz* (Berlin: Philo, 2002), 125-56; M. Schiller, *'Es war ein harter Kampf um meine Erinnerung'. Ein Lebensbericht aus der RAF. Mit einem Nachwort von Osvaldo Bayer*, ed. Jens Mecklenburg, 2nd edition (Hamburg: Konkret Literatur Verlag, 2000). Ruprecht-Karls Universität Heidelberg/Fachschaftskonferenz der Uni Heidelberg/Fachschaft MathPhys, '"Aus der Krankheit eine Waffe machen!" Wo aus Psychiatrie-Patienten Revolutionäre werden sollten – das Sozialistische Patientenkollektiv SPK (1970/71)', *ruprecht*, no. 35, 16 May 1995 (*http://ruprecht.fsk.uni-heidelberg.de/ausgaben/35/ganz.htm*).

90. Schiller, *op. cit.* (note 89), 31f., 34 (ch. 'Abschied vom bisherigen Leben').

91. For a contemporary study, see D. Kerbs (ed.), *Die hedonistische Linke. Beiträge zur Subkultur-Debatte* (Neuwied: Luchterhand, 1970). See also: A. Schildt and D. Siegfried (eds), *Between Marx and Coca-Cola. Youth Cultures in Changing European Societies, 1960-1980* (New York/Oxford: Berghahn Books, 2004).

92. *SPK – Aus der Krankheit eine Waffe machen. Eine Agitationsschrift des Sozialistischen Patientenkollektivs an der Universität Heidelberg. Mit einem Vorwort von Jean-Paul Sartre* (München: Trikont-Verlag, 1972).

93. See, summarizing: Brink, 'Psychiatriekritik', *op. cit.* (note 89), 172f.

94. *Ibid.*, together with Ruprecht, *op. cit.* (note 89), 4f.; M. Overath, *Drachenzähne. Gespräche, Dokumente und Recherchen aus der Wirklichkeit der Hochsicherheitsjustiz* (Hamburg: VSA-Verlag, 1991), 82 (memoirs of Klaus Jünschke).

95. Kisker had already left Heidelberg at the time of the SPK conflict. In 1966, he received the chair for psychiatry at the newly founded medical university in Hannover (as director of the department for clinical psychiatry).

96. See the memoirs of Walter Ritter von Baeyer, in L.J. Pongratz (ed.), *Psychiatrie in Selbstdarstellungen* (Bern: Huber, 1977), 9-34: especially 29ff.

97.   Kersting, *op. cit.* (note 4), 492f.; *Idem*, '"Unruhediskurs". Zeitgenössische Deutungen der 68er-Bewegung', in M. Frese, J. Paulus, K. Teppe (eds), *Demokratisierung und gesellschaftlicher Aufbruch. Die sechziger Jahre als Wendezeit der Bundesrepublik* (Paderborn: Schöningh, 2003), 715-40: 735ff.

98.   H.-L. Siemen, 'Die chronisch psychisch Kranken "im Abseits der Psychiatriereform"', in Kersting (ed.), *op. cit.* (note 20), 273-86 (including some data with regard to the regional example of Bavaria).

99.   R. Forster, *Psychiatriereformen zwischen Medikalisierung und Gemeindeorientierung. Eine kritische Bilanz* (Opladen: Westdeutscher Verlag, 1997), passim.

CHAPTER 9

'Misery'[1] and 'Revolution'[2]

The Organisation of French Psychiatry, 1900-1980

*Jean-Christophe Coffin**

This paper will focus on the debates which have orientated the transformation of the framework of psychiatric care in the public sector throughout the twentieth century in France. It will give a general overview of the French public psychiatric sector between 1910 and 1980. One may say that this sector has dominated the scene over that period but was not the sole generator of this history. Though university and private sectors have not been included here, these should not be forgotten.[3] The analysis will focus on a group of psychiatrists who were particularly active in the care of patients after World War 11. This group of men have been seen largely as the founders of a psychiatric revolution in contemporary times. Although much praised, their history remains largely unwritten. The epistemological issues in the field, mainly between Foucauldian versus anti-Foucauldian thinking, have been passionate and produced a vast literature.[4] Paradoxically, though, French psychiatry remains virtually unexplored by French historians, which has favoured presentist narratives of the medical profession. The aim here is not only to reflect on French psychiatry and its history, to paraphrase Porter and Micale's title,[5] but also to combine individual, intellectual themes with broader institutional and political perspectives. It also attempts to review two major aspects: changes in psychiatric theory and practice, and efforts by psychiatrists to promote the reform of public mental health policies.

The years preceding World War 1 were marked by the loss of influence of the theory of degeneration, by reconciliation between neurologists and alienists, and by several attempts at reforming the law on asylums, which dated back to 1838, during the reign of Louis-Philippe, the last king of France. For some years the asylum system had been at the centre of debates and had sustained much criticism. At the end of the nineteenth century, it had been subjected to violent press campaigns which had exposed the poor conditions of patients, whilst members of parliament were tabling bills aimed at a better protection of patients and at better definition of the legal framework for confinement. The 1838 law was no longer perceived as a legal and political model and did not appear to unite legislators with the professional community of psychiatrists, as it had done in the past. However, this law still had many supporters, most particularly amongst certain psychiatrists.[6] It forced the departments, which constituted an important entity in the governmental administrative organisation – administratively and politically –, to fund either an asylum or at least a ward in a general hospital dedicated to this type of patient. The department therefore played a major part in the care of asylum residents. Though doctors working in the asylums were recruited via national entrance examinations and could be posted anywhere in the country, the budget of each asylum was voted by a local assembly of elected representatives. Moreover, the law outlined two types of admission: voluntary and certified. The former could be requested by the patient himself, or any other relative, in particular an immediate family member. The latter could be enforced by a public authority (Mayor, Prefect) where law and order were threatened or 'in the case of impending danger', the latter being left to the judgement of the individual. Until about 1900 criticism had centred on these latter aspects, whilst the general architecture of the system had not been questioned.

There was a consensus among psychiatrists as they felt they were under attack for their management of patients, but also in admitting that the asylum system faced a number of problems. In 1902, the psychiatrist Paul Sérieux had written an exhaustive report on the status of asylums and the mentally ill, both in France and other European countries. In this he clearly outlined the numerous difficulties faced by these institutions. One of these was overcrowding, which made it more and more difficult to provide any treatment. It was partly for this reason that the Department of Seine, which administered Paris and its suburbs, had actively supported the creation of two family settlements at the end of the nineteenth century. In rural surroundings, they were aimed at patients whose condition did not require an enclosed ward – something close to the colony at Gheel in Belgium. On the other hand, 1910 saw the creation of a special unit for the most dangerous patients in Villejuif, a working-class suburb of Paris. For several years, the psychiatric profession had been concerned about the question of asylums dedicated to specific types of patients. Several public reports had discussed the creation of facilities for alcoholics or criminals, without any decision being made. These proposals and few new achievements demonstrated that, as defined in the nineteenth century, the asylum system was entering a new phase. The progressive transition from the word 'alienist' to the word 'psychiatrist' together with the evolution from 'mental alienation' towards 'psychiatry' were an illustration, at least symbolically, of the changes that were taking place.

If the 'golden age'[7] of the asylum already seemed in decline, promising developments of the discipline seemed to lie ahead.[8] To achieve this, though, it was necessary to reorientate the study and conception of psychiatric knowledge. At the beginning of the twentieth century, many members of the new generation wanted to pull psychiatry out of the isolation in which it found itself, by comparison with other medical disciplines. One of the most obvious signs of this was the

'Misery' and 'Revolution'

coming together with neurologists[9] as well as considering mental pathology as a 'pathology of the cortex', to use the words of Professor Gilbert Ballet (1853-1916).[10] The influence of the hereditary model, deriving from the theory of degeneration, which had such an impact on mental medicine in the second half of the nineteenth century, was again proof of the determination to be part of the flow of new knowledge stemming from biology and general pathology.[11]

In spite of the development of psychotherapeutic trends, more particularly from the work of Pierre Janet (1859-1947), adhesion to an organic model of mental illness remained strong at the beginning of the twentieth century. Belief in a determinism, not only of organs but also of the transmission of mental problems based on the 'constitution doctrine'[12] introduced in particular by Ernest Dupré (1862-1921),[13] Professor at the Paris Faculty of Medicine, was still shared by many psychiatrists, notwithstanding eventual disagreement over matters of classification, expertise or treatment.

The Inter-wars Period

The beginning of the 1920s was marked by an increasing preoccupation with hygienism and individual health protection. The death toll during the war and the large numbers of injured and invalid people amongst the French population were directly linked to this concern with prevention, which quickly acquired the overtones of a new crusade. It was under the nationalistic and conservative government of Alexandre Millerand (1859-1943), formerly a member of the republican left, that the creation of a new ministry was decided in January 1920: the Ministry of Social Hygiene, Assistance and Prevention. This decision followed findings made during the war: the sanitary provisions proved to be inadequate, and this was unacceptable in Pasteur's country!

From then on, the mentally ill and public asylums were managed from this new ministry to the detriment of the Department of Internal Affairs, whose sole responsibility it had been since the beginning of the nineteenth century. This new ministry often changed directions and with the latter came changes to its name. It was only from the 1930s that it was named the Ministry of Public Health. Amongst the different ministers who held the post, several were medical practitioners or philanthropists who had previously been involved with child protection or the fight against tuberculosis or alcohol. Without major resources, the ministers made speeches to explain the political and social dimensions of health and the necessity for it to be organised by public authorities. Thus, the ministry was the background for one of the very first meetings of a new association, the Ligue de prophylaxie et hygiene mentales (League for Mental Prophylaxis and Hygiene), created in December 1920 by the psychiatrist Edouard Toulouse. Taking its inspiration from the leagues against cancer and tuberculosis that were already active but also from the American mental hygiene movement, the ambitions of this new League were immense, and the stakes were high. Toulouse shared the views of the Minister of Hygiene, Paul Strauss (1852-1942), who declared that: 'after a war which killed so many people, it is necessary to save as many human lives as possible', and he concluded: 'there is a lot to do all over France as far as prophylaxis is concerned'.[14] Toulouse settled down to the task by creating study committees and projects within the League. Mental health was the stepping stone to national health since an abnormal life was no help to the general community. He campaigned for deep transformations in mental medicine, as well as for an increased role of psychiatry within society. In his eyes, the contribution of psychiatry lay mainly in a precisely targeted policy of prevention and selection. The new impulse he wanted to give stemmed from a constantly repeated hypothesis: 'we start from this principle, scientifically established, that madness, in many cases, is an avoidable and curable illness'.[15]

Toulouse was not unknown amongst French psychiatrists at the beginning of the 1920s. Born in 1865, he entered the public network of asylums at the beginning of the 1890s. Creator of a *La Revue de Psychiatrie* (Psychiatry Review) open to all opinions in psychology, psychiatry and neurology, he often criticized his colleagues for their stand on the causes of madness and above all for the too frequent ease with which they decided to have their patients hospitalised. But he did more than criticize, since he also carried out some research on different policies of management in other European countries, and published several texts suggesting alternative solutions. After World War 1, with the support of several politicians – mainly from the centre left and freemasonry – he dedicated himself to the reorganisation of the care given to the mentally ill. He succeeded in convincing the elected representatives of the Seine authority to attempt a new experiment: the creation of an open-door service, which was set up near Sainte Anne Hospital. Its name was the Henri Rousselle Hospital and was directed by Toulouse himself. Patients were free to come and leave the hospital grounds. It was initially organised for all mentally ill subjects, but in practice, only non-residents of asylums were accepted. Thus, it was for patients who were not confined under the procedures of the 1838 Law.

This measure was debated for several decades by French psychiatrists and its implementation continued to being discussed on a regular basis between the two wars because of the lack of unanimity. Toulouse's character irritated several of his colleagues, and his points of view on a whole variety of topics only contributed to emphasize his singularity within a professional community, which had traditionally been conservative.[16] More generally, this experiment and several others that were timidly put to the test in the 1930s[17] reawakened the discussion of an amendment to the 1838 Law. However, the psychiatric community remained divided on the necessity for it and on the breadth it should have. Whilst during the 1920s several bills had been tabled by members of parliament, the

'Misery' and 'Revolution'

one hundredth anniversary of the law was again an occasion for relaunching the debate, as well as for psychiatrists to celebrate that milestone.

The Popular Front

In the summer of 1936, France was governed for the first time by a Popular Front administration which brought together all the left-wing political forces: radicals,[18] socialists and communists. The latter were not part of the government but supported it in the National Assembly, where this coalition had a majority, though it did not in the Senate. The Health Minister of this government led by the socialist Leon Blum (1872-1950) was Henri Sellier (1883-1943). Mayor of a town in a working-class suburb close to Paris, Sellier had been the founder of the *Office Public de la Seine pour l'Hygiène Sociale* (the Seine Public Department of Social Hygiene) in 1918. This body, which was initially mainly dedicated to the fight against tuberculosis, gradually turned towards a policy of detection and struggle against 'social ills', including mental disorders. Sellier was also renowned for his expertise on the question of low rents and had become an active spokesman for the welfare services. He followed the work of several medical practitioners including E. Toulouse, whom he appointed as one of his technical advisers. Sellier had conceived the establishment of 'health centres' set up at the local level and developing activities of prevention, care and social support for a specific territory.[19] However, because of the short time spent in his ministry, he was unable to carry through this vast project. Under the circumstances, his legacy remained a policy of intentions, rather than of achievements. For example, in the spring of 1937, he passed a decree transforming 'asylums for mentally disturbed people' into 'psychiatric hospitals'. His successor was Marc Rucart (1893-1964), who had previously been the Justice Minister. A freemason, coming from Radicalism, he managed to head the ministry longer than Sellier, who had stayed just over a year, whilst the left-wing coalition was starting to experience very serious internal tensions. At the end of the 1939 winter, after taking advice from a committee of experts, Rucart tabled a bill aimed at reforming the 1838 Law. At this time, though, political instability and the urgency of some of the government's choices with regard to both internal and external policies were delaying action on social projects.

Psychiatrists and the ministry had slowly reached the common conclusion that the asylums needed reform. These institutions were generally overcrowded; although this was not a new situation, the extent of the phenomenon was becoming a real worry. In less than thirty years, the number of resident patients had almost doubled, whereas the number of available beds had lagged behind this trend, and the building of new institutions had not gathered any significant speed. On the contrary, there still remained a dozen departments without a real psychiatric infrastructure, although it was legally required to provide it. Following H. Sellier's work, Rucart's objective was to contribute to a more general reform of psychiatric services, alongside the amendments to the law. Thus, in October 1937, he had passed a decree recommending the establishment of 'open wards' on a very similar basis to that initiated by Toulouse 15 years earlier. Similarly, the outpatient dispensary, as the model used in the fight against tuberculosis, became a ministerial policy to prevent and identify mental disorders. These recommendations, however, which encompassed proposals made by some psychiatrists,[20] were still a long way off from changing the institutional landscape of French psychiatry on the brink of World War II.

The Psychiatric Landscape on the Eve of the War

The psychiatric landscape looked diverse. Several initiatives had been started, and criticisms were being expressed more and more forcefully on both theoretical and clinical work. Many scientific associations had been created since the beginning of the 1920s; as well as the League for Mental Hygiene, associations had been formed dealing with sexology, crime prevention and labour psychology. Not only did they gather psychiatrists together but they were also proof of deep changes in the profession whose social and expert role was playing a new and unprecedented part. In this new perspective, child psychiatry began to develop. In the middle of the 1920s, the psychiatrist Georges Heuyer (1884-1977) opened a child guidance clinic, run first by a voluntary association and then by the Paris Faculty of Medicine, which welcomed young female psychoanalysts. This organisation was quite similar to that of contemporary American child guidance clinics. Approximately at the same period (1926), the *Société de Psychanalyse de Paris* (Paris Psychoanalytic Society) was created, a year after the foundation by psychiatrists of a *Société de l'Evolution Psychiatrique* (Society for Psychiatric Development). These initiatives indicated the diffusion of new ideas, but the fragility of these associations threatened their development. The *Société de l'Evolution Psychiatrique* centred around Eugène Minkowski (1885-1972), a psychiatrist with a phenomenological orientation who came from Russia and had been trained in Germany and Switzerland. Until the 1930s, it encountered many problems in consolidating the publication of its review, entitled *L'Evolution psychiatrique*. The Paris Psychoanalytic Society quickly became dependent on the funds received from an extraordinary person, Marie Bonaparte (1882-1962), great-grand-niece of Napoleon I, as well as a royal princess through her marriage to Prince George of Greece. Psychoanalysts and young phenomenological psychiatrists could also be found in the Sainte-Anne Hospital, where several prominent psychiatrists of that time practised, amongst whom was Henri Claude (1865-1939). Between the two wars, Claude held the Chair of Psychiatry at the Paris Faculty of Medicine;

'Misery' and 'Revolution'

he was a practitioner more expert in neurology than psychoanalysis, but welcomed the ideas of this new generation.

These 'think tanks' remained strictly Parisian and had little impact on asylums throughout the century. For example, in the Isère Department, near Lyon, the superintendent welcomed the ministerial initiative recommending the creation of open wards, yet in his own establishment one was not opened until the 1950s, because the local elected representatives opposed it.[21] Other superintendents were struggling primarily with another decision of the first Popular Front government: the reduction of the working week which obliged hospital doctors to revise the working pattern of nurses, with whom they often had conflictual relationships.[22] Finally, in France, the question of sterilisation of mentally ill patients was debated on several occasions; it was the opinion of part of the mental hygiene movement that early detection was paramount, since there would be no solution at a later stage.[23] In a way, it was this mix of determination and pessimism which defined this period and personalities such as E. Toulouse.

From the Vichy Regime to the Foundation of the *Information Psychiatrique* Group

After the declaration of war against the Nazi government and the marked difficulties of the French army in 1940 in fighting the German troops, a vote of confidence was given to Marshal Pétain, who became the dominant figure of a new administrative system and was determined to turn his back on the Republic. From Vichy, a spa town in the centre of France, Pétain headed several governments up to 1944, when the Resistance forces led by General de Gaulle, formerly an undersecretary of state in the last republican government, gradually gained power. During the Vichy years, the Health Minister was in charge of the family, a political focus of the Vichy regime. During this period, thousands of mentally ill patients died. Apart from several psychiatric hospitals being bombed, provoking casualties amongst patients and staff and creating heavy material damage, the main causes of these deaths were malnutrition and the generalised destitution to which many inmates were subjected during those years. In the 1930s, the average annual death rate was about 10 per cent. By 1945, it had tripled, according to the figures from hospitals where enquiries had been possible. Where patients had survived, their condition was close to absolute deprivation. In a report commissioned by the French Home Office, the author wrote: 'altogether patients are extremely underweight. One is struck by their paleness, their state of deep asthenia and advanced decay. Asylums are clearly overcrowded.'[24]

It was in this troubled atmosphere that, at the end of the 1945 winter, with World War II not over yet, the *Union Médicale Française* (Union of French Doctors) organised a meeting whose agenda was to consider a national health service, once France had been freed from Nazi occupation. This gathering was organised by the Resistance Doctors' Committee, and the chairman was the psychologist Henri Wallon (1879-1962), the founder of the *Front National Universitaire* (National University Front), a resistance group. Another participant was Professor Robert Debré (1882-1978), a pillar of the medical establishment as well as a Resistance activist. Parallel to this meeting of doctors who were to become the French medical elite, the *Journées Nationales de Psychiatrie* (National Psychiatry Days) were held, bringing French psychiatrists together. What was at stake was psychiatry itself and the influence psychiatrists would have on their own profession and its institutions. A committee was set up on these questions, and their work resulted in a 24-point programme. It was demanded that the specificity of psychiatric programmes be better considered and that psychiatrists should play a bigger role, notably in the social arena. The notion of mental health care was clearly stated, and it was argued that this should extend beyond the walls of hospitals, whose administration should be reviewed, too. Psychiatrists should be more involved in decision-making about general health. Such an enlargement of competencies required a massive recruitment campaign, which they demanded, emphasising that there had been only one during the whole Vichy period.[25] Finally, 'an increased intervention of the authority of the State at central level' was strongly requested.[26]

In the reformist atmosphere of the time, *Les Journées Nationales* took the opportunity to tackle the major issue of the 1838 law. Xavier Abély (1890-1966), chief doctor at Sainte Anne Hospital in Paris, unveiled the first elements of a possible new law. One of the major innovations in his draft was to foresee different types of management depending on the patients' mental state and reaction to society.[27] Confinement in an asylum would no longer be the sole possible strategy.

Along with the case for reorganisation of the institutions, some psychiatrists advocated the total restructuring of psychiatric thinking. Henri Ey (1900-1977), a public health service doctor at a psychiatric hospital 100 kilometres from Paris, asserted that French psychiatry had failed to perform its duties for several years and that it lacked doctrinal depth.[28] He also accused his colleagues of 'taking refuge in a scalpel and microscope psychiatry'.[29] But his attacks also targeted the State, which had failed to take an interest in psychiatric matters and the fate of mental patients; public provision to them had been neglected by those in charge of social policies. It was to curtail this negative cycle of 'decadence'[30] in which French psychiatry was imprisoned that professionals ought to mobilise themselves. As Ey saw it, the mobilisation of the psychiatric profession should be articulated in two directions: the design of a new institutional framework and the elaboration of a new doctrinal corpus. On the institutional framework, in agreement with X. Abély he proposed that admission to hospital should come last in the set of options offered by psychiatrists. There were several alternatives

'Misery' and 'Revolution'

such as outpatient services, social readaptation units and care at home. The accepted categories of patients such as 'chronically disordered', 'dangerous', and 'incurable' were disputed.[31] Compassion was not the motive here. Rather than emphasizing the strange, frightening or inexplicable character of mental illness, Ey pointed to what he considered an 'immanence of human nature'.[32] This reflected his position: that by integrating madness into human destiny, it allows one to understand it better and therefore to treat it better. On the basis of this postulate, psychiatry would find its true value and ethical dimension. It was important to consider the pathological aspect fully, to avoid presenting as normal something which was not. To dispute this was to be dangerously naive and was as reprehensible as considering madness a simple brain malfunction. Ey concluded that insanity could not be understood and dealt with either by biological or social psychiatry alone. Anthropological psychiatry was what was needed.

Ey was not the only psychiatrist willing to do away with some of the old practices and conceptions. For instance, the communist practitioner Lucien Bonnafé (1912-2003) had written the previous year that 'madness is as curable as tuberculosis'.[33] And even earlier, before World War II, he had declared that psychiatric care in France had to 'be fully revised'.[34] In his 1945 speech, Ey mentioned young colleagues who, like himself, were willing to offer 'their experience and good will to the nation'.[35] A few months later, some psychiatrists founded a professional union, the *Syndicat des médecins des hôpitaux psychiatriques* (Psychiatric Hospital Doctors Trade Union).[36] The team was headed by Georges Daumézon (1912-1979), clinical director at an asylum near Orléans some 130 km from Paris. It comprised Paul Sivadon (1907-1992), Paul Bernard (1909-1995), Jean Lauzier, Louis Le Guillant (1900-1968), Lucien Bonnafé, X. Abély and H. Ey.[37] This organisation recruited psychiatrists from the public mental health service, created in the nineteenth century. They had started their careers in the 1930s as chief doctors of their institutions, away from urban centres.[38] Most of these men knew what isolation meant.

The choice of the word 'trade union' was meant to underscore that association and community life had not really been possible under the Vichy regime. It was also meant to mark a discontinuity with the pre-war *Amicale des médecins aliénistes des établissements publics d'aliénés* (The Medical-Alienists Circle of the Public Mental Hospitals). The team also founded a new review, the *Information psychiatrique*.[39] None of the members of the Union was nostalgic for the 1930s. In 1950, Daumézon stated that 'in 1938 the situation of French psychiatry was characterised by the extraordinary overcrowding of the different hospital units. The number of mental patients rose to 120,000. Hospitals in Paris had beds in the middle of the dormitories, not to mention the mattresses in the corridors'.[40] Sivadon wrote in his memoirs : 'When I took charge of my department, I was gripped by the sight, the smell and the buzzing of this crowd with grim faces, some on their beds sometimes even tied to them.'[41]

We can understand from this that the creation of the trade union and the journal was one way to inculcate the spirit of reform and to put pressure on the state representatives to obtain their commitment to action. A telling example was the removal in the review's title of the word 'alienist', which dated back to the nineteenth century and was still very much in use in the 1930s. Daumézon explained that: 'we thought the word "alienist" was too restricted compared to the centres of interest of our review. We agreed that the review should widen the scope and cover not only mental patients but all questions dealing with the country's mental health both at the individual and social level.'[42] The team's membership reflected the tripartite political composition of the government, sharing the post-war hope and willingness for change with the new political elite. For the first time in their history, psychiatrists were governed by a Health Minister, François Billoux, who was a member of the French Communist Party. In the autumn of 1945, he declared : 'Nowadays, it's all or nothing... a person suffering from mental disorder is either confined or left at home ignored. We feel this needs to be changed, and a decree is being prepared by the government which will ensue that mentally sick people will be treated at home and in care centres, and patients needing confinement will stop being treated as mere convicts.'[43]

It seemed that for once, the State representatives and practitioners agreed on the need for ambitious changes, yet the situation just after the war was very difficult. Several hospitals had been badly damaged by bombings and others were used as camps for American soldiers. A sharp decrease in hospitals revenues had rendered the financial situation even more catastrophic; the number of resident patients had halved since 1939. It was therefore a matter of urgency to undertake a major renovation programme, but what would this imply? In fact, the renewal of thinking was far more dynamic than the institutional renovation in these years.

The Post-war Years: A New Start

By 1946 every sector in French society sought to close the Vichy chapter. France was then back under a regime with republican values. The Ministry of Health, which had been suppressed during the Vichy years, was re-established. L. Le Guillant became technical adviser on mentally deficient infants to the new ministry in 1944. L. Bonnafé joined in March 1947 and became responsible for mental health and social readaptation questions. The *Conseil supérieur d'hygiène publique* (Higher Council for Public Hygiene) was also reorganised; it comprised several committees including one on mental health.[44] Several psychiatrists such as X. Abély, P. Bernard and L. Bonnafé were invited to join. Finally, Eugène Aujaleu (1903-1990) became the head of the Social Hygiene Department and maintained close ties with those doctors. It created a stability which contrasted

　　　　　　　　　　　　　　　'Misery' and 'Revolution'

with the political instability of the Fourth Republic, replaced by the Fifth in 1958. The *Chaire de Pathologie Mentale et de Maladies de l'Encéphale* (Chair of Brain and Mental Pathologies) at the Faculty of Medicine of Paris was awarded to Jean Delay (1907-1987), after the death in a concentration camp of the former head, J. Lévy-Valensi. The Psychiatric Evolution Society, whose activities had been interrupted during the war, started again, run by Eugène Minkowski and Ey.

Along with the political and administrative reorganisation came new thinking and practices. In addition to their union and review work, the IP Team embarked on the publication of a series entitled the *IP Documents*. Also, two important books were published between 1945 and 1950, providing a programme for post-war public sector psychiatry, from both institutional and theoretical perspectives. The first was *Au-delà de l'asile* (Beyond the Asylum) and the second, *Le malade mental dans la société* (The Insane within Society),[45] both offering a harsh criticism of the asylum as it was then run. One of the strongest attacks was on the principle of patient isolation. Contrary to Esquirol (1772-1840), who had influenced the 1838 law and who regarded isolation as the one guarantee for recovery, the new authors claimed quite the reverse. Their personal experience as practitioners in isolated locations had convinced them that care centres should be located in the cities and not outside.[46] They did not propose to close down the mental hospitals[47] but to change their function. As J. Lauzier put it: 'For the old concept of the asylum being synonymous with refuge and confinement, one may substitute the notion of care centre and social readaptation.'[48] Insanity was no longer perceived as a social plague, but as a public health problem.

These views were rooted in several theoretical trends. The first post-war issue of *L'Evolution Psychiatrique* was dedicated to what psychiatry could become and the main research subjects that ought to be explored. Social psychiatry and British experiments were much praised,[49] notably by Jacques Lacan (1901-1981), psychiatrist, psychoanalyst and friend of Ey during their training years in the 1920s. At his Bonneval hospital, Ey organised a meeting entitled *Le problème de la psychogénèse des névroses et des psychoses* (The Psychic Causality of Mental Disorders).[50] For three days in 1946, the participants exchanged their views. Today, one is still struck by the absolute difference in the approach to insanity at that time, compared with the one prevailing just a few years before, which would have privileged organic perspectives. Bonnafé and Follin declared: 'By no means should psychiatry be reduced to a simple medical speciality (...) Psychiatry is a social science which evolves along with the progress of all the other social sciences.'[51] The first post-war meeting at Bonneval inaugurated a tradition of regular gatherings where psychiatrists and psychoanalysts shared information and experiences.

The articles published by the IP Team contained indications that these practical psychiatrists were keen to test their theories in the daily care of patients. One of the first experiments was Sivadon's in 1947. He created a care and social readaptation centre inside the Ville Evrard asylum in a Paris suburb (Seine).[52] This experiment quickly became a model, proving that a dynamic team could change a nineteenth-century asylum into a revitalised structure. Ey followed suit in his own hospital.[53] These practitioners had created a structure inside the existing asylum that could become tomorrow's mental health care organisation with new resources and increased staff to allow follow-up of patients. In addition, difficult patients were no longer segregated from more manageable ones; in a common unit, all patients were treated according to their specific illness. The objective was to create what Sivadon and Daumézon both called a 'therapeutic community'.[54] Sivadon was eclectic, using psychotherapy, games, occupational-therapy[55] or standard medication.[56]

Also in the Seine Department, the Public Office of Social Hygiene supported an experiment in 1950. The initiator was Philippe Paumelle (1929-1974), a young psychiatrist who was the former assistant of G. Daumézon. He was supported by the senior doctor of this Office, Henri Duchêne (1915-1965), a close friend of Ey's. Paumelle set up a team of doctors and social workers who were to provide care for alcoholics outside the hospital. They concentrated their action on a limited territory, the 13th arrondissement of Paris, a poor neighbourhood at the time. The project received a grant from the City of Paris for whom prevention of alcoholism was high on the political agenda.[57] But Paumelle and his team wished to expand the scope of the experiment to other categories, such as the insane, since the pattern of care that included tracking down, caring and following up could be applied also to them as well. The team set up an association, *Mental Health in the 13th District*, and provided care to individuals in the area who needed it. This initiative had some similarity to Doctor Querido's in Amsterdam via the Municipal Mental Health Department, which had started 20 years earlier. Sivadon praised Querido in an article entitled 'Hope'.[58] In 1952 Daumézon and Paumelle wrote an article entitled 'Contemporary French Institutional Psychiatry' which was published in a Portuguese review.[59] This text can be considered as the foundation of a new psychiatric trend.

Another experiment was tried in 1954 in the 13th District at the Alfred Binet care centre, another child guidance clinic, with psychoanalysis playing a larger part, due to the special staff training. The medical team was composed of both child psychiatrists and psychoanalysts. This experiment became famous on two accounts: it was undeniably innovative, since very few child guidance clinics existed at that time in France, and it benefited from a unique status for many years.[60] A new generation of practitioners gave visibility to their orientation at the *Congrès mondial de psychiatrie de Paris* in 1950 (World Congress of Psychiatry), largely organised by Henri Ey.[61]

All these experiments benefited from favourable circumstances, such as money and the support of civil servants of the Health administration. Since they needed to fit into a legal framework which had remained unchanged since the

'Misery' and 'Revolution'

nineteenth century, only the creation of subsidiary structures – such as the Paumelle's association – could allow the experiments to be carried out.[62] Finally, close co-operation was required between different administrative departments, the political authorities and medical researchers. The 1950s were marked by this genuine co-operation between practitioners and government departments; they were united by a true spirit of public service. Ey, who succeeded Daumézon at the head of their Professional Union in the 1950s, was on good terms with the high ranking civil servant, E. Aujaleu,[63] one of the directors at the Health Minis-try. In 1951, the Health Minister announced a ten-year plan for the refurbish-ment of old hospitals and the building of new ones, and increased space for both patients and staff. An appendix was more specifically targeted to mental health care and to prevention and services.

These proposed measures were decidedly ambitious, but the reality proved to be stubborn. In the mid-1950s, contrary to article 1 of the 1838 law, one quarter of French territory was still without any asylums.[64] At Saint-Yon Hospital, where L. Bonnafé was superintendent from 1947 to 1958, the buildings, damaged during the war, were still not yet fully rebuilt when he left, despite his continuous demands. Nationally, the number of admissions had started to increase again from the end of the 1940s, so that several hospitals located 300 kilometres from Paris were required to take in 'surplus patients' who could not be admitted to the overcrowded Paris asylums. This made it impossible for the ministerial recom-mendations to be fully applied concerning a reduced number of patients per practitioner which had been forcefully demanded for years by doctors. In Bon-nafé's hospital, for instance, every practitioner was responsible for 461 patients in 1948, and this rose to 606 in 1956.[65] At mental hygiene clinics[66] attendance increased to a point where staff found it difficult to cope.

It seems that the real efforts on the part of both political leaders and practi-tioners were not enough to trigger a true change. This led Daumézon to declare in 1960 that 'the psychiatric revolution has been betrayed', referring to the 1945 programme that he and his colleagues had prepared.[67]

The 1960s: A New Frustrated Start

Daumézon's declaration was a bitter reminder that all was not well. Yet at the same time, the *Journal officiel de la République française* (Official Journal of the French Republic) published a circular on a 'Programme for the organisation and provision of resources in the departments in matters of prevention of mental diseases'. The theoretical and therapeutic innovations in France in recent years were said to have allowed for a clearer and more tolerant interpretation of insan-ity. Thus, nobody could consider the asylum as the only possible solution; it was only one step in the process. The circular was intended to provide these scientific advances with an organisational framework to ensure their general implementation: 'From now on departments will be subdivided into geographical zones inside which the same social-medical team will be in charge of the implementation of the whole treatment of tracing and provision of care outside the hospital, treatment within the hospital, and follow-up for all sick people, male and female.'[68] Whenever possible, the rule now was to avoid separating the patients from their families and environment.[69] Mental hospitals were to be integrated in a larger extramural network, comprising a centre for mental hygiene, a day-care unit, and a sheltered workshop where patients could perform paid work.[70] The need for one mental hygiene centre in each Department was emphasized. A decree of 1955 had made it compulsory for the State to pay a grant to each Department to cover the cost of this facility. The circular praised British, Dutch and American achievements in day treatment, while France was lagging behind in this respect. The concept of a psychiatric *secteur* (sector) was given official recognition.[71]

The circular had actually drawn on many subjects put forward by the IP Team. Unfortunately, the close partnership between the administration and practitioners was not to last, and some deterioration in the relationship started to show in the following years. Paradoxically, the state seemed to lose interest in the fate of public sector psychiatry at the time when the economy was picking up, public money was available, and national reconstruction and modernisation were well advanced. In 1964, the new Minister of Health abolished the *Commission des maladies mentales* (Committee on Mental Diseases) – a consultative body created at the end of the 1940s. He imposed a reorganisation of the public health administration, which resulted in the resignation of E. Aujaleu, who in 1956 had been nominated *Directeur général de la Santé* (Director General of the Health Department), the highest position in the ministry. This left behind a leaderless department, a move which was resented by the unionised practitioners, who were used to dealing with it. Moreover, other obstacles emerged, notably the special status of public sector psychiatrists and the place allocated to psychiatry in medical studies. These serious questions mobilised the unionist doctors, led at that time by Jean Ayme (born in 1924), and more particularly Henri Ey.

These questions and others concerning the organisation of the profession were at the centre of what has become known as the *Livre blanc de la psychiatrie* (White book on psychiatry). This label is applied to three volumes of discussions, debates and proposals published by the *Society of Psychiatric Evolution* between 1965 and 1967 under Ey's supervision. They stemmed from forums organised in those years. The 1960 government circular had failed to bring about a true reorganisation of psychiatry along the lines of the sector model which it encouraged. Psychiatrists estimated the magnitude of the reorganisation and renovation work still needed, and showed that a wide range of interpretations of the sector concept existed. The IP founding fathers were at the forefront of this debate, but the forums were not dedicated solely to the sector issue; they included the organisation of psychiatric practice as a whole. One aim was to renew the university teaching of psychiatry by giving it true autonomy, clearly detached from neurology. The number of psychiatrists would have to be considerably increased to implement the sector model. The 1838 law was declared obsolete, and L. Bonnafé proposed a new one consisting of a single article: 'The 1838 law is abolished.'[72] In the end, though, that law was not abolished but the procedures were somewhat clarified, thanks to a new law passed in 1968 which concerned the protection of 'adults who are declared handicapped'. Judicial situations such as tutelage were created to control legally aberrant situations which had never been dealt with before and to protect the property of mentally handicapped and psychiatric patients. A better framework was established for the protection of patients' civil rights.

On matters of professional status, though, psychiatrists were quite successful. They gained inclusion in the general framework of hospital laws and a new status almost similar to that of hospital practitioners in other branches of medicine (July 1968). Thus, psychiatry became part of what the sociologist R. Castel has named the 'medicalization of mental health'.[73] Finally, the Minister of Public Education, Edgar Faure (1908-1988), an influential figure of the Fifth Republic although not a Gaullist, accepted one of their main demands: the creation of a university degree for psychiatry (December 1968). This was to be distinct from the degree normally delivered by the medical schools, for which university neurologists rather than psychiatrists would teach. Since the reorganisation of medical teaching in 1958, psychiatrists had been fighting for that measure.

The 1970s : Psychiatry and Its Ambiguity

This decade will be remembered as the period when the sector model was truly implemented and, as in other countries, psychiatry was highly criticized. It was a highly paradoxical situation. Just when the spirit of renovation was gaining momentum, mental health fell victim to very radical questioning, though the lack of thorough studies renders an analysis of the situation complex and risky for the historian today.[74] In March 1972, Robert Boulin (1920-1979), appointed Health Minister in 1969, published two circulars on the implementation of the sector model. Being respected and close to the social Christian Democratic movement, he was able to renew a dialogue with the psychiatrists' union. The geographical approach was chosen, leading to the distribution of psychiatric care over the whole country. The sector was thus organised according to the map drawn up for the law on hospital provision voted in 1970.[75] Thus, the administrative or rather public service point of view seemed to have prevailed over the medical one.[76] This did not contradict the psychiatrists' wishes elaborated in the 1950s, but little was said about the role of the hospital, which in fact remained central for the sector. The unionist psychiatrists had pointed out that the sector should be an opportunity for equal access to care by everyone, as well as for reinforcing partnership between the educational, social and judicial sectors. It was seen as a possibility for the public to choose from a variety of treatments, though this did not seem to be the case. The public did not in fact have much choice, given that the psychiatric hospital still remained the overwhelming central provision within the care structure.

Another circular concerned the child psychiatry sector. This was larger than the one for adult patients, but more importantly, its medical team was to be distinct from the one caring for adults. However, several psychiatrists wanted the same team to be in charge of all individuals in the sector with no distinction as to sex or age. Innovation in treatments was not left out, particularly for the child and adolescent sectors. It was expressly stated that notions such as 'incurability' or 'intelligence' level were not to be the primary criteria in practitioners' intervention. This was to be based on dynamic psychiatry and child psychoanalysis which had been developing in the preceding years.[77]

At the same time, 'psychiatric power' was questioned.[78] Movements emerged such as the *Groupe Information Asile* (Asylum Information Network), modelled on the *Groupe Information Prison* (Prison Information Network) to which the philosopher Michel Foucault (1926-1984) belonged. New reviews were published such as *Les psychiatrisés en lutte* (The Mental Patients in Revolt) or *Les cahiers de la folie* (Insanity notebooks), supervised by Félix Guattari (1930-1992), psychiatrist at the Borde private hospital, together with Jean Oury,[79] promoter of institutional psychotherapy – a different movement from Daumézon's.[80] Among the numerous publications on anti-psychiatry, there was a special issue of the review *La Nef*[81] edited by Lucie Faure (1908-1977). She was the wife of Edgar Faure, the minister who had supported the demands of public health service psychiatrists in 1968. Contributors to this special issue were psychiatrists and psychoanalysts who were considered avant-garde, but not supporting the anti-psychiatric movement because they believed it neglected the concept of mental diseases. In psychiatric reviews, there was a critical and sometimes even hostile posture towards anti-psychiatric ideas, particularly in the *Evolution psychiatrique*. Despite health problems, Henri Ey himself had come out of his retirement and published a series of extremely harsh articles on this movement.[82] His former companions followed suit and were shocked at being considered 'jailers'[83] when throughout their careers they had never ceased to free the mentally ill from asylums, as Philippe Pinel (1745-1826) is said to have freed them from their chains. A rift had appeared between successive generations of psychiatrists, as well as between psychiatrists and certain psychoanalytic trends. Anti-psychiatry is likely to have had some impact on the perception of the asylum and on the notion of 'psychiatric power'; the arbitrary nature of this has remained in people's minds,

'Misery' and 'Revolution'

while public opinion did not perceive the sector model as being particularly innovative.

Thus, it was parallel to these innovations that in the late 1970s, the sector model was finally implemented and its existence acknowledged. By then, some 800 sectors had been set up all over the country; this was not yet adequate, but in 1960, after the circular was published, only a dozen had been opened.[84] The 13th district project located in Paris can be considered as the first example. Several sectors were also initiated in small cities or rural areas. This time, the sector psychiatrists were financially advantaged, compared with the non-sector ones. However, it was necessary to assess the complete chain of care, the capacity of the socio-medical team to work coherently. Contrary to expectations, it seemed that the level of provision remained variable. For example, there were many instances where outpatient and day-care services could not be provided because they had not been set up. The psychiatrist Hubert Mignot (1910-1982) wrote that sector policy needed few heavy investments, but implied important expenditures on staff.[85] Nonetheless, sector teams were rarely staffed to the theoretical levels. The sector policy had been thought out in rational, logical terms, but with no allowance for the unexpected problems that would be inherent in any implementation. As early as the 1970s, some psychiatrists and sociologists published *L'Histoire de la psychiatrie de secteur ou le secteur impossible* (History of the Psychiatric Sector or the Impossible Sector).[86] Now that it was the official policy of the successive governments, it was not perceived anymore as an innovative doctrine but primarily as the administrative organisation of psychiatric treatment. Moreover, it became clear that the hospital had maintained its predominant role within the whole network and that a growing number of people were still treated there. Although the average length of hospitalisation had shortened, the number of chronic patients remained high. 'De-institutionalisation' did not appear to have had a great impact on the whole organisation of psychiatric practice. If the reduction in hospital beds had not provoked opposition when supported by psychiatrists themselves as a necessary step in the rejection of 'hospitalocentrism',[87] reactions were different when the same measure was promoted by the State. In 1980, the Health Minister of the current conservative government of that period announced a reduction programme of about 40,000 beds. Some years later, the ixth Economic Plan (1984-1988) promoted a reduction of a similar number of beds when the socialist government decided to cut expenditure because of a growing persistent economic crisis. Moreover, increasing difficulty in curtailing health costs and the re-emergence of conservative political forces made it less and less legitimate to maintain the welfare state as it was.

Conclusion

Unlike other public services, psychiatry was managed from the nineteenth century at the departmental level. Although the French State dictated the duties and general objectives, the responsibility laid with the elected representatives of the department. This led to variations in terms of admissions, budgets and the political will to create a local mental health service. Daumézon, Bonnafé and others had often protested against this situation. Secondly, one cannot but note the intellectual vivacity and production of the IP psychiatrists. Except for the most committed inside the French Communist Party during the cold war,[88] they were rarely dogmatic but on the contrary were open to all opinions, whether it involved sociotherapy or psychotherapy. They were genuinely interested in psychoanalysis and supported the creation of therapeutic centres. They also introduced occupational therapy and showed an interest in H. Simon and others such as Moreno and psychodrama. On the whole, Henri Ey's organo-dynamism and institutional psychotherapy, whether of Marxist psychology or Freudian orientation, evolved side by side for many years. The political plurality which existed alongside the intellectual, as well as the presence of different religious beliefs need to be remembered.

The founders of the IP created a public service for a greater number of people and closer to the population; this is their great achievement. It is what kept them together during the post-war years, in spite of their political and doctrinal differences, but the paradox was contained in their will to create an institution outside the official health service framework. They wanted to be public sector doctors, but not necessarily civil servants or part of the administrative machinery. They did not de-institutionalise mental health, but rather created new structures outside the hospital in the hope of seeing a more adequate structure of care emerge. Their purpose has been to give psychiatry a real social function. By giving psychiatry such a specific role, however, they transformed the image of mental health into something separate from other disorders, which was the opposite of what they wanted to achieve. In 1980, the sector model did not obtain a clear legal framework, while the 1838 law had still not yet been substantially modified or abolished. Despite their truly reformist intentions, they were left out in the cold by the other members of the psychiatric profession.

The scope of this article has unavoidably been limited. Little has been said about psycho-pharmacology for instance and its impacts on the care provision as well as the relation between psychiatry and psychoanalysis within the psychiatric hospital. It has also revealed to what extent we are still ignorant about some aspects of French psychiatry. The stigmatisation of the madman and the 'ideologisation' of madness seem to have favoured the marginal place of psychiatry in the French historical literature. There are still questions to be asked about the 'psychiatric revolution', as well as about French psychiatry as a whole.[89]

And it has to be done in a way that approaches psychiatry as an element of scientific thought rather than a mere social construction.

Notes

*   This article has benefited at various stages from the helpful comments of the editors and especially J. Vijselaar and H.L. Freeman. I would like to extend my thanks to I. Brunois, E. Seince and C. White.

1.   'Misère de la psychiatrie', *Esprit*, 20 (1952), 777-944.

2.   G. Lanteri-Laura, 'Modes et révolutions en psychiatrie', *L'Evolution psychiatrique*, 57 (1987), 79-84.

3.   Robert Castel, 'La psychiatrie dans notre société', *L'Evolution psychiatrique*, 49 (1984), 719-31; Robert M. Palem, 'La pratique privée', *Informations sociales*, 11, (1979), 99-105; and also Françoise Tétard, 'La psychiatrie 'associative' en mouvement', in J.P. Arveiller (ed.), *Cinquante ans de psychiatrie sociale* (Ramonville Saint-Agne: Erès, 2002), 14-35.

4.   See for instance: P. Raynaud, 'La folie à l'âge démocratique', *Esprit*, 51 (1983), 93-110; R. Castel, 'Les aventures de la pratique', *Le Débat*, 41 (1986), 41-51; M. Gauchet, 'A la recherche d'une autre histoire de la folie', in G. Swain (ed.), *Dialogue avec l'insensé* (Paris: Gallimard, 1994), IX-LVIII.

5.   R. Porter and M.S. Micale, 'Introduction: Reflections on Psychiatry and Its Histories', in R. Porter and M.S. Micale (eds), *Discovering the History of Psychiatry* (New York & Oxford: Oxford University Press: 1994), 3-36: 3.

6.   G. Ballet, *Leçon d'inauguration de la chaire de clinique des maladies mentales* (Paris: Impr. Tancrède, 1909).

7.   R. Castel, *L'ordre psychiatrique. L'âge d'or de l'aliénisme* (Paris: Les Editions de Minuit, 1976).

8.   G. Ballet, 'Discours d'ouverture', in *XIth Congrès des médecins aliénistes et neurologistes de France et des pays de langue française* (Limoges: H. Charles-Lavauzelle, 1902), 343-50.

9.   'Avis aux lecteurs', *L'Encéphale*, 1 (1906), 1.
Société de Neurologie de Paris and Société de Psychiatrie, 'Du rôle de l'émotion dans la genèse des accidents névropathiques et psychopatiques', *Revue neurologique*, 17 (1909), 1551-687.

10.   G. Ballet, *Traité de pathologie mentale* (Paris: Doin, 1903), 1.

11.   J.C. Coffin, *La transmission de la folie 1850-1914* (Paris: L'Harmattan, 2003).

12.   A theory mainly based on the congenital origins of mental disorders.

13.   E. Dupré, *Pathologie de l'imagination et de l'émotivité* (Paris: Payot, 1925).

14.   P. Strauss, *Allocution prononcée dans la salle d'honneur de l'hôpital civil* (Bayonne : Impr. Foltzer, 1923), 11-12.

15.   E. Toulouse, *Ligue de prophylaxie et hygiène mentales. Son but. Son organisation*, Paris, National Archives, F22-529.

16.   M. Huteau, *Psychologie, Psychiatrie et Société sous la Troisième République: la biocratie d'Edouard Toulouse* (Paris: L'Harmattan, 2002).

17. An open door system, for example, had been created earlier at the mental hospital near Orléans. It was run during the 1930s by G. Daumézon, who failed to extend the open access to a greater number of patients.

18. The French radicals do not precisely constitute a radical movement. The Radical Party was created at the beginning of the twentieth century, regrouping some moderates and representatives of the centre left. It was an important element of political life in France in the first half of the twentieth century and participated in several governments. Deeply attached to the republic, in turn patriotic and pacifist, its leaders were anti-clerical; it supported the development of hygienism, but was not in favour of too big a development of the State. Except during the Popular Front period, it has always stood out in its declared hostility to the Communist Party and in its difficult relationship with the Socialists, who were its direct competitors.

19. H. Sellier and R.H. Hazemann, 'La santé publique et la collectivité (hygiène et service social)', L'infirmière française, 14 (1936), 437-47.

20. Conseil Supérieur de l'Assistance publique, Sur les dispensaires d'hygiène mentale et leurs généralisations (Paris: Imprimerie Nationale, 1937). In 1940, a practical guide to mental health facilities listed about 30 dispensaries in France (Paris included). L. Viborel, Savoir prévenir. Guide pratique de santé et de lutte contre les maladies sociales, (Paris: L.V., 1939), 263-4.

21. S. Odier, De l'asile Saint-Robert à l'hôpital Saint-Egrève. Progrès thérapeutiques et malheurs de la guerre 1930-1960 (Saint Egrève: Saint Egrève Hospital Publication, 1997).

22. L. Le Guillant, Compte rendu moral et administratif et rapports médicaux pour l'exercice 1936 (La Charité: R. Thoreau, 1937).

23. Psychiatrists did not usually support eugenics measures like forced sterilisation, but they did not condemn it either. Some of them discussed the Swiss law passed in 1928 and gave a positive interpretation of it.

24. Rapport sur l'asile de Cadillac, Paris: National Archives, F60-601, 1943. See also: O. Bonnet and C. Quetel, 'La surmortalité asilaire en France pendant l'Occupation', Nervure, 4 ; 2 (1991), 22-32; I. von Bueltzlingsloewen, L'hécatombe des fous. La famine dans les hopitaux psychiatriques français sous l'Occupation, forthcoming 2005.

25. In standard French, the 'Vichy period' refers to the time when Marshall Philippe Pétain was head of the State (1940-1944).

26. L'Information psychiatrique, 22 (1945), 20. From now on : IP.

27. X. Abély, 'Avant-Projet de loi sur l'assistance et l'hospitalisation des malades mentaux', IP., 22 (1946), 104.

28. A printed version of Henri Ey's speech has been published in Etudes psychiatriques. Historique, méthodologie, Psychopatholgie générale, vol. 1 (Paris: Desclée de Brouwer, 1948), 13-9. I use one of the hand-written versions from H. Ey private fund kept in the Perpignan's municipal archives (France). On Ey, see: R.M. Palem, Henri Ey, psychiatre et philosophe (Perpignan: Ed. Rive Droite, 1997) ; P. Clervoy, Henri Ey 1900-1977. Cinquante de psychiatrie contemporaine (Paris: Les empêcheurs de penser en rond, 1997); J. Garrabé, Henri Ey et la pensée psychiatrique contemporaine (Paris: Les empêcheurs de penser en rond, 1997).

29. Ey, op. cit. (note 28), 6.

30. This is Henri Ey's own term.

31. Ey, *op. cit* (note 28), 8.

32. *Ibid.*, 9.

33. L. Bonnafé, 'Assistance et prophylaxie psychiatriques', *Le Médecin français*, 4 (1944), 7.

34. These terms are used in the forewords of his Medicine Phd.: L. Bonnafé, *Psychoses chez les diabétiques* (University of Toulouse, 1939), 7.

35. Ey, *op. cit.* (note 28), 11.

36. For more details see: J. Ayme, *Chroniques de la psychiatrie publique. A travers l'histoire d'un syndicat* (Ramonville Saint-Agne: Erès, 1995).

37. On these authors, see: L. Le Guillant, *Quelle psychiatrie pour notre temps* (Toulouse: Erès, 1984); L. Bonnafé, *Désaliéner: Folies et societés* (Toulouse: Presses universitaires du Mirail, 1991); P. Sivadon, *Psychiatrie et socialités. Récit autobiographique et réflexions théoriques d'un psychiatre français* (Toulouse: Erès, 1993).

38. This is the case for instance of P. Sivadon or L. Le Guillant who were 30 when they were appointed.

39. The prewar structure had its review too, the *French Alienist*.

40. G. Daumézon and Ph. Koechlin, 'La psychothérapie institutionnelle française contemporaine', *Anais portugueses de psiquiatra*, 9 (1952), 272-311: 277.

41. P. Sivadon, *op. cit.* (note 37), 35.

42. G. Daumézon and J. Lauzier, 'Ce que sera L'Information psychiatrique', *I. P.* 22 (1945), 6.

43. François Billoux, 'Esquisse d'une politique de la renaissance sanitaire française', *IP.*, 22 (1945), 30-32: 32.

44. Decree of Feb. 28th 1945.

45. The titles in French are: *Au-delà de l'asile d'aliénés et de l'hôpital psychiatrique* (Paris: Desclée de Brouwer, 1946) and *Le Malade mental dans la société* (Paris: Desclée de Brouwer, 1946). Desclée de Brouwer was an openly Christian orientated publisher.

46. Mental hospitals were often located in towns with small populations, as was the case for Ey's and Le Guillant's before the war.

47. They were not 'anti-esquirolian'-orientated, though.

48. *Au-delà de l'asile, op. cit.* (note 45), 10.

49. J. Lacan, 'La psychiatrie anglaise et la guerre', *L'Evolution psychiatrique*, 14 (1947), 293-318.

50. L. Bonnafé, H . Ey, S. Follin, J. Lacan, J. Rouart (eds), *Le problème de la psychogénèse des névroses et des psychoses* (Paris: Desclée de Brouwer, 1950).

51. *Ibid.*, 162.

52. P. Sivadon, 'Le Centre de traitement et de réadaptation sociale de Ville-Evrard', *Annales medico-psychologiques*, 107 (1949), 166-69.

53. Louis Le Guillant also set up a C R T S in 1950 inside his asylum in a nearby Paris suburb.

54. P. Sivadon, *op. cit.* (note 37), 83.

55. Occupational therapy was also named 'ergotherapy'. Daumézon has praised Hermann Simon's work in his article previously mentioned. Daumézon, *op. cit.* (note 40).

56.   *Ibid.*, 71. Henri Ey shared the same approach; he declared during a conference: 'in our unit, we use all kinds of therapies'. 7S 51, Municipal archives, Perpignan. One version of his handwritten manuscript has been published in 'la psiquiatria francesa de 1900 a 1950', *Actas luso-espanolas de neurologia y psiquiatria*, 9 (1950), 73-82.

57.   A law was voted a year later.

58.   P. Sivadon, 'Espoir', *Esprit*, 20 (1952), 926-27.

59.   G. Daumézon and Ph. Koechlin, *op. cit.* (note 40).

60.   For more details see: *Serge Lebovici raconté par lui-même et ceux qui l'ont connu* (Paris: Bayard, 2003), 35-60.

61.   Many more comments could be made on this congress, but it would require a full separate presentation. For more details, see: R.M. Palem, *Henri Ey et les congrès mondiaux de psychiatrie 1950-1977* (Perpignan: Trabucaire, 2000), 7-22.

62.   Paul Sivadon set up another private institute in 1948, *L'Elan retrouvé*, which grew in the 1960s without becoming a public body, although its functions were to provide therapies in a day-care centre, a dispensary, etc. On this history, see: E. Diebolt, *De la quarantaine au quarantenaire: histoire du foyer de postcure psychiatrique de l'Elan* (Paris: L'Elan retrouvé, 1997).

63.   Private correspondence between E. Aujaleu and H. Ey reveals no doubt about their good relationships and mutual appreciation. Aujaleu came regularly to visit Ey at Bonneval at weekends. Aujaleu joined the Resistance groups in London after the establishment of the Vichy regime and was former head of the cabinet of a communist Health Minister. After leaving the Health Ministry, he became Health General Director, then director of the new National Research Centre for Health and Medical Research (Institut national de la santé et de la recherche médicale, INSERM).

64.   In 1955, 96 mental hospitals were listed; no more than ten were private institutions with a religious character; 107,976 patients were registered. In 1960, 155 day-care units and 72 dispensaries were listed, and the number of mentally ill patients was about the same.

65.   M.T. Magnaval, *L'hôpital psychiatrique de Seine-Maritime. Rapport de stage* (Paris: Ecole nationale d'administration, Nov. 1957), Annexe 11.

66.   From the 1960s onwards they will be called prevention centres more and more often.

67.   *L'Hygiène mentale*, 49 (1960), 352-72.

68.   *Journal officiel de la République française* (15 March 1960), 498.

69.   *Ibid.*

70.   *Ibid.*, 500.

71.   On the sector, see: M.C. George and Y. Tourne, *Le secteur psychiatrique* (Paris: Presses Universitaires de France, 1994). And for a testimony: M. Audisio, *La psychiatrie de secteur: une psychiatrie militante pour la santé mentale* (Toulouse: Privat, 1980).

72.   This request for the suppression of the law had been publicly made in an article entitled 'Does the 1838 law on insanity need changing ?' It was co-signed by H. Ey, P. Sivadon and L. Bonnafé. On that occasion, they wrote: 'any specific legislation on insanity would nowadays be considered as an historical heresy'. The article was published in the review *Le concours médical*, 89 (1967), 533-37.

73. R. Castel, *La gestion des risques* (Paris: Les editions de Minuit, 1981), 75-114. This measure was supported by the Unionists in 1968, but later on, the homogeneity of positions was not so clear anymore.

74. For instance, the sociologist M. Crozier thinks that anti-psychiatry may be a pathological deviation of the far-left movement which emerged from the May 1968 events, whereas the psychoanalyst and historian E. Roudinesco considers that the European anti-psychiatry movement has had no influence whatsoever in France. See R. Lefort, 'Antipsychiatrie et psychiatrie', *Encyclopedia universalis*, XIX (Paris: Encyclopedia universalis, 1989), 196-8: 198. And E. Roudinesco and M. Plon (eds), 'Antipsychiatrie', *Dictionnaire de la psychanalyse* (Paris: Plon, 1997), 54.

75. The law was mainly concerned with buildings and financial support.

76. It was actually already implicit in the 1960s circular.

77. The fact that S. Lebovici (1913-2000), child psychiatrist and psychoanalyst, was technical adviser at the Ministry is probably not coincidental.

78. M. Foucault, *Le pouvoir psychiatrique. Cours au Collège de France. 1973-1974* (Paris: Gallimard/Le Seuil, 2003), 293-300.

79. J. Oury recently declared that he did not share Guattari's option and talks today about the 'silliness of anti-psychiatry', in F. de Martinoir, 'Hommes en souffrance', *La Croix* (Feb. 20th, 2003), 20.

80. See: P.F. Chanoit, H. Chaigneau, J. Garrabé, 'Les thérapies institutionnelles', in *69th Congrès de psychiatrie et de neurologie de langue française* (Paris: Masson, 1971), 5-238.

81. 'L'antipsychiatrie', special issue, *La Nef*, 42 (1971).

82. Also: H. Ey, *Défense et illustration de la psychiatrie* (Paris: Masson, 1977).

83. L. Bonnafé, 'Lettre à un jeune psychiatre sur l'anti-psychiatrie', *La Nouvelle critique*, 53 (1972). Later published in: Bonnafé, *Dans cette nuit peuplée* (Paris: Editions sociales, 1977), 103-24.

84. Ministère de la Santé. Direction générale de la Santé. Sous Direction des Actions de Soins et de Rééducation, *Evolution de la sectorisation depuis octobre 1975* (Paris: 1977).

85. H. Mignot, *Note sur les besoins des secteurs en psychiatres*, (Paris: 1973) – Archives H. Ey, 7S 235.

86. F. Fourquet and L. Murard (eds), 'Histoire de la psychiatrie de secteur ou le secteur impossible', *Recherches*, 17 (1975), 10-575.

87. This neologism is supposed to have been coined by Bonnafé. See L. Bonnafé, *op. cit.* (note 37), 40.

88. L. Bonnafé, 'La psychanalyse, une idéologie réactionnaire', *La Nouvelle critique*, 7 (1949), 52-73.

89. J.P. Segade and O. Faure (eds), *Questions à la 'révolution psychiatrique'* (Lyon: La Ferme du Vinatier, 2001).

CHAPTER 10

Outpatient Psychiatry and Mental Health Care in the Twentieth Century

International Perspectives

Harry Oosterhuis[*]

This article is about the main similarities and differences between the twentieth-century history of extramural psychiatry and mental health care in the countries that are central in this volume: France, the Federal Republic of Germany, Italy, the Netherlands, the UK and the USA. My comparative analysis does more than switch back and forth between relevant general trends and specific national developments. It also has a double focus: the development of outpatient services and other facilities in society, also known as 'community care' in the Anglo-Saxon countries, and 'de-institutionalisation', the demise of the public system of mental institutions, or at least a considerable reduction of its size. First I outline the relevant developments in extramural mental health care during the first half of the twentieth century. Then I will explore the changing constellation of psychiatry and mental health care in the second half of the last century, which some scholars refer to as the third psychiatric revolution[1]: the different ways and degrees in which de-institutionalisation was implemented in the various countries and the accompanying shift towards outpatient or community care. Moreover, special notice will be taken of the tensions between ideals and realities. At the very end I shall again briefly consider the main differences and similarities between the six countries.

Histories of psychiatry largely centre on mental institutions; studies on the history of outpatient psychiatry and mental health care are still thin on the ground, and therefore the data at my disposal are incomplete and fragmentary. My comparative analysis relies on some available studies in English, Dutch and German, the preceding articles in this volume, and some papers presented at the Anglo-Dutch-German Workshop on Social Psychiatry and Ambulant Care in the Twentieth Century, which took place in London in 2002.[2]

Outpatient Psychiatry and Mental Health Care before De-institutionalisation

In the post-World War II era, it was hardly a new view that it was better to keep psychiatric patients as much as possible outside mental institutions and establish alternative care facilities for them. In the nineteenth and early twentieth centuries, mental institutions were not by definition isolated, total institutions. British, Dutch, Italian and Japanese studies show that many patients stayed in them for only a limited time-period, not so much because of their illness in itself as their disturbing behaviour. Also, their relatives played a central role in the decisions over admission and discharge, and often they or non-related households took care of patients. The walls of the mental asylum were not impregnable barriers separating the insane from society.[3]

Nor was the aim of prevention through early treatment of essentially healthy individuals troubled by psychosomatic and mental symptoms or behavioural problems a product of new insights. Already in the last decades of the nineteenth century, some psychiatrists extended their professional domain beyond the walls of the asylum, not only by treating psychosomatic complaints, nervous disorders, addiction, sexual deviance, 'moral insanity' and criminal psychopathology, but also by presenting themselves as experts in the field of social hygiene in society at large. The first national psycho-hygienic movement was established in 1909 in the USA on the initiative of the ex-psychiatric patient C.W. Beers and the psychiatrist A. Meyer. After the First World War, the American National Committee for Mental Hygiene began to spread its doctrine internationally, and in 1930 it organised an international conference in Washington. Mental hygiene organisations were founded in the UK (1918), France (1920), Belgium (1924), Italy (1924), the Netherlands (1924) and Germany (1925). Besides the USA, France stimulated international developments in this area: in 1922, 1927 and 1937 international conferences on mental hygiene were held in Paris. While laypersons played a major role in the American Mental Hygiene movement, in Europe psycho-hygiene was mainly promoted by professionals – psychiatrists and other doctors in particular – but also by psychologists, educational experts and social workers.[4] Various mental health services were also set up, such as pre- and aftercare facilities, outpatient clinics, and prevention-orientated counseling centres for children and adults. These small-scale facilities mainly depended on scattered local or private initiatives, though. Centrally co-ordinated national networks of services still barely existed during the first half of the twentieth century.

The first social-psychiatric facilities originated in Germany, dating back to the early twentieth century. The so-called *nachgehende Fürsorge*, a form of aftercare with facilities where discharged psychiatric patients could work, was aimed at reducing their chances of regression and subsequent re-admission. This project, set up by psychiatrist G. Kolb from the psychiatric institution of Erlangen, received international attention, as did H. Simon's occupational therapy in the 1920s, which in part aimed at enhancing the social rehabilitation of the mentally ill through work. In the early 1920s, there was also a pioneering initiative by the psychiatrist F. Wendeburg in Gelsenkirchen, who, independently of the mental asylum and as part of public health care, developed a form of social psychiatry that sought close collaboration with social and juridical agencies. This project comprised the monitoring of discharged patients, their aftercare, their social reintegration, as well as the registering of mental disorders among the population at large so as to be able to provide immediate care if necessary.

Apart from these forms of social psychiatry, during the Weimar Republic psychotherapeutic institutes and counseling centres for psycho-social problems emerged in some cities, especially in the fields of family, marriage, sexuality and education, staffed by psychologists, psychoanalysts, sexologists and educational experts. They were inspired by reformist ideals and were occasionally supported by social-democratic local authorities. Psychiatrists, who in general followed a medical approach and rejected psychoanalysis, hardly played a role in these activities on the borderland of mental health and social work. In fact, social psychiatry struck out on a very different course. The protection of public order and the improvement of people's mental health already played an important role in pre-World War 1 German social psychiatry, a tradition that became strongly influenced by eugenics in the 1920s. From the start, social psychiatry was not only extramural care for psychiatric patients, but it also implied a preventive regime as a way to monitor the overall population's mental health. In this light, some psychiatrists argued in favour of a prohibition on marriage for mental patients, their sterilisation or long-term institutionalisation, and even euthanasia, so as to prevent the mentally ill from procreating. Proposals of this sort suggest there was at least some continuity between German social psychiatry and the murder of psychiatric patients in the Third Reich, despite the fact that the Nazi regime had banned all mental hygiene associations in Germany in 1935.

The Third Reich and the Second World War signified a radical break in the development of extramural psychiatry in Germany. Until the mid-1960s, when initiatives from innovation-minded psychiatrists could count on more support, the various social-psychiatric and other outpatient services remained minimal. Psychiatrists who worked outside mental hospitals, like those in university psychiatry, were mainly geared toward medical science, neurology in particular. The social aspects of care provided to the mentally ill received little attention, and extramural facilities for chronic patients, like special housing and work facilities, were scarce. Preventive and aftercare services aimed at psychiatric patients, as well as other social-psychiatric activities such as those involving admission, were co-ordinated by the *Gesundheitsämter*, local public health services that were not allowed to perform medical interventions, such as the prescription of medication. Before the mid-1970s, with the exception of university psychiatric hospitals, there were hardly any outpatient clinics for emergency psychiatric care. The largely privately established medical sector closely guarded its monopoly on treatment. By and large, private psychiatrists and neurologists dominated mental health care outside the walls of mental hospitals. They almost exclusively practised in urban centres and were medically orientated, treating psychiatric disorders and neurological complaints in tandem, a practice with roots in the late nineteenth century. This medical focus was in part stimulated by the medical insurance system, which discouraged time-consuming forms of counseling and psychotherapy. Furthermore, psychotherapy in Germany did not so much develop as part of psychiatric practice, but more in general health care, as part of psychosomatic medicine.

In Great Britain, a Mental After-Care Association was founded already in 1879, but until the 1930s, it did not provide any services to support mental patients in society. The frequently large-scale and overcrowded asylums mainly functioned as shelters rather than as hospitals, and they were closely linked up with the poor relief tradition and the juridical procedures that were necessary for admission. Although many of the mentally ill were cared for in the community by their own families, in non-related households (in Scotland), or in other institutions and were never hospitalised or only for a short period, outside of the asylum, psychiatric treatment could only be found in private practice. By the 1910s, however, in part because of the attention given to soldiers who suffered from shellshock, this situation began to change. Some of these soldiers were treated according to new psychotherapeutic principles in the Maudsley Hospital, which opened in 1916 and offered both intramural and outpatient treatment of acute psychiatric disorders. In the 1920s, psycho-dynamic psychiatry, which undermined degeneration thinking and the therapeutic pessimism tied to it, was also applied in the Tavistock Clinic, established in 1920. Starting in the late 1920s, under the aegis of the mental hygiene movement, Child Guidance Clinics were established in some British cities. Extramural mental health care was further stimulated by courses in psychiatry offered to nurses and general practitioners, and by training facilities for psychiatric social work, the first of which started in 1929 at the London School of Economics. A major impetus for such developments was the Mental Treatment Act of 1930, which marked a first step toward the integration of psychiatry in medicine. This act not only provided for voluntary admission in what were now called mental hospitals instead of asylums, it also enabled the establishment of some public outpatient clinics, voluntary aftercare services and convalescent homes. However, their scale and numbers were small, and only in London did a few psycho-analysts in private practice offer psychotherapy. On the eve of World War II, there was certainly no comprehensive extramural network in place.

World War II, like the first one, brought a number of psychiatric innovations. Army psychiatrists, for instance, who tried to address the problems of soldiers traumatised by the war's violence applied new forms of treatment, like brief psychotherapy and group therapy. After the war these innovations challenged psychiatrists to work more with psychotherapy and to experiment with therapeutic communities. Moreover, that psychiatry became part of the National Health Service in 1946 was of the utmost importance. This collective health provision made it possible for people with more or less serious mental disorders to receive treatment outside of psychiatric hospitals. After the number of inpatients peaked in the mid-1950s, the application of anti-psychotic drugs in particular, but also electro-convulsion therapy, shortened the average time of hospitalisation and led to a larger turnover of patients. The new medication also enlarged the opportunities for psychotherapeutic and social-psychiatric treatment of patients, as well as for helping them outside mental hospitals in outpatient clinics, day hospitals and general practice. Some psychiatrists and psychiatric social workers began to visit patients at home, emphasizing the importance of the social environment and integration in society. In the 1950s, British psychiatry gained an international reputation with its approach aimed at breaking the barriers between mental institutions on the one hand and somatic medicine and society on the other. It was argued that psychiatry had to be integrated into general medicine as much as possible, which implied, among other things, that acute mental disorders should be treated in the psychiatric wards of general hospitals. Furthermore, there was increasing interest, also at the level of government, in new ideas about what was termed 'community care', which would make patients less dependent on mental hospitals.

Even earlier than in Great Britain, the legislative conditions in France were favourable to the development of forms of outpatient psychiatry. Already in the second half of the nineteenth century, the French government permitted asylums to spend as much as a third of their budget on activities aimed at reintegrating patients in society. In practice, however, for a long time little was accomplished. Although in the 1920s, on the initiative of the psychiatrist E. Toulouse, the first outpatient facility for the treatment of psychiatric disorders was established in Paris, such facilities continued to be scarce in France until the 1950s. The centres for mental hygiene, which were set up in the 1930s under the aegis of the *Societé d'Hygiène Mentale*, were tied to *dispensaires* (outpatient clinics) for social hygiene that targeted children and, from 1937, adults as well. During the reign of the leftist *Front Populaire*, the government was positively interested in social hygiene, as well as in open wards of psychiatric hospitals and social casework, as a method for managing discharged patients.

After the Second World War, the preventive activities in general health care that were funded by local, regional and national governments, co-ordinated by the *Office Public d'Hygiène Social*, provided the framework for developing an aftercare system aimed at early discharged psychiatric patients, which helped to reduce the average length of their hospitalisation. Both psycho-tropic drugs and the increased role of psychotherapy were instrumental factors. In the mid-1950s, the fight against alcohol addiction provided a reason to increase the number of social-hygienic *dispensaires,* of which the psychiatric counseling centre became a mandatory unit. In medical psychiatry, however, little changed at first: around 1960, the mental hospitals still existed basically in isolation from the rest of the medical world, and to the extent that general hospitals had psychiatric departments they were fairly small and operated on a policy of selective, limited admission. In the late 1950s, several psychiatrists in Paris took the initiative to organise a first form of community psychiatry that consisted of a local clinical facility and various outpatient services for treatment, care and support. This local project would serve as a model for the reforms that were launched in the 1960s and beyond.

In Italy, some local extramural psychiatric facilities were set up in the early twentieth century, but more important was the widespread practice of various forms of family care in several provinces. Mental asylums saw little modernisation. The 1904 Insanity Act stipulated that the mentally ill who were dangerous to themselves, other people or the public order had to be confined in public asylums. Patients who were not considered dangerous could also be cared for in society by their families or in other facilities. Voluntary admissions were only possible in private hospitals and university clinics. The fascist regime, stressing that the insane were dangerous to society, expanded the number of public asylums so that the number of inpatients doubled during the first four decades of the twentieth century. It also introduced the provision that a person's psychiatric admission was registered by the police. Even though the Italian asylums were renamed 'hospitals' after the war, in comparison to the other countries discussed here, the quality of the care they offered was low, in part because of these institutions' overcrowding and the lack of qualified personnel. Although the government paid lip service to the desirability of outpatient facilities, in practice little changed, with the exception of local experiments that were set up from the 1960s onwards in some cities in the north and middle of Italy. A notable example was Trieste, where the isolation of the psychiatric hospital was brought to an end, and patients received much more freedom of movement. These innovations were inspired by *Psichiatria Democratica,* developed by a group of left-orientated psychiatrists, social workers and sociologists under the direction of F. Basaglia. They turned against medical psychiatry and argued for the socialisation of care and treatment of psychiatric patients. This would allow psychiatry to cater to their needs more effectively, which in turn would improve their ability to cope with their problems on their own.

In the Netherlands, several social-psychiatric pre- and aftercare services, counseling centres for alcoholism as well as Child Guidance Clinics and other mental health facilities for children were set up during the first four decades of the twentieth century. Pre- and aftercare, organised by psychiatric hospitals, was first modelled after German examples, but in the 1930s, a Dutch version of social psychiatry emerged in the sense that its facilities developed more or less independently of mental institutions. The Child Guidance Clinics in the Netherlands, which combined a psycho-dynamic and social approach, were a copy of the American ones. Already before the Second World War, many psychiatrists were working in general hospitals and public outpatient clinics as well as in private practices. In the early 1940s, two new types of outpatient facilities emerged: the public clinic for psychotherapy and the Centre for Marriage and Family Problems. The next three decades saw a vast expansion of the various extramural services. A striking feature of mental health care in the Netherlands was its broad orientation. It comprised not only social psychiatry in the sense of outpatient care for psychiatric patients, but also counseling centres for problem children, marriage and family related issues, social adjustment, and alcohol addiction. This broad orientation is accounted for in part by the fairly early differentiation between institutional psychiatry and the outpatient mental health sector in the Netherlands, and the moral-didactic and, increasingly, psychosocial focus of the latter. In other European countries the institutional and public mental health sectors were more exclusively geared toward psychiatric patients, while there was also a closer link with the domain of clinical psychiatry. From the start, Dutch psychiatrists working in outpatient facilities joined forces with other, non-medical mental health workers: social-psychiatric nurses, psychiatric social workers, clergymen, psychologists, educational experts and various specialist therapists.

In the USA the first form of outpatient psychiatry took shape at the end of the nineteenth century, when the growing professional group of neurologists in private practice, who dissociated themselves from asylum psychiatry, started to treat not only patients with neurological problems but also those with mental and psychosomatic difficulties. Several psychiatrists too began to dissociate themselves from the asylums and established their own practices. In part because of the rise of psycho-dynamic psychiatry, which downplayed the boundary between mental health and mental illness, psychiatrists focused on new categories of patients, which until then had remained outside psychiatry's scope. In the early twentieth century, this broadening of the professional domain not only occurred in private practice, but also became manifest in the social-hygienic focus of psychiatrists. Some of them stressed the need for social-economic reforms, while others emphasized the desirability of eugenic measures as a way to counter unwanted immigration, alcohol abuse and various forms of deviant behaviour. In the USA, as in Germany, there was an overlap between the mental-hygienic aim of prevention and eugenics. From 1896, in various states, the mentally ill were not allowed to marry anymore and from 1907, as many as 30 states adopted laws that made it possible to sterilise without consent feeble-minded and mental patients.

American psychiatrists, however, were divided on eugenics, and many opposed compulsory measures. In the 1920s and 1930s, they became more interested in developmental psychology – in part through the influence of psychoanalysis – and began stressing the impact of education and the social environment. In the mental hygiene movement, the two divergent orientations – eugenics and psycho-dynamic approaches – existed side by side; both fitted the aspirations of psychiatrists like A. Meyer to expand the psychiatric domain. The National Committee for Mental Hygiene moved away from the problems of institutional psychiatry and geared its effort towards alcoholism, juvenile crime, feeble-mindedness, venereal diseases and deviancy. It supported in particular the prevention of juvenile crime through its Child Guidance Clinics, which were established in the 1920s and later copied in several European countries. Their approach was characterised by a combination of psycho-dynamic and psychosocial approaches.

The psychiatric expansion from intramural to extramural care and from treatment to prevention was stimulated, in the USA even more than in Great Britain, by the experiences of army psychiatrists during the Second World War. They developed new methods of treatment for soldiers who suffered stress and nervous breakdowns from their battlefield experiences. These mental afflictions, the origin of which was traced to social-environmental factors, might strike any soldier, and the forms of treatment applied near the battlefront had a strong psychotherapeutic element and took place in groups. After the war, psychiatrists working in mental institutions lost their dominance in American psychiatry, giving way to the advocates of psychoanalytic and social-psychological approaches. At this point, it was of key importance that innovation-minded psychiatrists found support with the federal government, which, until then, had never involved itself with psychiatry because the care of mental patients in public asylums had always been a responsibility of the state governments.

The mounting influence of the American federal government in the domains of health care and social services after World War II gave a strong impetus to outpatient psychiatry. Federal policy-making and advisory facilities for mental hygiene and public health were set up, and they developed elaborate plans and an effective lobby. The National Mental Health Act of 1946 allocated federal funds to research in the social and behavioural sciences, professional training in mental health care (for psychiatrists but also clinical psychologists, psychiatric-social workers, and mental health nurses), and experimental facilities that served as an alternative to the large-scale, socially isolated mental institutions and were aimed at treating mild mental problems, to prevent them from growing worse. In the mid-1950s, there were almost 1,300 psychiatric outpatient clinics, most of them in the states of the Northeast, the North-Midwest and in California. Moreover, in the 1950s, partly as a result of the American middle classes' openness toward psychological and psychoanalytical approaches of feelings and social behaviour, there was also a significant growth of the treatment offered by psychotherapists in private practice. These practitioners not only included psychiatrists but also other doctors, clinical psychologists and social workers. Although there were indications that these services primarily met the needs of people with mild problems, instead of those of serious and chronic mental patients, in the 1950s the notion caught on that the need for alternatives to mental institutions was concrete and compelling. The results of treatment with new psychiatric drugs nurtured this optimism. Far-reaching proposals for a more extensive extramural psychiatric care system, including facilities for people who sought help for their psycho-social problems, fell on fertile ground during the years of the Kennedy administration.

Bold Plans

In the second half of the twentieth century, the role of extramural mental health care in Western Europe and North America grew more prominent. For a large part, this development was connected with the introduction of psycho-pharmacological drugs, growing criticism of institutional psychiatry culminating in anti-psychiatry, the striving for reform of the care and treatment of psychiatric patients, and the expansion of mental health care from mental illness to a variety of psycho-social problems. Although new forms of treatment had been introduced in the preceding decades and the care and living conditions of the patients had improved, mental hospitals still stood in bad repute among the general public. These institutions, often dating from the nineteenth century, were isolated from the rest of society as well as from the general health care system, and many of them were massive and overcrowded. In the 1950s, the largest mental hospitals in Europe – with around 4000 beds – were to be found in France. In Germany and Great Britain, the average number was over a thousand. In the USA, state mental hospitals were even larger: some had around 10,000 beds. Only in the Netherlands did most of them not surpass a thousand beds.[5] In all countries, mental hospitals were often seen by the public at large as secluded shelters for the chronic and incurable mentally ill that belonged in a tradition of social care or poor relief, rather than to the health care system.

Reform efforts aimed at a renewal of psychiatric hospitals by reducing their size and breaching their isolation on the one hand, and an organisational shift to new or already existing alternative intramural and, especially, extramural facilities on the other. The alternatives included special institutions for demented elderly and the mentally handicapped, psychiatric wards of general hospitals, outpatient clinics, day hospitals, night shelters, half-way houses, social-psychiatric services, general practitioners, Community Mental Health Centres, counselling centres, and rehabilitation and work facilities. This reorganisation was motivated by the aspiration to separate the functions of therapeutic treatment, care, custody and social rehabilitation. Closely connected to this was the wish to differentiate between the facilities for various categories of patients, such as chronic cases and emergency cases, or mentally handicapped and demented elderly. The alternative facilities were no longer merely conceived as complementing psychiatric hospitals but also, at least partly, as replacing them. It was strongly felt that treatment and care for psychiatric patients should be integrated into the overall health and social care-providing system, while their social integration came to be seen also as a priority. Moreover, the medical character of psychiatry increasingly became an issue of debate; in hospitals, psychiatrists and nurses were in charge, but in the outpatient sector, other professional groups, including clinical psychologists, social workers and social-psychiatric nurses, claimed responsibilities as well. Finally, especially in the closing decades of the twentieth century, there was a growing emphasis on volunteer aid and self-help, partly because of efforts to reduce public spending on mental health care.

New ideas about the treatment and care of the mentally ill had been developed from the late 1940s onwards and sometimes had been put into practice on a small scale, but it was only from the 1960s that they could be realised on a broader scale. Growing prosperity made it possible to increase budgets for mental health care and thus expand provision and employ rapidly increasing numbers of psychiatrists, as well as psychologists and other mental health professionals.[6] Three other new developments were of no mean importance in all of the countries discussed here: greater interference by the government in a period characterised by democratisation and social emancipation, growing attention to a variety of mental health problems that did not require hospitalisation, and acknowledgement of the rights of individual psychiatric patients. The nationally designed plans for new mental health networks were meant to bring care-providing facilities closer to the people, enlarge their accessibility, and ensure an efficient interconnection between the various psychiatric and psycho-social services for the mentally ill, as well as clients with minor complaints or behavioural difficulties. The combination of growing supply of and demand for mental health care entailed an extension of its domain.

In the first half of the twentieth century, social-psychiatric services were set up mainly for pragmatic reasons, such as cost-effectiveness and to relieve the overcrowded asylums. However, the interests of individual patients were clearly secondary to those of society. In the post-war period and especially since the 1960s, when ideals concerning better, more humane care, a greater autonomy of psychiatric patients, and discouraging prejudices against them played a major role, psychiatry was brought up for public debate, often with strong political overtones. (Financial concerns, however, made a comeback from the mid-1970s.) In nearly all countries, the legislation on insanity, which often dated back to the nineteenth century, was amended. This reflected the shifting emphasis from legal procedures associated with maintaining law and order as well as protecting citizens against arbitrary detention to voluntary admission, patients' civil rights, and their right to receive adequate care and therapeutic treatment. This recognition became concrete in the Netherlands in 1916, 1929, and 1994, in the UK in 1930, 1959, 1983 and 1995, in several German states from the early 1950s on and from the second half of the 1970s, in France in 1968, and in Italy in 1968 and 1978.[7] However, the increased rights to self-determination of the mentally ill, in combination with de-institutionalisation, would enlarge the friction between the freedom of the individual and public safety. At the end of the century, there was a growing concern over the risk posed by those who neglected themselves or who were dangerous to themselves or other people.

Most national governments played an active part in the renewal of the mental health care system. After World War II, Western Europe and the USA saw greater government involvement in and more collective funding of health and social care, whereby mental health became increasingly integrated into these two domains. (This is not to deny that mental health care still received less funding, compared with somatic care, in nearly all countries. Even after de-institutionalisation took off, only a small portion of the health care budget ended up in the publicly organised mental health sector, while most of that budget – 80 per cent on average – went to psychiatric hospitals.)[8] In the UK, for example, the establishment of the National Health Service (1946) and the National Assistance Act (1948) caused the management and funding of intramural and outpatient psychiatry to become part of a centrally co-ordinated collective health care and welfare sector.[9] In France, where the central government had administered asylum psychiatry since the nineteenth century, the extramural facilities were publicly funded as part of the public health care system and co-ordinated by the national *Office Public d'Hygiène Social*. While in the United States institutional psychiatry was traditionally a responsibility of the governments of the individual states, after World War II, the federal administration actively involved itself in mental health and increased national funding substantially.

In the federally organised system of West Germany, the situation was rather complicated. The responsibilities and financing of both intramural and extramural care were distributed between the national government, the governments of the individual states, and local boards and voluntary organisations, but here too the federal government relied on legislation and increased funding to become a more active player in this sector. However, with the exception of the *Gesundheitsämter* for public health, the carrying out of health care was largely left to (subsidised) voluntary organisations and doctors in private practice. Although the Netherlands had a more centralised political system, until the 1970s their mental health sector had more in common with that of Germany than with that of France or the UK. Both in Germany and the Netherlands, a central principle of welfare and health care was 'subsidiarity' – a basic preference for organising provisions at the lowest organisational level possible. The Dutch government issued regulations, provided subsidies, and monitored mental health care, but left the responsibilities for actual care-providing in the hands of the (partly religiously based) voluntary organisations and local and regional authorities, while funding tended to be scattered. Not until the late 1960s did the central government begin to play a more active role, especially by introducing uniform, collective funding regulations. The Italian government was even slower in adopting a more active stance. Only in the late 1970s did it propose nation-wide initiatives for renewing Italy's mental health sector, and psychiatry was included in a national health insurance.

Decisions to reform mental health care and pursue de-institutionalisation were taken at the national level, although local experiments and voluntary initiatives sometimes served as the model. In Europe, the UK led the way, whose psychiatric sector was internationally regarded a model in the 1950s. After a Royal Commission voiced its preference for community care, in 1959 parliament passed a new Mental Health Act, which replaced the older legislation. To bridge the gap between hospital and society and to promote community care, the juridical procedures for admission and discharge were simplified, and medical criteria were given priority. Two years later, the conservative Minister of Health, E. Powell, pointed to a drastic reduction of the number of beds in psychiatric hospitals. Psychiatric wards of general hospitals would take care of acute cases, while outpatient facilities should provide care to chronic psychiatric patients in society.

In the United States, under the Kennedy and Johnson administrations, inclined as they were to social reform and the expansion of the welfare state (the 'Great Society'), the government took an active stance in reforming the mental health sector, in part thanks to an effective lobby of the National Institute of Mental Health under the leadership of R.H. Felix. In the early 1960s, the mental health lobby aimed for the establishment of the Community Mental Health Centre that should serve as an alternative for mental hospitals. This easily accessible facility would offer outpatient mental health services to a broadly composed clientele, and also provide public educational programmes aiming at prevention. Throughout the country, 2,000 of these centres were deemed necessary, to be supported by the federal government in the initial phase. This plan constituted the core of the Mental Retardation and Community Mental Health Centres Construction Act of 1963. Also, the expansion of federal medical insurance and assistance programmes (Medicare and Medicaid) as well as social security benefits for the indigent formed a driving force behind the decline in the number of patients in mental hospitals. Many of the elderly patients moved to nursing homes, while others were able to live in the community and could be treated in the short-term and outpatient psychiatric clinics of general hospitals.

In France, changes in governmental policies were associated with several reform-minded hospital directors and officials of the Ministry of Public Health.

In 1960, in a ministerial memo, they launched an ambitious plan aimed at both the improvement of institutional care and the building of a uniform system of extramural facilities on a regional basis, the *psychiatrie de secteur*. France was supposed to be divided into 750 geographical regions, with an average population of 70,000, in which multidisciplinary teams were granted the responsibility for running mental health care on a local basis. Social-psychiatric outpatient clinics, day centres and work facilities together with psychiatric hospitals would contribute to a coherent care system based on preventive activities, early detection and intervention, curative treatment, and aftercare. For the time being, however, all of this did not get beyond the planning stage. In the mid-1960s, a group of progressive psychiatrists led by H. Ey, who favoured a social orientation of psychiatry rather than a strictly medical one, argued for the actual implementation of the reform plans, as well as for a larger budget to enable this reform to take place.

Around 1960, bold plans were launched in the UK, the USA, and France at the level of the central government. By contrast, the reform proposals in Germany and the Netherlands were less drastic, less promoted by the government, and formulated somewhat later. After critical and reform-minded psychiatrists had organised themselves in pressure groups, like the German Society for Social psychiatry and the Mannheim Circle, a special investigative commission of the German parliament, established in 1971 on their instigation and mainly consisting of medical and academic experts, published a report in 1975. Painting a bleak picture of Germany's large-scale, overcrowded and isolated mental institutions, it concluded that there were not enough preventive, outpatient and rehabilitation facilities. It called for a decrease in the size of mental hospitals, more psychiatric wards in general hospitals, a sustained effort in prevention and social reintegration, and the establishment of regional networks – *Standardversorgungsgebiete* of about 250.000 inhabitants – of integrated extramural services. Moreover, in addition to the care provided by psychiatrists in private practice, there was a need for more psychiatric outpatient clinics and multidisciplinary social-psychiatric services in public health centres.

Starting in the mid-1960s, the first plans for reorganising mental health care in the Netherlands came from the sector itself, rather than from the government. Although mental health care was increasingly funded by national health insurance schemes, and the outpatient sector expanded rapidly, psycho-therapeutic facilities in particular, only in the early 1970s did the Dutch government begin to formulate policies in this area. The Ministry of Health presented a plan for a new system that would provide public inpatient as well as outpatient facilities on a regional basis to all citizens. The plan aimed at a reinforcement of the outpatient sector by forging a more coherent ensemble of all the various facilities that had developed since the 1920s, and establishing Regional Institutes for Ambulatory Mental Health Care, which were modelled on the American Community Mental Health Centres.

A striking similarity in the French, German and Dutch government policies was the absence of sweeping plans for large-scale de-institutionalisation. They aimed at a reform of mental hospitals – reducing their size, ending their isolation, and improving care and psychiatric treatment – and an expansion of extramural services, not so much as a substitution of hospitals, but as an extension of a more or less integrated mental health care system. This rather cautious approach contrasted with developments in Italy. Although Italy had been slow to develop new policies, none of the countries discussed proposed such drastic plans. Perhaps it was precisely Italy's antiquated institutional psychiatry that led to the formulation of radically new policies in the late 1970s. It was only in 1968 that the 1904 Insanity Act was amended, certification was abolished, and voluntary admission became possible. At the same time, in the wake of the 1960s protest movement, psychiatry and the mental hospital in particular became the subject of heated public debates. In 1978, the Italian government, in order to avoid psychiatry becoming the subject of a referendum for which the activist groups were lobbying, ensured that parliament passed a law that contained far-reaching provisions. This prohibited the building of new hospitals and the admission (and, from 1981 on, also re-admission) of patients to public mental institutions. Furthermore, it was decided that psychiatric wards of general hospitals could have no more than 15 beds, that compulsory admissions were subject to restrictive rules, and that multidisciplinary extramural facilities, *Servici d'Igiene Mentale*, had to be set up to offer a broad range of services – not just medical treatment, but also counselling, social care and public information.

Stubborn Realities

The modernisation of mental health care through de-institutionalisation and the promotion of community care were frequently accompanied by high expectations and much enthusiasm, but nearly everywhere, this commitment met with financial, political, organisational, or professional obstacles. In most countries, the reform plans were developed in the 1960s and early 1970s when the economy was booming, public expenditure rose sharply, and there was a euphoric, change-minded, even revolutionary political climate. When, in the ensuing decades, plans had to be implemented, the economic tide had turned and, in many cases, the political tide as well. As a result of the economic crisis that started in 1973, there were fewer funds available, and governments cut back on collective services – a policy to which especially the public facilities for mental health care fell victim. A community care policy appeared to create the possibility of cutting costs in a way that institutional care did not allow. The assumption that community care was cheaper than hospital care – in itself doubtful if hospitals were to be replaced by extensive outpatient facilities that would offer good quality substitute care – was now realised in some countries, just by shifting the emphasis from public to voluntary and informal care. Moreover, the ideals of the 1960s movement paled, confidence in the steering power of central government diminished, and the political spectrum as a whole, especially in Anglo-Saxon countries, moved toward the right: smaller government and more free market was the motto of both the Thatcher government and the Reagan administration. Their example, albeit in a more moderate form, reverberated on the European continent. The pace of reform slowed down, and the distinction grew more pronounced between widely accessible public care facilities and private facilities that were only available for people of means. One of the negative results was that chronic and long-stay institutional patients in particular were sometimes neglected.

Besides changing external circumstances, organisational problems put a brake on innovation. Policies that were designed at a central level proved not always easy to implement in actual local and professional contexts. It turned out to be hard to distribute the forms of care provided by the various intramural and extramural facilities effectively, in part because both health care and welfare officials were in charge of their supervision, and in part because these facilities could have a public, voluntary and/or commercial status. Moreover, innovation did not always agree well with the divergent interests of the therapeutic professional groups involved. Psychiatrists in particular succeeded in opposing some measures that would negatively affect their dominant position or because the prevailing medical approach threatened to be sidelined. Psychiatric hospitals did not automatically co-operate in de-institutionalisation; after all, in general, the extramural sector could only be expanded at the expense of their own funding and influence.

As the available data suggest, in the period 1950-1980, the total number of beds in psychiatric hospitals substantially declined only in the UK, the USA and Italy. While in the UK, the USA and the Netherlands the mental hospital population peaked in the mid-1950s, this happened in the Italy around 1960, and in France and Germany in the early 1970s.[10] In the last two countries and in the Netherlands, the subsequent decline in beds was slower and less drastic than in the first three. Until the early 1970s, there was still a serious increase of the number of beds in mental hospitals in France and Germany, to be followed by only a slight decrease, but there were still more beds in 1980 than in 1950. Moreover, the relatively small loss of beds in mental hospitals in these countries was more or less compensated for by the creation of new beds for psychiatric patients in general hospitals and for the elderly with dementia in nursing homes. The Netherlands saw a slight decrease of the number of beds in psychiatric hospitals, as well as a slight increase of provision in the psychiatric wards of general hospitals between 1950 and 1980. Around 1980, the number of psychiatric beds (in psychiatric hospitals and psychiatric wards of general hospitals) for each 1,000 inhabitants varied from 1.2 in the USA, 1.5 in Italy, around 1.9 in Germany, the Netherlands, and the UK to 2.3 in France.[11] It should be added that fewer beds did not automatically imply more community care: many demented elderly and mentally handicapped individuals who used to be in psychiatric hospitals were increasingly housed in nursing homes and other specific institutions. In this respect, 'trans-institutionalisation' rather than de-institutionalisation would be a fitting term.[12] In this period, though, the average length of a psychiatric patient's hospital stay did go down in all the countries discussed.

To what degree was community care in fact accomplished in the various countries discussed? In Germany, it ran up against institutional obstacles: the split responsibilities between federal and state governments in particular, the funding systems in health care and social care, and the established medical interests. The implementation and funding of federal policies were largely left to the individual German states, as the central government only funded specific model experiments temporarily, and their willingness to implement changes varied substantially, depending on the political colour of their governments. The individual states generally responded rather slowly to the 1975 parliamentary report. Day and night hospitals as well as facilities for emergency care were set up, but in general, these did not replace a large number of hospital beds. Radical de-institutionalisation was not pursued in Germany. Although between 1975 and 1981 the number of beds in psychiatric hospitals dropped by 13 per cent, this drop was mainly caused by removing older and chronic patients to other (cheaper) living and nursing facilities.[13] Germany's states tended to spend more money on improving and reducing the size of mental hospitals than on building and expanding extramural facilities.

The latter was also complicated by the fragmented financing and management systems in mental health care. The distribution of responsibilities among federal government, state governments, private organisations, medical professional associations, health insurance companies, social security boards and hospital organisations conflicted with the promotion of community care. Mental health care in Germany was funded by health insurance (inasmuch as medical treatment aimed at curing patients was concerned) and by collective social insurance (inasmuch as the care and rehabilitation – mainly of chronic patients – were involved). The strict distinction between medical treatment and (social) care hardly favoured the building of new services for psychiatric patients, like special housing or work facilities that were geared toward providing social assistance to patients rather than 'curing' them. While such provisions were not eligible for funding from health insurance, the criteria for funding from social insurance frequently did not apply to the care needed by chronic psychiatric patients. As a result, not enough services were put in place to facilitate community care for these patients. Furthermore, the projected expansion of outpatient clinics in psychiatric departments of general hospitals for emergency cases did not work out as planned. Both psychiatrists in private practice and general practitioners feared competition from these clinics, and their professional organisations succeeded in restricting their spread. Before an outpatient service could be established, it had first to be demonstrated that there was a shortage of private office psychiatrists. Private practitioners even strengthened their dominant position as their number went up significantly; in the early 1980s, 45 per cent of all psychiatrists were in private practice.[14]

In part because social psychiatry and psychotherapy received little attention in the academic training of psychiatrists, German extramural psychiatry continued to have a solidly medical focus. This emphasis was also encouraged by the fact that psychiatrists in private practice were inclined to have patients hospitalised rather than refer them to social-psychiatric facilities, because of the limited options provided by the health insurance system. This meant that the public social-psychiatric services – with their emphasis on emergency care, aftercare and social care – were basically left to service chronic psychotics, addicts with mental problems, and the mentally handicapped. When, starting in the early 1980s, the German government's policies in the area of health care and welfare became dominated by cost-control, it was the public outpatient mental health sector in particular that was hurt. Many chronic patients who were not hospitalised were to a large extent dependent on family care and had little contact with psychiatric services. In general, the reform process of the German health care system continued in the 1980s and 1990s at a slow pace. At the end of the century, the integration of psychiatry into general hospitals was accomplished, and many of the chronic and elderly patients had been moved from mental hospitals to other institutions. Psychiatrists were divided over the question of whether all inpatient mental health care should be transferred to general hospitals, but in general, there was a strong reluctance against radical de-institutionalisation. The availability of community services, which have to compete with private psychiatrists, varied by federal state or region.

Funding and organising mental health care were less complicated matters in centralised France. Each year, the Ministry of Social Affairs, which was responsible for this policy area, decided on a total budget and issued five-year plans. Around 1980, in the light of a decentralisation effort, the responsibility for the actual activities was handed over to the provinces and regional agencies for health care and welfare. The organisation of public extramural facilities was assigned to local governments, which either took charge or – the option that was chosen by most – conferred their authority to voluntary organisations and psychiatric hospitals. Patients could go to the public facilities but also to their family doctor and, in large cities, to the growing number of psychiatrists – and psychotherapists – in private practice. Mental health care was basically funded in three ways: health insurance companies paid for medical treatment in hospitals and treatment by psychiatrists in private practice; as part of its preventive effort, the government subsidised most of the public extramural facilities for both mental patients and alcohol and drug addicts; finally, the provinces paid for most of the care and re-integration of chronic psychiatric patients.

Although the idea had been launched already in 1960, the *psychiatrie de secteur*, in which regional teams for outpatient care – each consisting of some 15 members (one senior psychiatrist, four to five junior psychiatrists, seven psychiatric nurses, one social worker and one secretary) – played a major role, did not develop until the 1970s. In addition, outpatient clinics saw strong growth, with the number of patient visits increasing fivefold between the mid-1960s and the mid-1980s.[15] Furthermore, new extramural facilities were established: for child and adolescent psychiatry, and housing and nursing facilities for the mentally handicapped and chronic psychiatric patients. Despite these innovations, a government commission concluded in 1980 that only a minority of the regions had enough facilities and that day centres and housing facilities for chronic mental patients were especially lacking. As a result, the expansion of community care had not contributed to a reduction in the number of hospital admissions; the new services largely served another, less seriously ill clientele. Psychiatric hospitals, which fulfilled a major role in the organisation of extramural care, also proved to be an obstacle for its realization; to ensure their continued existence, their discharge policies tended to be conservative.[16]

The socialist government that came to power in 1981 developed plans to fund extramural facilities at the expense of hospitals, but starting in 1984, the emphasis shifted towards controlling expenditure, in which the community care for chronic patients especially suffered. It was apparent, moreover, that private practice and commercial initiatives for those of means were outperforming the public mental health system. In France, as in Germany, psychiatrists – their number rising fourfold in the 1970s – continued to play first fiddle in mental health care. Frequently, they combined a position in hospitals with extramural work, but gave priority to their intramural responsibilities; it was not uncommon for them merely to pay lip service to community care. Psychiatric nurses, who saw their number double between 1975 and 1985 and whose training in the 1970s became directly tied to the general training for nurses, continued to have a subordinate position.[17] By and large, their career opportunities remained tied to psychiatric hospitals. In France, clinical psychologists and social workers played only a minor role. As a result of this overall situation, many regional teams were not multidisciplinary but consisted mainly of psychiatrists and nurses, which carried the risk that the outpatient sector merely became a copy of the hospital model. In the 1980s, innovation-minded mental health workers began to doubt the feasibility of the once ambitious reform plans. However, compared to Germany, Italy and the Anglo-Saxon countries where extramural services were often patchy, in France, with its strongly centralised health policy, a uniform mental health framework was realised on a national scale. In the early 1990s, more than

800 sector teams were in operation, each covering areas with around 70,000 people and providing care for psychiatric patients in hospitals as well as in out-patient clinics and day and rehabilitation centres.

If large-scale de-institutionalisation did not happen in France and Germany, it did not take place in the Netherlands either. Certainly, the medical model and the powerful position of psychiatrists were increasingly questioned, but the medical-psychiatric establishment averted polarisation or a radical break by adopting a co-operative and accommodating stance and by integrating new prac-tices into the existing institutional framework. Experiments with new psycho-therapeutic and social-psychiatric forms of treatment, like the therapeutic com-munity, were supported, and the democratisation of internal professional rela-tions made it possible for nurses and patients to voice their views. In the 1980s and 1990s, the isolation and large size of psychiatric hospitals were broken down, and outpatient clinics and half-way facilities, like sheltered housing, were expanded. Increasingly, psychiatric patients lived and worked outside treatment facilities, so as to raise their sense of self-responsibility. The number of long-term admissions, although still significant, dropped because of this process, for which policy-makers introduced the term 'socialisation' (*vermaatschappelijking*) rather than 'de-institutionalisation'. That no priority was given in the Nether-lands to more radical forms of de-institutionalisation became clear in the early 1980s, when plans to build new psychiatric hospitals, aimed at downscaling, substituting old institutions, and a more even regional spread were pursued, despite protests. In fact, some new psychiatric hospitals were built.[18]

Changes were implemented in the Netherlands on the basis of gradual, well-prepared and extensive deliberations with those involved and with respect for the structures that were in place. Thus, it took more than ten years before, at the government's initiative, most of the existing outpatient facilities were com-bined into about 60 Regional Institutes for Ambulatory Mental Health Care in the early 1980s, each covering catchment areas of between 150,000 and 300,000 residents. Continuing the tradition of some of the older extramural fa-cilities, in these new institutes psychiatrists constituted a minority among other mental health professions, while various forms of psychotherapy and counsel-ling set the tone. They were not so much geared towards (chronic) psychiatric patients as toward clients suffering from minor mental complaints and psycho-social problems. Fuelled by a generous budgetary system, compared with that in other countries, they developed into the main providers of outpatient mental health care, and despite the crisis of the welfare state in the 1980s, they and other extramural and half-way facilities saw further expansion in subsequent years.

In actually achieving de-institutionalisation, the UK, Italy and the USA clearly distinguish themselves from France, Germany and the Netherlands. The first three countries saw a drastic reduction of beds in psychiatric institutions, but at the same time, their organisation of alternative community care facilities did not live up to their intentions and were not up to the standards of those in France and the Netherlands. The UK was the first country in Europe that put de-institutionalisation on the agenda. From the late 1950s, pragmatic concerns constituted a major incentive. De-institutionalisation was inspired by optimism about the new pharmaceutical options for treating mental illness, rather than by a decided preference for a social-psychiatric approach. Although the British government stressed again and again the importance of community care, it did not actively pursue policies in this area. The responsibility for its organisation was largely left to local authorities in the field of health care and welfare, which had insufficient funding to compensate for the reduced number of psychiatric beds by aftercare services, day centres, special housing, work and re-integration facilities. In the 1970s, the de-institutionalisation effort became increasingly mixed up with efforts to control expenditure, a trend that grew even stronger under the Thatcher government. Moreover, a gap continued to exist between psychiatry and social care, and this hardly contributed to the development of extramural care for chronic psychiatric patients. Psychiatrists and nurses mainly looked to the medical world because it meant more professional status; as a result, they basically operated independently of social work and other social services. Great Britain developed a combined form of community care: a social-psychiatric service by community mental health teams of psychiatric departments of general hospitals, and basic care provided by general practitioners in collaboration with social workers and community psychiatric nurses. Compared to Germany, France, the Netherlands and the USA, Great Britain had only a few psychiatrists and psychotherapists in private practice, most psychiatrists being employed by the National Health Service. Moreover, the number of clinical psychologists in British mental health was fairly small until the 1970s.

In the mid-1970s, the British government launched plans for a regionally organised and multidisciplinary mental health care system, whereby the proposed size of each region varied from 60,000 to 250,000 inhabitants. However, the policies of the Thatcher government, aimed at the primacy of the free market and the downsizing of the welfare state, conflicted with this plan. While the number of psychiatric beds continued to decrease – of the 130 hospitals in 1960 only 41 were left in the early 1990s[19] – the public community care services were facing serious cutbacks, while market forces were introduced into mental health care. Voluntary initiatives, commercial facilities and volunteer aid had to take over public tasks in part, without there being much co-ordination between them. The overburdened community mental health teams increasingly concentrated on acute mental patients who were considered dangerous to themselves or others and who made up a large part of the so-called 'revolving door' group. Consequently, more and more chronic psychiatric patients ended up in commercial boarding-houses and nursing homes, or became dependent upon their relatives. In 1985, a parliamentary commission referred to the United States and Italy, where radical de-institutionalisation had produced a situation in which psychiatric patients were entirely left to their own devices and ended up on the streets – a development that could also be witnessed in the UK. Chronic mental patients, it seemed, were discharged from mental hospitals without there being sufficient alternative forms of care available.

In 1979, a year after de-institutionalisation was formally enacted in Italy, the accessibility of (mental) health care facilities was enlarged by the introduction of national health insurance. These two measures, in theory at least, offered a favourable condition for the development of the public *Servici d'Igiene Mentale*, the Italian version of the Community Mental Health Centre that was meant to replace the psychiatric hospital as the basic mental health facility. These centres, staffed by psychiatrists, nurses, psychologists and social workers, had to provide accessible and flexible psychiatric care and be fully integrated into society. It was only when hospitalisation could not be avoided that small psychiatric wards of general hospitals had to bring relief. Around 1980, the Italian experiments with community care received much international attention and were frequently seen as a model. This positive response, however, was mainly prompted by some more or less successful local projects in regions and towns in North and Central Italy, including Trieste, the home base of Basaglia. In the rest of Italy, notably the southern part, community care remained basically a pipe dream, and mental hospitals remained dominant. The Italian government, even more than its British counterpart, did not set out a tough policy, hardly allocated funds, and left the actual organisation of care facilities in the hands of local initiative. This caused the remaining patients in the public psychiatric hospitals – around 40 were still in operation at the end of the century – to be neglected, while in many regions, there were hardly any alternative forms of care available, in part because local authorities ignored or even resisted the mental health law of 1978. The out-patient clinics, more often than not the only extramural facilities, were overburdened with acute patients, so that psychiatrists and nurses were driven back on methods of coercion and pharmacological treatment. They could not prevent many chronic patients from being left to their own devices. Half-way houses and sheltered accommodation were in short supply, while relatives were not always able or willing to take care of them. In addition to the often poorly organised and under-funded public facilities, in large urban areas there were also private hospitals, university clinics, and private psychiatrists and psychotherapists, but in general, they only treated patients with acute disorders or less serious mental problems from the middle and upper classes. Not surprisingly, de-institutionalisation stagnated and became controversial in Italy, not only among members of the professions involved, but also with the general public.

The trend towards de-institutionalisation developed in the United States more drastically than in any other country. Since the mid-1960s, the number of patients and their average stay in American public mental institutions declined quite rapidly. Between 1970 and 1990, the number of beds decreased from more than 410,000 to around 120,000.[20] Alternative residential accommodation (half-way houses, group homes and nursing homes for elderly chronic patients and other people with long-term psychiatric disorders) and psychiatric departments of general hospitals (for emergency cases) took over some care or treatment, but in the 1970s, more and more of the mentally ill ended up in society for shorter or longer periods of time. The Community Mental Health Centres, set up after 1965, were supposed largely to replace intramural care for mental patients by offering a broad supply of outpatient services. Yet, in the course of the 1970s, it became apparent that they failed to do so. First, too few facilities were in fact established: the 754 centres that were put in place by 1980 lagged far behind the total of 2,000 that had been planned in the early 1960s.[21] In part because of the war in Vietnam and the economic crisis of the 1970s, there were not enough financial means, while in the 1980s the Reagan administration even discontinued the federal involvement and financing of the extramural mental health care sector. Second, most Community Mental Health Centres were not geared to providing social care and the rehabilitation of chronic psychiatric patients; rather, they catered to the needs of another clientele with less severe problems, who were offered psychotherapy; thus, they overlapped the substantial private psychotherapeutic sector. The social-psychiatric care for the first group suffered, also because psychiatrists, influenced by biological psychiatry, increasingly retreated from outpatient facilities, with psychotherapy-minded psychologists taking their place. Given these circumstances, de-institutionalisation could hardly have been successful. Although many older discharged mental patients, who previously were hospitalised for long periods, managed to cope with their problems because of the support of family and neighbours or some other form of community care, the limitations of the extramural care system became visible once more, and more individuals with psychiatric disorders (who were often young and who might also be addicted to alcohol or drugs) joined the growing army of homeless people in the metropolitan areas of the United States.

Conclusion

In the last three decades of the twentieth century, there was clearly a general trend away from reliance on long-term hospitalisation towards a more varied and more extramural pattern of care and treatment. However, between countries and regions, considerable variations in policy and implementation as well as timing can be found. My comparative account suggests that in terms of de-institutionalisation, France, Germany and the Netherlands lagged behind the UK, Italy and the USA, but also that the gap between reform plans and their implementation was smaller in the first three countries than in the last three.

Whereas in France, Germany and the Netherlands de-institutionalisation was pursued in a more gradual and moderate form, at the same time, France and the Netherlands especially succeeded in building and maintaining a network of alternative outpatient facilities and community services on a national scale. In the Netherlands the public outpatient sector was well established already from the 1940s – earlier than in other countries – and it also showed a great degree of continuity. The French *psychiatry de secteur* and the Dutch outpatient sector, as well as the policy of 'socialising' mental health care were rather successful compared with the fragmented and understaffed situation in Germany, Great Britain, Italy and the USA, which sometimes lacked community care facilities. In France and the Netherlands, more money was spent on health care and social provision than in the other countries.[22] The Dutch welfare state and the French centralised health funding system guaranteed that public mental health care facilities were available and accessible to all citizens and that they functioned fairly well. However, the end of the twentieth century saw a growing differentiation between the public mental health sector and private practices, which had occurred earlier on in other countries. In Germany and the United States in particular, private practice had held a prominent place in extramural psychiatry for a longer time.

In another way, the United States and the Netherlands stood apart from France, Germany, Great Britain and Italy. Whereas in the other countries the expansion of public community care facilities was concomitant with de-institutionalisation and they focused on psychiatric patients, in both the United States and the Netherlands, the development of extramural public mental health care was only partly linked to what happened in institutional psychiatry. In both countries, the emphasis on prevention and a multidisciplinary approach in outpatient services during the second half of the twentieth century ultimately resulted in the wide expansion of the mental health domain, as well as a strong psychological orientation. The psychologising approach and the prestige of psychotherapy in both countries contributed to the situation where many mental health workers in public extramural care focused their attention on psycho-social problems rather than on psychiatric disorders. In the 1970s and 1980s, there was a clear parallel in this respect between the development of the American Community Mental Health Centres and the various Dutch counselling centres, psychotherapeutic institutes and, later, the Regional Institutes for Ambulatory Mental Health Care.

What was a unique Dutch development was that from the late 1960s, psychotherapy developed as a separate, interdisciplinary profession and that it was practised not only by private therapists but also in public mental health institutes. This ensured broad accessibility of this treatment. The major role of psychotherapists – psychologists among them in particular – in Dutch mental health since the 1960s sets the Netherlands apart from other European countries, where psychotherapy largely remained limited to more or less elitist private practices or, as in Germany, was part of psychosomatic medicine. In this respect and probably also in the more general psychologisation of society, developments in the Netherlands were more similar to those in the USA than to those in its neighbouring countries. However, since the last decade of the twentieth century, these differences have decreased. With the return of a stricter biomedical and pharmaceutical approach, many Dutch psychotherapists have withdrawn into private practice. As in other European countries, public mental health care in the Netherlands focused more and more on medical treatment, as well as on the social rehabilitation of psychiatric patients.

At the beginning of the twenty-first century, some convergence may be taking place between the six countries. Apart from the dominant biomedical and pharmaceutical approach, it is recognised more and more in all countries that de-institutionalisation has its limits. Community care partly depends on a great deal of social tolerance for mentally ill patients, if their behaviour is disturbing or risky, but it is questionable whether people in modern society are able to meet this ideal. De-institutionalisation and community care have clearly not improved the quality of life of all psychiatric patients; for some of them, who are not able to cope with life in society, these may have resulted in a deterioration of their living conditions. The emphasis has often been more on the treatment of acute patients and clients with minor mental problems than on the social support and rehabilitation of the chronic sufferers. Some categories of the mentally ill still need and perhaps prefer the overall protection and care of a mental hospital in order to lead reasonably secure and untroubled lives. Also, there is a growing anxiety over the mentally disturbed who are (possibly) violent or who cause public nuisance. In the countries where de-institutionalisation has been carried through extensively – the United States, Great Britain and Italy – there is evidence of increasing use of hospital beds and some movement towards re-institutionalisation.

Notes

*   I am indebted to Hugh Freeman, Marijke Gijswijt-Hofstra, Gerald Grob, Patrizia Guarnieri and Joost Vijselaar for their comments on earlier drafts of this article, and to Ton Brouwers and Hugh Freeman for correcting the English.
1.   See R. Castel, F. Castel and A. Lovell, *The Psychiatric Society* (New York: Columbia University Press, 1982). They refer to the emergence of psychiatric asylums since the early nineteenth century and the rise of dynamic psychiatry since 1900 as the first and second psychiatric revolution, respectively. The third revolution marks the diffusion of mental health care facilities and a psychological approach of problems in society.

2.   Comparative overviews are provided by S.P. Mangen, 'Psychiatric Policies: Developments and Constraints', in S.P. Mangen (ed.), *Mental Health Care in the European Community* (London: Croom Helm, 1985), 1-33; H.L. Freeman, T. Fryers and J.H. Henderson, *Mental health services in Europe: 10 years on* (Copenhagen: World Health Organization, Regional Office for Europe Copenhagen, 1985); S. Goodwin, *Comparative Mental Health Policy. From Institutional to Community Care* (London: Sage, 1997).

For France I rely on the article by Coffin in this volume; S.P Mangen and F. Castel, 'France: the "psychiatrie de secteur"', in Mangen, *op. cit.* (above), 114-47; P. van Lieshout and P. Meurs, 'Geestelijke gezondheidszorg in Frankrijk. Principes en praktijk van de "psychiatrie de secteur"', *Maandblad Geestelijke volksgezondheid*, 42 (1987), 282-93.

For Germany: the articles by Roelcke and Kersting in this volume; S.P. Mangen, 'Germany: The psychiatric enquete and its aftermath', in Mangen (ed.), *op. cit.*, (above), 73-113; H.-P. Schmiedebach and S. Priebe, 'Social Psychiatry in Germany in the Twentieth Century: Ideas and Models', *Medical History*, 48/4 (2004), 449-72; V. Roelcke, 'Psychotherapy between Medicine, Psychoanalysis, and Politics: Concepts, Practices, and Institutions in Germany, c. 1945-1992', *Medical History*, 48/4 (2004), 473-92; M. Cramer, 'De Duitse GGZ op bezoek in Nederland', *Maandblad Geestelijke volksgezondheid*, 38 (1983), 296-303; W. Schaufeli, 'Psychologie, GGZ en crisis in de Bondsrepubliek', *Maandblad Geestelijke volksgezondheid*, 39 (1984), 703-08; F.-W. Kersting (ed.), *Psychiatrie als Gesellschaftsreform. Die Hypothek des Nationalsozialismus und der Aufbruch der sechziger Jahre* (Paderborn: Ferdinand Schöningh, 2003); and some unpublished papers for the Anglo-Dutch-German Workshop *Social Psychiatry and Ambulant Care in the 20th Century*, London, 4-6 July 2002: C. Brink, 'Precarious Attitudes: social psychiatry and the public in the Federal Republic of Germany, 1960-1980'; M. von Cranach, 'The Complex Dynamics of Change: thirty years of psychiatric reform in Germany' and C. Vanja, 'Psychiatry in Hesse: Between institutional treatment and outpatient care, 1900-2000'.

For Italy: the contribution by Guarnieri in this volume; S. Ramon, 'The Italian psychiatric reform', in Mangen (ed.), *op. cit.* (above), 170-203; P. Guarnieri, 'The history of psychiatry in Italy', *History of Psychiatry*, 2 (1991), 289-301; H. van der Klippe, 'Het Italiaanse voorbeeld na tien jaar', *Maandblad Geestelijke volksgezondheid*, 44 (1989), 429-34.

For the Netherlands see the articles by Blok, Gijswijt-Hofstra, Oosterhuis and Vijselaar in this volume; H. Oosterhuis, 'Between Institutional Psychiatry and Mental Health Care: Social Psychiatry in The Netherlands, 1916-2000', *Medical History*, 48/4 (2004), 413-28; G.J.M. Hutschemaekers and H. Oosterhuis, 'Psychotherapy in The Netherlands after the Second World War', *Medical History*, 48/4 (2004), 429-48.

For the UK: the article by Freeman in this volume; S.P. Mangen and B. Rao, 'United Kingdom: socialised system – better services?', in Mangen (ed.), *op. cit.* (above), 228-63; J. Busfield, 'Restructuring Mental Health Services in Twentieth-Century Britain', in M. Gijswijt-Hofstra and R. Porter (eds), *Cultures of Psychiatry and Mental Health Care in Postwar Britain and the Netherlands* (Amsterdam: Rodopi, 1998), 9-28; K. Jones, *Asylums and After. A Revised History of the Mental Health Services: From the*

Early 18th Century to the 1990s (London: Athlone, 1993); J. Welshman, 'Rhetoric and reality: community care in England and Wales, 1948-74', in P. Bartlett and D. Wright (eds), *Outside the Walls of the Asylum. The History of Care in the Community 1750-2000* (London: Athlone, 1999), 204-26; S. Payne, 'Outside the walls of the asylum? Psychiatric treatment in the 1980s and 1990s', in *ibid.*, 244-65; E. Jones, 'War and the Practice of Psychotherapy: The UK Experience 1939-1960', *Medical History*, 48/4 (2004), 493-510; some papers for the Anglo-Dutch-German Workshop *Social Psychiatry and Ambulant Care in the 20th Century*, London, 4-6 July 2002: P. Barham, 'The English Mental Patient in the Twentieth Century: continuity and discontinuity', V. Long, '"Often there is a great deal to be done, but socially rather than medically": the psychiatric social worker as social therapist, 1945-1970' and T.H. Turner, 'The Return of the Private Madhouse: the rise and fall of community care in Britain over the last 50 years'.

For the USA: the contribution by Grob in this volume; G.N. Grob, *The Mad Among Us. A History of the Care of America's Mentally Ill* (Cambridge (MA): Harvard University Press, 1994); E. Shorter, *A History of Psychiatry. From the Era of the Asylum to the Age of Prozac* (New York: John Wiley, 1997); A. Scull, 'Social Psychiatry and Deinstitutionalization in the USA', unpublished paper for the Anglo-Dutch-German Workshop *Social Psychiatry and Ambulant Care in the 20th Century*, London, 4-6 July 2002.

See also: *Acta Psychiatrica Scandinavica*, 104 (Suppl. 410) (2001), which contains articles on psychiatric reform in Europe during the last quarter of the twentieth century. See: T. Becker and J.L. Vázquez-Barquero, 'The European Perspective of Psychiatric Reform', in *Ibid.*, 8-14.

3.   Bartlett and Wright (eds), *op. cit.* (note 2) and the articles by Vijselaar, Guarnieri and Suzuki in this volume.

4.   On international developments in the field of psycho-hygiene, psychiatry and mental health care and the growing impact of the USA and the UK, see: M. Thomson, 'Mental hygiene as an International Movement', in P. Weindling (ed.), *International Health Organisations and Movements, 1918-1939* (Cambridge: Cambridge University Press, 1995), 283-304; M. Thomson, 'Before Anti-Psychiatry: "Mental Health" in Wartime Britain' in Gijswijt-Hofstra and Porter (eds), *op. cit.* (note 2), 43-59; K. Angel, E. Jones and M. Neve, *European Psychiatry on the Eve of War: Aubrey Lewis, the Maudsley Hospital, and the Rockefeller Foundation in the 1930s* (London: The Wellcome Trust Centre for the History of Medicine at UCL, 2003); H. Pols, 'Preventing Mental Disorder, Fostering Mental Health, and Diagnosing Society: Mental Hygiene in the United States', unpublished paper for the Workshop *Cultures of Psychiatry and Mental Health Care in the Twentieth Century: Comparisons and Approaches*, Amsterdam, 18-20 September 2003.

5.   Goodwin, *op. cit.* (note 2), 9.

6.   Freeman et al., *op. cit.* (note 2), 60-65.

7.   Mangen, *op. cit.* (note 2), 28.

8.   *Ibidem*, 9-12.

9.   This, however, hardly ensured generous funding. In fact, the portion of the national income that was spent on health care in Britain – six per cent – was lower than in the other EU member states. Mangen and Rao, *op. cit.* (note 2), 236.

10.   Goodwin, *op. cit.* (note 2), 105. The information on the Netherlands has been provided by Marijke Gijswijt-Hofstra on the basis of publications by the Dutch Central Bureau of Statistics.

11.   The data on the various European countries are derived from the World Health Organisation statistics as listed in Mangen, *op. cit.* (note 2), 21-22 and in Goodwin, *op. cit.* (note 2), 50-51, and the data on the USA are based on Grob, *op. cit.* (note 2), 291 and C.A. Taube and S.A. Barrett (eds), *Mental Health, United States 1985* (Washington, D.C.: Government Printing Office, 1985), 30. Taking the substantial decrease in psychiatric bed space in Britain over the past decades into consideration, these figures suggest that, at least until the mid-1950s, this country must have had more beds in mental hospitals than France, Germany and the Netherlands, and probably also than the USA and Italy.

12.   See Grob in this volume.

13.   Mangen, 'Germany: The psychiatric enquete and its aftermath', in *op. cit.* (note 2), 96.

14.   *Ibid.*, 108.

15.   Mangen and Castel, *op. cit.* (note 2), 136.

16.   However, recent information on France reveals that between 1989 and 2000, 40 per cent of the beds in psychiatric hospitals were closed. NRC *Handelsblad*, 20 December 2004. See also: Dominique Provost and Andrée Bauer, 'Trends and Developments in Public Psychiatry in France since 1975', *Acta Psychiatrica Scandinavica*, 104 (Suppl. 410) (2001), 63-68: 65.

17.   Mangen and Castel, *op. cit.* (note 2), 134.

18.   H. van de Beek, *Tussen zorgen en behandelen. Ontwikkelingen in de sociaal-psychiatrische hulpverlening* (Utrecht: Nederlands centrum Geestelijke volksgezondheid, 1991), 4.

19.   Busfield, *op. cit.* (note 2), 22.

20.   Grob, *op. cit.* (note 2), 291; Goodwin, *op. cit.* (note 2), 12.

21.   *Ibid.*, 262.

22.   Mangen, *op. cit.*, (note 2), 10.

Psychiatric Patients

CHAPTER II

Out and In: The Family and the Asylum

Patterns of Admission and Discharge in Three Dutch Psychiatric Hospitals 1890-1950

Joost Vijselaar

In March 1917, a 22-year-old Dutch serviceman was sent from his barracks to a psychiatric hospital by a medical officer, with the rare diagnosis of insania moralis. The young man already had a history of alcoholism, vagabondage, stealing, blackmail and promiscuous behaviour. Being forced by his father to enter the army as a way to quell this irresponsible behaviour, he turned out to be a sergeant's nightmare, a lazy, undisciplined man, insubordinate, drinking, laughing at his superiors, etc. Since he was unresponsive to punishment or imprisonment, it was decided to refer him to an asylum. Within a month's time, during which he behaved childishly and was described as an imbecile, he was discharged as 'improved' and returned to a military hospital.[1]

Colourful stories like these of a dissolute, unsociable soldier who was discharged from the asylum within a couple of weeks shed a special light on the (social) function of the psychiatric hospital at the beginning of the twentieth century. It is especially in patients' records that this illuminating information about actual reasons for the admission and discharge of individuals from mental institutions can be found.

The often-massive collections of case histories from psychiatric hospitals have up till now hardly been used for the study of twentieth-century asylums, Braslow's *Mental ills and bodily cures: psychiatric treatment in the first half of the twentieth century* being one of the exceptions.[2] That these medical archives can be a source of new perspectives on the workings of psychiatry has amply been demonstrated by authors like Anne Digby and Charlotte MacKenzie, who analysed these sources for the nineteenth century at The Retreat and Ticehurst, respectively.[3] It is largely owing to the strict rules for the protection of the privacy of the patients involved that this type of historical research has been mostly limited to the period before 1900.

Official records, whether they consist of archival material or publications, offer a digested, selective and considered account that has often been influenced by an ideological or scientific agenda or else by institutional and professional interests. Contemporary statistics often lack continuity, cannot be correlated with each other, or do not correspond to the needs of the modern historian. Patient files on the one hand create the possibility of individualising both the experience and careers of particular groups of psychiatric patients whilst on the other hand, proffering the essential descriptive and quantitative data that allow the social history and dynamics of the psychiatric institution, its population and its role within society to be analysed. They provide raw data that are open to new questions and methods. That these records do have their own structural limitations and are biased as a consequence of their purpose and being authored almost exclusively by doctors has been argued convincingly by Guenther Risse and Jonathan Andrews, amongst others.[4]

In the Netherlands, continuous series of case histories have been kept in psychiatric hospitals ever since the first lunacy legislation in 1841, which obliged the hospitals to keep a file for every individual patient. The law prescribed the proper content of the case history, consisting of daily, monthly and annual accounts of the patient's state, as well as official declarations as to the reasons for a prolonged stay in the asylum. Usually, these files also contained various forms or admission certificates regarding the future inmate's personal history and illness. It was only in the course of the twentieth century that the files gradually lost their uniform structure as a result of the introduction of a procedure for uncertified admissions, which obviated the legal regulations concerning the form of the file. Thanks to growing historical awareness during the last twenty years, it has become a custom among psychiatric institutions in the Netherlands to preserve at least a random sample of their files for future research. Many have transferred their older medical archives to public record offices.

In the present research, case histories were studied of patients who had been admitted to a psychiatric hospital between 1892 and 1992, some of the most recent notes even dating from the new century. The main focus of the study is on the social process leading to the admission, the character of the stay in the institution, and the social mechanisms related to discharge. It concerns questions like: how long did people cope with the individual's aberrant behaviour and what made them decide to send him/her to an asylum; how was it to be in hospital, and to what extent did therapeutic considerations influence the life within it; which criteria played a role in the decision to discharge someone, and was there any interaction between the hospital and families at this point?

At a higher level, the study aims to examine whether the general picture of the development and function of the psychiatric hospital, as described in recent historiography, is corroborated by the information from patients' records. This is especially true for the older but still influential idea of the asylum being a static, total institution, used to repress 'deviancy' and creating lifelong dependency on the part of its inmates. The study also tries to assess whether data like these can be used to approach more general questions about the development of culture and mentality, following the example set by Michael MacDonald in his book *Mystical Bedlam* on the patients of a physician in early seventeenth-century England.[5]

For this study, three psychiatric hospitals were selected as being representative of both the denominational segmentation and geographic distribution of asylums in the Netherlands. The oldest of these, Voorburg, was a large Roman Catholic institution (with around 1,400 beds in 1955, when it was the second largest in the Netherlands), catering for men and women of all classes from the southern province of Brabant.[6] Next, Endegeest, the municipal psychiatric hospital of Leyden and closely affiliated with Leyden University, had a public character and took only indigent patients, mostly from the urban west of the country (and almost half from Leyden itself).[7] The third, Wolfheze, situated in the middle of the country, belonged to a strictly Calvinist organisation and was, like Endegeest, a medium-sized institution (500-600 beds in its heyday) for indigent men and women.[8] Both Voorburg and Wolfheze had a mixed urban-rural catchment area. A random sample was taken from the medical archives of these three institutions: every five years (1892, 1897, 1902, 1907, etc.), the first five files from a sample of one in ten were selected, amounting to a total of 300 records for the whole century or 30 per decade.

All of these files were transcribed (almost in full) into a qualitative database (Nvivo by QSR, Australia), which allows the material to be analysed from a range of perspectives by creating demographic attributes, coding of specific themes, textual and Boolean searches, simple statistical counts and refined selections of groups of patients.[9] With this database it is possible to master the huge volume of information contained within the files, once the time-consuming clerical job of transcribing and coding has been finished. At the time of writing, the files from the first 50 years have been analysed, and part of the result will be presented in this article.

Care in Society

Before 1950 the family, taken in a wider sense, constituted the background of the majority of admissions to a psychiatric hospital. According to the records, about 18 per cent of the patients were on their own prior to their hospitalisation. Almost 60 per cent of all cases came from a family – 75 per cent of the patients of Endegeest and Wolfheze. Even in the case of people living on their own, family members or relatives were generally involved in the process of admission.

The often incomplete information from the files proves that long-term care in the family was not uncommon in the first half of the twentieth century. Some 30 per cent of the patients at least had been attended to by family members at home, sometimes for a considerable number of years. A clear indication of this is the fact that 17 per cent of the newly admitted patients had been ill for more than five years, most of them staying with their families during this period. It was mostly parents, spouses, brothers and sisters, children or sons- and daughters-in-law who had been looking after them.

The majority of these people belonged to the category of chronic patients, suffering from dementia (almost 50 per cent), other neurological complaints or mental retardation. Many of the others had milder psychopathological symptoms like nervousness, apathy and indifference, melancholy, fear, restlessness or irritability. But there are also examples of men and women showing really disturbed, psychotic behaviour who had been cared for by their next of kin for years, even for decades.[10]

In quite a number of files there is evidence of patients and their family turning for help to a third party or to an institution other than an asylum. Interestingly enough, representatives of the clergy are almost missing: there are only two references in files from the Roman Catholic asylum of Voorburg: one about the use of confession as a means to alleviate mental problems, and the other being a vague allusion to exorcism.[11] Unorthodox or irregular healers are absent, save what was indicated by patients as a possible source of the mental disturbance. One lady from The Hague claimed to have been 'spoiled' by a quack, while another woman thought she was possessed by the devil, after having consulted a fortune-teller.[12]

It was to ordinary doctors and medical specialists that most of the future inmates had had recourse. In one-fifth of the records, it was a family doctor who had been seen. The material suggests that in the course of the 1920s and 1930s, these GPs became more active in actually treating their mental patients. The therapy of choice seems to have been medication, bromide being the most popular, while opiates or somnifen were used at times. But apart from these drugs, an occasional practitioner prescribed rest, conversed with his patient and in a unique case even used persuasion and hypnosis. Nevertheless, it was quite normal for a GP to admit that he did not do anything.

Already at the beginning of the century, psychiatrists, or 'nerve-doctors' as they were commonly called in the Netherlands, were seen by one or two of these psychiatric patients. As seen from the perspective of these records, it was only after 1925 that consultations with psychiatric specialists became more frequent, and even quite common during the 1930s. Psychiatrists in private practice are mentioned in 15 per cent of the files. They played a double role – as expert in the admission procedure and as therapist. Clues as to their way of treating their private patients, 70 per cent of whom suffered from psychosis or mood disorders, are hard to find in the files. A number of these psychiatrists worked within the setting of a general hospital.

The asylum does not seem to have been the institution of choice for a significant number of people looking for a place for their disturbed relative to stay. The files bear witness to the existence of a number of alternatives to hospitalisation

Out and In: The Family and the Asylum

in a mental institution. In Brabant, a province in the south of the country, a sizeable number of patients had a history of care in general guesthouses or workhouses, some of them with a religious character. These seem to have catered primarily for elderly people with mood disturbances (1/4) and the mentally retarded (1/3). Sanatoriums specialising in the care of nervous disorders and the 'overstrained nerves' had a more marginal function.

It was the general hospitals in particular that appear to have played a significant role in the care for the mentally ill – a fact that has been left unnoticed by recent Dutch historiography. Some 16 per cent of the psychiatric patients in this study had been treated in a general hospital before entering the asylum. So already before the Second World War, the general hospital seems to have developed an autonomous psychiatric function to a certain extent. In some of the larger cities (like Arnhem in Gelderland or Tilburg in Brabant), this materialised in the form of specialised wards, like the 'zenuwpaviljoen' (nerve-pavilion) in the municipal hospital in Arnhem.[3] As pointed out, psychiatrists did part of their work in these wards or in the early outpatient clinics of these hospitals. The general hospital looked after a particular group of patients, mostly with milder types of psychopathology, some 40 per cent suffering from mood disorders. Depression and melancholia were also amongst the conditions seen at the psychiatric clinics of the university hospitals, together with hysteria and neurological syndromes like dementia paralytica. The academic clinics, having their own tasks of observation, research and treatment, acted to a certain extent as a selection filter, transferring the more disturbed patients to the asylum.

So even at the beginning of the twentieth century, a number of doctors and institutions outside the mental hospital could be involved in the care of a disturbed individual. The records show that it was during the 1920s and 1930s that the patterns of referral grew more complex, patients being sent by a general practitioner to a psychiatrist, who referred them to a general hospital, that eventually had to hand them over to an asylum. After 1950, these patterns of referral grew ever more intricate and dense.

Reasons for Admission

The Dutch psychiatrist Henk Jelgersma, working at Endegeest asylum and one of the first to introduce the theory and practice of social psychiatry, made an elucidating distinction between psychosis and insanity. For him psychosis meant an illness that in itself did not imply the necessity of hospitalisation. However, when a psychosis was complicated by disturbed, unsociable behaviour that hampered the social integration of a person and made hospitalisation inevitable, one should talk about insanity.[4] To a certain extent, patient records provide the information for studying the social boundary between psychosis and insanity and the actual reasons for sending someone to an asylum. For practical purposes, four main motives for hospitalisation can be distinguished: 1) social annoyance or disturbance, 2) endangering others, 3) being a danger to oneself, and 4) being in need of care or treatment. Apart from the behaviour of the identified patient, another element that could provoke a committal to an asylum has to be reckoned with: a change in the social environment that weakened the power or aptness of those around to cope with this behaviour.

Thus, mildly disturbed and pathological behaviour seems to have been tolerated for quite some time in domestic settings, even if it gradually became worse. It was often a sudden escalation in the conduct of the patient towards agitation and excitement, confusion and aggression that triggered a request for admission to a hospital. Agitation was by far the most common behavioural characteristic of those sent to a psychiatric hospital, some 45 per cent of those admitted being described in these terms, regardless of age or diagnosis. What could be an insidious process of escalation with chronic types of mental illness could develop within weeks and even hours into acute cases. The shorter the duration of the mental disorder before admission to hospital, the more agitation, confusion, anxiety and suicidal tendencies dominated the patient's behaviour. Dementia and delusions, being more characteristic of those with a long history of family care, seem to have been borne by those around for a longer period of time.

It was disorder and confusion, interpreted as nuisance and annoyance without danger being involved, that constituted a major reason for referral to the asylum in almost 37 per cent of the cases. The behaviour of these patients was overtly being designated by those around as troublesome, annoying or irritating, and said to be intolerable, impossible to deal with or to be influenced, ungovernable, intractable, etc. It often seemed to mark the end of a family's ability to cope or to endure. It was indeed family members who were mentioned most often in these situations as the ones being annoyed, whereas there is mention of neighbours in only eight files. It was only once in a while that public order seemed to have been at stake, with an old demented lady causing a row on the street or an alcoholic upsetting a theatre.[15] In general, annoyance caused by people suffering from psychosis or other kinds of psychopathology seems to have had a more 'intimate', domestic and a less public character than might have been expected.

Like social 'nuisance', posing a threat to others was a factor in the admission of somewhat more than a third of all patients. However, in around half of these records, 'being a danger to others' amounted to nothing more than a verbal argument that was not substantiated by a description of any material danger posed by the patient. In many cases, it was an assessment made by those around, especially by the doctor, based on either the presumed syndrome or the previous history of the person in question. With others, it was their intimidating conduct or speech, e.g. a threat to kill or harm someone or actually brandishing some sharp instrument, that constituted the risk. Most concrete were those cases in which

Out and In: The Family and the Asylum

someone hit or bit somebody else. But it was only in 14 per cent of the case histories that actual harassment was presented as an argument for committal, real life-threatening behaviour being mentioned only once. Victims were never mentioned; in all, the actual danger posed by these patients should not be overestimated.

Most often the people at risk, if mentioned at all in the clinical record, were either the partner or relative of the alienated person. Being dangerous to others as a reason for admission occurred more frequently and had a more concrete character in family settings than with single people. This phenomenon can perhaps be explained by higher levels of tolerance within families towards aberrant behaviour than amongst other people, the disturbance, agitation and risks escalating more before hospitalisation was considered and realised. This is supported by the tendencies towards domestic coping and care identified above. In general, the records show men and people suffering from psychoses, epilepsy and alcoholism to have been the most aggressive and dangerous among this population.

In about 20 per cent of all cases, patients were admitted to the asylum because of the danger they constituted towards themselves, most of them by showing suicidal inclinations. Being a danger to oneself was among the most important occasions for a hasty admission to the asylum, it being a chief reason for admission in half of the cases of people being ill for less than two months, and of 40 per cent of those ill for less than six months. However, even with presumed self-destructive behaviour, in many cases it was a formal motive for referral without the specific acts or conduct being made explicit in the documents. As with possible peril for others, it often was a deduction based on the diagnosis or a fear of relapse. 'Being a danger to oneself' could be used, of course, as a very effective and urgent argument for hospitalisation, because of the risks involved in delay.

Many were the thoughts, wishes or threats to do away with oneself that have been recorded in the files. But apart from these conscious expressions of self-destructive ideas, the refusal of food is described in at least ten records (6 per cent). Deluded ideas of sin, a presumed ban on eating or about the deformation of the bowels motivated this type of self-annihilating behaviour. In only ten records were actual attempts at suicide recorded, the majority by drowning, but others did try to cut their veins or hang themselves. One patient even asked his doctor for assistance in his attempt to kill himself.[16] As could be expected, almost half the people with suicidal tendencies were being diagnosed as depressive or suffering from some other mood disorder. Patients from a Calvinist background were over-represented within this group, and there were more men than women who made an actual suicide attempt.

A more or less urgent need for care was mentioned in approximately 25 per cent of the records as a reason for admission. In general, this need could stem from two different origins: the distressed condition of the patient or the incapacity of those who had been looking after him/her. It was mostly mentally retarded or elderly, demented patients who were sent to an asylum for the first reason, some 38 per cent of them being older than 70. Often, it was changes within the family context that impaired its caring ability, e.g. the ageing or death of the main carer or the marriage, moving or new occupation of concerned children or other relatives. In other cases, the burden of care exhausted those involved, unsettling the family and leading to a request for admission of the identified patient.

It was in only two instances that therapy was mentioned as a motive for hospitalisation. The first had to do with a patient with general paralysis who needed to be treated for malaria, the second with an addict who would only abstain forcibly.[7] The relative unimportance of cure as an explicit reason for admission to the psychiatric hospital is symbolical of its function before the 1950s. It was care not cure that characterised the main goal of this institution.

Diagnosis

Looking at the people who ultimately entered the three asylums, the diagnoses they received were reduced to the following broad categories (N = 160):

Cognitive disorder / dementia	28	17.5%
Mood disorders	34	21%
Psychotic disorders	35	22%
Neurological disorders (epilepsy)	9	6%
Addictions	7	4.5%
Mental retardation	15	9.5%
Personality disorders	5	3%
Unknown	16	10%

However, there did exist considerable differences between the three hospitals:

	Voorburg	Endegeest	Wolfheze
Dementia	10%	25.5%	18%
Mood disorders	18%	18%	29%
Psychotic disorders	13%	22%	33%
Neurological disorders	5%	9%	2%
Addictions	5%	9%	2%
Mental retardation	18%	4%	2%
Personality disorders	3%	3.5%	2%
Unknown	23%	-	4.5%

Out and In: The Family and the Asylum

Some of these differences seem to have an obvious, institutional explanation. In Brabant, where almost all of the patients in Voorburg came from, there still existed a considerable number of charity hospitals or guesthouses that, among others, accommodated the elderly destitute. Brabant too was a largely agricultural province, whereas the hospitalisation of the demented seems to have been an urban phenomenon, as demonstrated by the example of Endegeest. A disproportional number of the patients in Endegeest suffering from dementia came from a large town. The low numbers of mentally retarded who entered Endegeest or Wolfheze likewise can be attributed to the existence of specialised institutions for this group within their region; in Endegeest, this was a separate institute within the premises of the asylum.

The striking number of patients who did not receive any diagnosis in Voorburg (almost a quarter) will have something to do with the relatively slender resources of this hospital. Compared with the other two hospitals, its records are sparse, lacking not only diagnoses but also reports of any medical examination or psychiatric interview. The lax attitude towards diagnosis may offer part of the explanation for the conspicuously low number of patients suffering from a psychotic disorder in this hospital.

In all, almost 45 per cent of the population of these three hospitals consisted of people with dementia, neurological complaints or mental retardation. Considering the fact that a similar percentage of those admitted to the asylum was older than 50 (apart from those with dementia, mostly with mood disorders), it will be clear that to a large extent, the asylum had of necessity the role of a (geriatric) nursing home.

Only some 43 per cent of those entering these psychiatric hospitals were thought to be suffering from one of the classical psychiatric illnesses: mood disorders or psychotic disorder (in general, dementia praecox or schizophrenia). The figures from Wolfheze, where some 62 per cent belonged to these two main categories, anticipated the common situation after World War ii, when the feeble-minded and demented were transferred to specialised institutions.

Leaving the Asylum

How long did these people stay within the asylum, under what circumstances did they leave, and how many lived in the institution for the rest of their life and died in it? The statistics provide part of the answer to these questions:

Length of stay	All asylums		Voorburg		Endegeest		Wolfheze	
< 1 year	76	48%	27	45%	32	58%	17	38%
1-5 years	50	31%	19	32%	15	27%	16	36%
> 5 years	32	20%	13	22%	8	15%	11	24%

Ways of discharge	All asylums		Voorburg		Endegeest		Wolfheze	
Cured	34	21%	12	22%	10	18%	11	25%
Improved	24	15%	9	15%	11	22%	4	9%
Cured & improved		36%		37%		40%		33%
Unimproved	11	7%	3	5%	4	7%	4	9%
Against advice	2	1%	2	3%	-	-	-	-
Transferred	20	13%	12	20%	3	6%	5	11%
Deceased	65	41%	20	33%	25	46%	20	44%

No less than 36 per cent (58 patients) of those who were sent to the asylum left it cured or improved, most of them (81 per cent) before a year had passed. Around half (53 per cent; almost one-fifth of the whole group) went home within six months, 36 per cent of them within three months. Those who were discharged in a 'healthier' condition were on average younger (some 60 per cent younger than 40, as against 41 per cent in the whole group) and more often had a family network in society (69 per cent against 59 per cent). Their illness did have an acute character more frequently, whereas 55 per cent were diagnosed as having mood or psychotic disorders.

A fifth of those recorded as 'cured' or 'improved' did not receive any treatment during their period in the asylum, while most of the others (72 per cent) had only done some work or 'occupational therapy', in addition to bed rest for some time. From 1925 onwards, somatic treatments were used for eight of these patients (14 per cent), sometimes resulting in an immediate alleviation of symptoms and early discharge. On the whole, the natural course of the disorder seems to have been the most important factor in the patients' improvement.

Among the first to be discharged from the asylum were those who did not seem to be mentally disordered at all. Apart from a woman with a psychiatric history who was actually suffering from decompensatio cordis, there was a girl of 18 living in a kind of fleeting trance and a young homesick conscript who had made a suicide attempt, said to be of a feigned character.[18] Another man of a good family had only been a little troublesome and refused to work for his father. Failing to show any 'abnormal' behaviour in the asylum, he was discharged from Voorburg within three months.[19]

Another group of patients who left within a few weeks or months were those that entered in a state of vehement agitation and confusion, so that they had to be restrained, isolated or sedated at once. A number of them suffered from what in contemporary jargon was called amentia (or delirium), while others were said to be in the manic phase of a manic-depressive disorder. Prominent among this group were women with puerperal insanity and alcoholics who were admitted in a state of delirium tremens. Without any specific therapy, this extreme behaviour abated in the short term, the patients being sent home, except for one who was transferred to a detox clinic. Two women, one of them pregnant, who had

Out and In: The Family and the Asylum

experienced an epileptic furor just preceding their admission, remained completely calm once in the hospital and were sent away after two months.

Compared with these patients for whom their stay in hospital could be considered a kind of crisis intervention, those suffering from a short melancholic or schizophrenic episode stayed somewhat longer than five months on average. There was another group (six in all) of alcoholics and people with depression or schizophrenia who stayed in between 1.5 to 4 years, returning home improved.

The criteria used to assess the improvement of these patients seem to have been both constant and consistent; they were made explicit in many files by the psychiatrist commenting on the amelioration of the patient's behaviour. Besides calming down and a diminishing of overt symptoms, adjusting to the group and demonstrating a certain co-operativeness were important. Ability to enter a conversation and communicate were emphasized, as well as readiness to work; the fact that a patient was industrious was generally associated with an improvement of his mental state. Work was considered both a road to health and a sign of greater psychological stability. With communication, it was not so much its content as the mere fact of being able to have a coherent conversation that mattered. Next, the expression of interest in one's fellow human beings, and especially one's own family, and a longing for home were seen as indications of a regained mental balance.

Strikingly enough, the complete disappearance of positive symptoms (hallucinations, delusions) never seems to have been a precondition for discharge. From a number of records, it is clear that people left the psychiatric hospital who were still under the influence of a delusion. The same is true for the awareness of being ill. In general, this awareness was interpreted as strong evidence of recovery or improvement, the patient distancing himself from his morbid thoughts or feelings. Nevertheless, people who denied the pathological character of their former behaviour were allowed to leave the institution. Thus, purely medical criteria for recovery did not seem to have been in the foreground; social phenomena like communication, work and social integration were more important.

Permission to leave was almost always given on a probationary basis. From the beginning of the twentieth century, probationary discharge was the customary procedure to put the improved patient to the (social) test. In a legal sense, the person involved still was a rightless, involuntary patient, but he was permitted to live outside the walls of the asylum. It sometimes started with a day or weekend at home, then a week or more, the patient eventually being discharged 'on parole' for months and, in the end, officially being 'taken off the list' as cured or improved.

It was not uncommon, even quite common, for the family or even for patients themselves to ask for a probationary release. The records suggest that psychiatrists were often quite willing to respond to these requests, provided that the patient was on the road to improvement. Discharge on parole was in many cases negotiated between the asylum and the family, constituting the primary scene of interaction between these parties. Patients not yet recovered would go home at the request of their relatives. The family had to report to the superintendent on the behaviour of the patient on leave, sending him/her back to the hospital when he/she disrupted normal life again. The probationary leave created an experimental situation, during which the 'sociability' of the former patient could be tested. Once a family informed the asylum that all was going well, that they could 'live' with the patient, the latter was usually discharged as 'cured' or 'improved'. The most important criterion here seems to have been social integration – a social assessment rather than a medical one. The discharge mirrored the admission procedure, when using the image of Jelgersma: the 'unsociable' behaviour which characterised insanity should become more sociable, regardless of whether or not some psychotic symptoms still remained. As families coped with their disturbed members until escalation triggered referral to an asylum, so they coped with those who were discharged early, often at their own request.

The influence of the family and its readiness to endure 'difficult' behaviour were clearly demonstrated in those cases where patients were discharged 'unimproved' or even against the explicit advice of the psychiatrist. In general, it was the family that pressed for their release, even with patients who were hard to care for or difficult to cope with. For example, children asked for a father to come home; he was a demented paralytic with many disabling neurological complaints. The hospital staff accepted this request even though they had the suspicion that the relatives only had an eye on their father's inheritance.[20] A man who had been very violent at home was discharged unimproved at the request of his children.[21] A mother asked for the release of her insane daughter, described in the records as excited, screaming and incontinent, on the grounds that she needed patience from those around – a kind of tolerance she thought an asylum unable to provide.[22]

Since families asked for their relatives back, they seem to have exerted a certain 'pull' on the hospital. This is demonstrated by the statistics: whereas some 58 per cent of all the patients under study came from a family, of those who were cured or improved, at least 74 per cent went back to their parents, partners or other relatives. (Of all those discharged cured, improved, unimproved or against advice, the figure was 76 per cent.) This does not seem to have been the effect of a better prognosis, which is hardly conceivable, but must partly be explained by the pattern of negotiation between the asylum and families. Those patients who did have a social network in society that could ask and receive them back home did have an advantage over those who had been living in isolation. At least to some extent, discharge was the result of a social process, of the interaction between the asylum and the family, and not the outcome of purely medical or custodial considerations.

The limited extent to which the asylum functioned as a 'repressive' institution that protected public order is paradoxically revealed by the way it handled people whose behaviour could be characterised as 'anti-social' or 'psychopathic'. In the files, at least six patients, mostly feeble-minded men, are described as having an outright criminal record: three had been committing thefts,[23] one was suspected of sexual abuse of minors, and the oldest among them had had an incestuous relationship with his daughter.[24] The sixth patient was the recalcitrant soldier described at the beginning of this article. All of them were discharged from the psychiatric hospital within a year: two were said to be 'improved', the mentally and morally 'defective' soldier among them, and three were released 'unimproved', again at the request of their relatives. One left the asylum at the insistence of his family and against the express will of his doctors, who thought him unfit for society.[25]

Twenty patients, 13 per cent of the sample, left the original asylum to be transferred to another institution. Most of them stayed within the psychiatric domain, being moved to a different asylum, with only a few being sent to an institution for the mentally retarded. In general, the reasons for this transfer were pragmatic; the other institution being cheaper or closer to the residence of the patient's family or belonging to the religious denomination of the inmate. A number of these people went to one of the new asylums that were built around 1900. The asylum Voorburg had the custom of moving chronic cases to its older 'mother-house', the Reinier van Arkel asylum, located in the nearby city of Den Bosch. Such an institutional split between a 'curing' and a 'caring' facility was generally uncommon in psychiatry in the Netherlands.

Staying and Dying in the Asylum

Because of the relatively large number of transferred cases, the actual figure of long-stay patients among the population under study is difficult to assess. At least 32 (20 per cent) were resident in one of these three asylums for more than five years (40 per cent more than two years). The majority of these people had been quite young (57 per cent <40 years) and unmarried at the time of their admission, many having a previous history of mental illness and almost a quarter having been hospitalised previously (in a workhouse, sanatorium, a general or a psychiatric hospital). Their diagnoses had a quite distinct profile: apart from a number of feeble-minded, they were mostly psychotic patients with a diagnosis of dementia praecox or schizophrenia (34 per cent) and older melancholic people (28 per cent). Their patterns of behaviour differed immensely: from a calm and ordered idiot who worked continuously and a patient in a stupor who lay motionless in his bed for years, to the man or woman suffering from chronic mania who was agitated and confused almost without interruption. There where those whose behaviour became more and more eccentric during their long years in the asylum, whereas others declined physically as well as mentally and developed a 'secondary' dementia, living a vegetative life in the ward for many years.

Apart from three patients who left the asylum against advice and three others who were moved from Voorburg to Reinier van Arkel, five of these chronic patients went home in an improved condition after having lived in the hospital for up to 11 years. With some of these, the transformation occurred quite suddenly and unexpectedly: a woman who thought herself to be sinful, mutilated herself and showed suicidal tendencies (she was diagnosed as hysterical) had been in the hospital, with only a short interruption, from 1928, then in 1943 her mood changed for the better within a month, no treatment having been applied. Within two months, she was sent to a boarding house, described as 'almost cured'.[26] Whereas three of the others also did not receive any systematic treatment, apart from some occupational therapy, the application of electroshock triggered a change in one young woman with schizophrenia after she had been in Voorburg for more than eight years. From being autistic, childish and at times aggressive, she became 'sociable' in a matter of months and was sent home under the supervision of the asylum.[27]

The striking finding in the discharge rates is the overall mortality of around 40 per cent: 65 patients in all. The actual number of deaths was even higher, the figures for Voorburg being flattered because of the relatively large number of hopeless chronic patients who were systematically transferred to the adjacent asylum of Reinier van Arkel. The majority of those who died in the asylum had been quite old at the moment of admission, 70 per cent being older than 50 and 46 per cent older than 65. Dementia was the most prominent symptom among this group (58 per cent); many of those who died eventually had been admitted because they needed care (40 per cent). Indeed, almost 50 per cent remained in bed for a considerable amount of time, only about a third being occupied with some kind of work. Mortality was spread unevenly between the different groups: of all those with the diagnosis of dementia, 93 per cent died in the asylum (26 patients); with general paralysis, this was 60 per cent, with neurological disorders (mainly epilepsy), 44 per cent; and of those with depression or other mood disorders, some 40 per cent expired in hospital.

A considerable number of patients (almost 11 per cent) died during their first year in the asylum. Apart from those who entered in an already hopeless physical state (TB, general paralysis), at least nine elderly patients, most of them over 70, died within two months of admission. Ageing, senile decay of both mental and bodily functions, together with somatic disease (of heart and lungs) combined to create a state of weakness, confusion or delirium and sometimes restiveness. Unable to care for them, their families had sought the help of the asylum, which acted for these often terminal patients as a nursing home and a hospice for the dying.

Out and In: The Family and the Asylum

Of the long-stay patients, 23 (72 per cent of the whole group) died during their stay in the asylum. Having grown old in the institution, many of them died a 'natural' death from exhaustion, marasmus, heart failure, apoplexy, etc., but some 22 per cent perished from the tuberculosis they seem to have contracted during their long stay. It was primarily those patients who had entered the hospital before the age of 40 who fell victim to TB. Pneumonia also caused the death of a number of fragile, enfeebled patients, both young and old. That the asylum was an 'unhealthy' environment and that the number of deaths as a result of tuberculosis and other conditions of the lungs was disproportionate was widely acknowledged at the time.

Epilogue

Studying a continuous series of patient records in great detail certainly changed my image of the history and character of the psychiatric hospital. Whereas I had been used to describe the development of the asylum as a succession of therapeutic regimes and changing anthropological or scientific paradigms (e.g. biological versus psychodynamic positions), reading the files drastically qualifies the meaning of therapy or shifting paradigms at the level of the individual patient, at least until the 1970s. Therapeutic or medical interventions, even in a wider sense, did not stamp life on the wards. Therapy, if it was used at all, was marginal and incidental. Even in the first half of the twentieth century, the asylum was a place in which to stay. It was characterised by a culture of care, not of cure, the regulation of disturbed behaviour dominating its daily practice. At the level of everyday life and routine, changes were slow, almost imperceptible, and continuities strong.

One of the important elements of this change of my image of psychiatry lay in the surprising discovery in these case histories of the dynamic interaction between families and the asylum. Case histories enable us to analyse step by step when, why, and by whom people were sent to an asylum and when, why and how they left it. The social patterns that can be traced in admission and especially in discharge show that the walls of the asylum were not as high as had been expected beforehand.

Paradoxically, the case histories show in the fragmentary information they contain about the life of the patient before admission that the asylum was just one of the possible responses to mental illness. Domestic care, consultations with general practitioners or psychiatrists, and care in workhouses, nursing homes or general hospitals were among the 'alternatives' to admission in an asylum. The mental hospital was part, maybe the most important one at a certain period, of a wider culture and social network to cope with mental illness. This conclusion is supported by recent epidemiological research which demonstrates that even today, only a fraction of those identified as suffering from mental problems or disease are in contact with official mental health services.[28] Future research into the history of psychiatry should widen its focus to encompass these different and wider societal responses to psychopathology. For that, we will also have to look to sources other than the institutional case histories if we are to trace these other 'strategies' beyond the confines of the asylum.

The patient records show that at least during the first half of the twentieth century, families did cope with and care for their disturbed relatives, sometimes for a considerable period of time and even when these individuals suffered from serious disturbances. In general, two major circumstances made them decide to refer their relatives to an asylum: changes in the conduct of the 'patient' or in his social environment. Mental illness as such (e.g. the delusion or depression) does not seem to have constituted the prime motive for admission. It was behaviour that disrupted the social integration of the patient (agitation, confusion, danger, etc.) that most often triggered an admission procedure. The fact that the danger constituted by those who lived in a family at the moment of referral was more concrete and grave suggests that families did tolerate even extreme behaviour. On the other hand, changes in the family that weakened its capacity to cope and to care, e.g. the death of a relative or the exhaustion of its social resilience, could provoke committal to a psychiatric hospital. The idea that families were eager to get rid of their 'deviant' or alienated relatives should certainly be questioned in the light of the stories told in these case histories. Families seem to have been hesitant in sending someone of their own blood to an institution; they waited, endured and looked for alternative solutions.

The patterns of discharge in a way mirrored the process of admission. First of all, the criteria for improvement seem primarily to have had a 'social' character: it was the patient's ability to communicate, to work and to integrate in a social environment that was thought to be more important than awareness of being ill or the disappearance of all positive symptoms. Secondly, families did exert a clear influence on the discharge of their relatives: they requested and negotiated release with the staff of the hospital. On the whole, doctors seem to have been quite willing to grant these requests, the probationary discharge (already in use at the beginning of the twentieth century) being their instrument of choice to try out the patient's ability to reintegrate in his social milieu and society at large. Families for their part showed a certain readiness to cope with relatives who had not been cured or relieved in purely medical terms – a fact underscored by the number of 'unimproved' patients who were sent home at the request of their relatives. Families did exert a certain 'pull' on the asylum, resulting in higher chances to leave the hospital for those inmates with an active family. This observation gainsays the idea of the asylum as a closed, high walled, custodial institution, impervious to interaction with the social milieu of its patients and society.

Out and In: The Family and the Asylum

Around 40 per cent of all patients left the hospital and went home in this way; cured, improved, unimproved or against the advice of the staff. Many of them did so in the first year after their admission and at the request of their families. Considering the fact that many of the other patients were really incurable (the mentally retarded, those suffering from dementia or debilitating neurological diseases) or terminal, for whom the hospital virtually had a different function (more of a geriatric nursing home), the asylum as such should be characterised in more dynamic terms than is commonly done. At the same time, its social function as a temporary asylum in the original sense of the word (a refuge, a 'time out' from society/family) needs to be emphasized, in contrast to its medical role as a real therapeutic institution.

Notes

1.   1917-3-16 END.
2.   J. Braslow, *Mental Ills and Bodily Cures: Psychiatric Treatment in the First Half of the Twentieth Century* (Berkeley: University of California Press 1997). There are some Dutch examples as well: Giel Hutschemaekers and Christoph Hrachovec (eds), *Heer en heelmeesters. Negentig jaar zorg voor zenuwlijders in het christelijk sanatorium te Zeist* (Nijmegen: SUN, 1993). Of a more statistical nature are: J.W.M. Jongmans, *Psychiatrisch Ziekenhuis Coudewater 1870-1970. Medisch-historisch verslag* (Rosmalen: Psychiatrisch Ziekenhuis Coudewater, 1971); H.F.M. Peeters et al., 'Historische veranderingen in aard en behandeling van geesteszieken. Een exploratief kwantitatief onderzoek in het psychiatrisch ziekenhuis Voorburg te Vught, 1885-1977'. (Unpublished internal report, Katholieke Hogeschool Tilburg, 1979); *idem*, 'Een historische analyse van een provinciaal psychiatrisch centrum over de periode 1885-1977', in: J.M.W. Binneveld et al., *Een psychiatrisch verleden. Uit de geschiedenis van de psychiatrie* (Baarn: Ambo, 1982), 154-80.
3.   A. Digby, *Madness, Morality and Medicine. A Study of the York Retreat 1796-1914* (Cambridge: Cambridge University Press, 1985); C. Mackenzie, *Psychiatry for the Rich. A History of Ticehurst Private Asylum, 1792-1917* (London: Routledge, 1992).
4.   G.B. Risse and J.H. Warner, 'Reconstructing Clinical Activities: Patient Records in Medical History', *Social History of Medicine*, 5 (1992), 183-206; Jonathan Andrews, 'Case Notes, Case Histories, and the Patient's Experience of Insanity at Gartnavel Royal Asylum, Glasgow, in the Nineteenth Century', *Social History of Medicine*, 11, 2 (1998), 255-81.
5.   M. MacDonald, *Mystical Bedlam: Madness, Anxiety and Healing in Seventeenth-Century England* (Cambridge: Cambridge University Press, 1981).
6.   H. Binneveld en R. Wolf, *Een huis met vele woningen. 100 jaar katholieke psychiatrie. Voorburg 1885-1985* (Vught: Algemeen Psychiatrisch Ziekenhuis Voorburg, 1985); Peeters, *op. cit.* (note 2: Historische veranderingen), *passim*; *idem, op. cit.* (note 2: 'Een historische analyse'), *passim*.

7.   Gemma Blok and Joost Vijselaar, *Terug naar Endegeest. Patiënten en hun behandeling in het psychiatrisch ziekenhuis Endegeest 1897-1997* (Nijmegen: SUN, 1998).

8.   G.A. Lindeboom and M.J. van Lieburg, *Gedenkboek van de Vereniging tot christelijke verzorging van geestes- en zenuwzieken, 1884-1984* (Kampen: Kok, 1984).

9.   Http://www.qsrinternational.com/; for general information about computer assisted qualitative data analysing software: http://caqdas.soc.surrey.ac.uk/index.htm

10.   1932-4-2 END; 1937-05-31 WOL.

11.   1922-5-10 VOO; 1932-03-17 VOO.

12.   1922-7-1 END; 1932-03-17 VOO.

13.   1937-02-19 WOL; 1937-01-06 VOO; 1937-1-6 WOL.

14.   H. Jelgersma, *Voorzorg verpleging en nazorg* (s.l.: s.p., 1928), 9-10; Blok and Vijselaar, *op. cit.* (note 7), 97.

15.   1912-04-04 VOO; 1902-05-03 END.

16.   1942-4-4 WOL.

17.   1932-7-19 END; 1941-12-31 VOO.

18.   1922-3-7 END; 1927-9-26 END; 1947-01-03 VOO.

19.   1902-2-1 VOO.

20.   1912-10-24 END.

21.   1942-2-11 VOO.

22.   1922-4-21 END.

23.   1942-01-19 VOO; 1942-6-10 WOL; 1892-3-8 VOO.

24.   1937-7-13 WOL; 1927-01-03 VOO.

25.   1892-3-8 VOO.

26.   1942-4-4 WOL.

27.   1937-2-12 VOO.

28.   R.V. Bijl and A. Ravelli, 'Psychiatric Morbidity, Service Use, and Need for Care in the General Population', *American Journal of Public Health*, 90 (2000), 602-7.

CHAPTER 12

Were Asylums Men's Places?

Male Excess in the Asylum Population in Japan in the Early Twentieth Century

*Akihito Suzuki**

Introduction

The subject of psychiatry and gender has attracted considerable scholarly attention in the last two decades.[1] From the late 1980s, the cultural history of women's madness has become an established sub-genre within the history of psychiatry and madness, through path-breaking works by Elaine Showalter and Mark Micale, to name just two.[2] More recently, the gender history of insanity has incorporated various approaches and historiographies, such as men's history and colonial history.[3] This chapter attempts to further expand the subject by bringing in the perspective of international comparison. Although it discusses mainly Japanese material, I have tried to go beyond a regional study and take a step towards a genuinely international social history of gender and psychiatry. Throughout, I will use one index that can be easily obtained for other countries: the ratio of male to female psychiatric patients (M/F ratio, or the number of male patients divided by the number of female patients).

In the first half of the twentieth century, Japanese psychiatric statistics presented a striking male excess. Between three-fifths and two-thirds of all hospitalised patients were men, M/F ratio fluctuating between 1.4 and 1.9.[4] Public and private patients shared roughly the same M/F ratio, despite their stark contrasts in many aspects.[5] Chronologically speaking, the national M/F ratio was roughly constant during the pre-war period of 1900-1940. Regional fluctuation existed, but in none of 47 prefectures did female patients outnumber male ones. This male predominance is supported by very robust evidence.

This characteristic of the Japanese psychiatric population deserves close attention, particularly because few, if any, countries in Europe and North America reported so large an excess of male 'lunatics' in the nineteenth and early twentieth century. In the 1830s and 1840, when Esquirol in France and Thurnam in England established asylum-based epidemiology as a genre of psychiatric research, psychiatrists did not obtain any clear-cut and uniform bias in the distribution of men and women in asylums.[6] When, in 1845, Thurnam claimed he finally found 'decided' evidence of a male excess in British asylums, he was talking about 13.7 per cent (M/F ratio being 1.14), a tiny excess if compared with the Japanese data that showed up to 100 per cent.[7] In 1899, in the 6th edition of his *Psychiatry*, Kraepelin maintained that 'statistical frequency does not reveal any considerable and reliable difference between both sexes'.[8] The Japanese M/F ratio of around 1.4-1.9 during the early twentieth century might well have been unique at that time, although the scope of my research into international comparisons is still very limited. The exceptionally large M/F ratio of Japan thus provides us with a solid and robust statistical basis for making a clear-cut analysis of the question of gender and psychiatric committal.

Psychiatrists in pre-war Japan were certainly aware of the disparity between their data and those reported in Europe. They knew, for instance, that Kraepelin and other German psychiatrists found that a decidedly higher proportion of manic-depressive admissions were female, and that men and women had roughly matched numbers in dementia praecox, while Japanese data almost invariably showed a substantial male excess in both diagnostic categories.[9] Seen from the viewpoint of present historians, these differences are very intriguing, inviting us to examine them and speculate on the causes that created them. In contrast, Japanese psychiatrists in the early twentieth century were more interested in finding Euro-Japanese similarities than studying their differences, being more comfortable in confirming what their German teachers had said. The large disparity between the M/F ratio of the European asylum population and that in Japan puzzled rather than interested pre-war Japanese psychiatrists. Moreover, they studied the statistics of psychiatric hospitals to investigate the prevalence of mental diseases and their causes, rather than to analyse the mechanism of committal to institutions. In other words, the psychiatric epidemiology of two sexes, not the analysis of gender-related factors underlying hospital statistics, was their major goal.

This chapter attempts to investigate what they failed to do. My focus will be on the gender-difference in the mechanism of committal of patients from their home to an institution. Although the M/F ratio may have been skewed in certain diagnostic categories because of the difference in the exposure to causal agents (e.g. addiction to alcohol and drugs), I will demonstrate below that the mechanism of committal was more important than the prevalence of mental disorders in creating the huge male excess in the early twentieth century.

Psychiatric Provision in Pre-WWII Japan

The treatment and confinement of the insane in Japan has a long history. By the late nineteenth century, a diversified system of care for the mentally ill already existed. On the eve of the Meiji Restoration in 1868, at least 29 medical and reli-

Were Asylums Men's Places?

gious institutions took care of the insane. Large cities had developed custodial institutions which housed the mentally ill together with vagrants, the physically sick, and the destitute. The most elusive but undoubtedly most important locus of care had been the family. They provided care and security by confining the patient in a cage ('sashiko') set up within the house, with the permission of the local authorities.[10] This indigenous system of provision for the insane was the background into which Western-style psychiatry was implanted from the 1870s.

'Modern' provision for the insane by the central government was provided through two Acts of Parliament – the Mental Patients' Custody Act (1900) and the Mental Hospitals Act (1919), both of which were repealed by the Mental Health Act in 1950. The Custody Act demanded that a lunatic be confined only by the officially appointed custodian, who was normally a family member, with the authority of the local government of city, town or village.[11] When a competent custodian could not be found, the administrative head of the local government would assume that status. The place of custody was usually the patient's own home, rather than a specialist institution. In 1905, about 12,000 patients were confined in their home, while about 5,500 were in institutions.[12] A cage with a heavy lock had to be set up in or close to the house, according to a detailed plan submitted to the local administrative office.[13] Perhaps to allow light and air into the cage and to facilitate vigilance over the confined person, a latticework seems to have been the norm. This meant extremely high visibility of the patient in confinement, and those now in their sixties or seventies still retain vivid memories of the chilling horror and fascination with which they watched a 'furious' patient through the lattice.

The Custody Act essentially left the care of the insane to the patient's family. The Mental Hospitals Act, on the other hand, assigned a more active role to the public authorities, particularly the state, and attempted to expand institutional confinement. To achieve this goal, the act empowered the central government to order the prefectures (a larger local governmental unit, comparable to counties in England) to build public asylums. Half of the cost of building and one-sixth of the cost for maintaining the patients would be covered by the central government, the rest being paid by the prefectures. This plan must have looked unrealistic, however, for the public sector in psychiatric provision was very small in Japan at that time. In 1918, there was only one public asylum, which was in Tokyo and housed about 450 patients. In contrast, in the same year, 57 private psychiatric hospitals already existed, which together housed about 4,000 patients.[14] Moreover, many of the private hospitals regularly admitted patients whose cost was paid by their local authority, either through the Custody Act or otherwise.[15] This large mixed sector of psychiatric provision was codified through the Mental Hospitals Act in 1919. Several private asylums were allotted a certain number of 'substitute' beds and accepted public patients up to that number. Private mental hospitals that were thus appointed were called 'substitute hospitals' and were to become a major provider of the care for the insane for the next couple of decades.

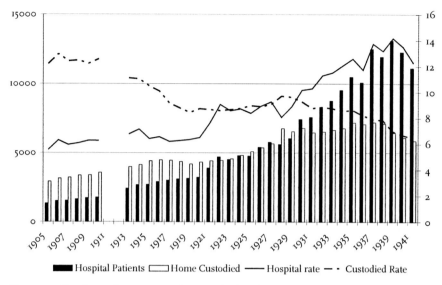

Figure 1   *Number and Percentage of Hospitalised and Home-Custodied Patients, 1905-1940*

The two acts structured pre-war psychiatric provision, which had somewhat contradictory aims, one centring on home custody and the other on hospitalisation. Figure 1 indicates a clear shift in the locus of confinement from home to hospital. The hospital, the cornerstone institution of the Mental Hospitals Act, was on its way to success, presenting the familiar picture of medicalisation and institutionalisation of the care for the insane.[16] On closer examination, however, the first point to be noted is the timing of the decline of home custody. In proportion to the total number of registered patients, this decline started around 1910, about ten years before the passing of the Mental Hospitals Act and before the significant rise in the number of hospitalised patients. Despite the image promoted of mental hospitals as the modernising institution against the evil of home custody, the latter had started to decline on its own, rather than being overwhelmed by the former. This is not very surprising if one recalls that the Custody Act imposed strict regulation on the private confinement of the insane, making it more official and difficult. The other point to be noted is the ambiguous impact of the Mental Hospitals Act. This act undoubtedly contributed to the dramatic rise in hospitalised patients after 1920: the number of public hospitals and substitute hospitals grew from 8 (one public and 7 substitute hospitals) in 1919 to 84 (7 public and 77 substitute ones) in 1940. However, neither the public nor the mixed sector bore the major burden of care for the insane. Table 1 shows the proportion of publicly supported and fee-paying patients in mental hospitals in total, taken from statistics in *The Annual Report of Hygiene*. While the proportion of publicly supported patients resident in private institutions actually *declined*, the purely private type of hospitalisation, i.e. patients who paid for their

Were Asylums Men's Places?

stay at privately run hospitals actually *grew*. The proportional growth of privately funded confinement reveals a hitherto little-noticed aspect of the rise of mental hospitals in pre-war Japan: the emergence of a large number of people who were ready to pay significant sums of money to be treated there. In other words, the growth of the *demand* for psychiatric services contributed significantly to the evolution of a society that segregated a large number of the insane. The demand for psychiatric services at hospitals became larger, but it was met only partially by public provision, the gap between the demand and the public supply being filled by private means.

Table 1 *Percentage of Public and Fee-Paying Patients in Public and Private Hospitals*

	Public Hospitals		Private Hospitals	
Year	Public Patients	Fee-paying Patients	Public Patients	Fee-paying Patients
1928	11.0	5.1	50.0	33.4
29	13.6	4.7	44.5	35.8
30	12.7	4.2	49.4	33.6
31	13.0	3.8	50.1	33.1
32	12.1	3.7	49.5	34.6
33	12.5	3.6	47.3	36.9
34	12.0	3.9	47.1	36.9
35	11.3	3.7	46.5	38.9
36	11.5	3.8	46.1	38.7
37	11.9	4.1	44.7	39.3
38	11.3	4.3	43.0	41.2
39	10.5	4.3	40.4	44.8
40	10.3	5.0	39.6	45.1

The importance of the demand side vis-à-vis the supply side suggests that to understand the mechanism of the growth of psychiatric provision in Japan in the early twentieth century, we should examine the role of the family as an important actor in institutionalisation. The family normally brought its insane member to a psychiatric hospital. It is true that there existed cases in which the police brought troublesome lunatics to the hospital, but such cases were few. Likewise, public authorities did occasionally organise a large-scale 'hunting' of wandering lunatics, but such forceful confinement was exceedingly rare.[17] Without denying the indirect influence of such activities of public authorities on the demands of families for psychiatric care, the initiative for confinement normally came from the patient's family. Moreover, the family continued to provide a major locus of care of the insane: thousands of patients were registered as lunatics but were not confined either at home or in a hospital – just remaining in their own home. Those patients were called 'non-custodied' patients, and they vastly outnumbered both home-custodied and hospitalised patients. For most of the period under review, about 80 per cent of the registered patients were 'non-custodied'. Although the figure became slightly lower in the 1930s, in 1941 about 70 per cent of registered mental patients still remained at home, nominally under no restraint. The family thus had a large pool of home-residing patients, from which psychiatric hospitals drew their inmates.

This account of the intersection of the family and the asylum illustrates the key role played by the families of patients in their institutionalisation. Psychiatric hospitalisation largely resulted from the family's decision, for one reason or another, to send the patient to an institution. In this context, the question of M/F ratio of Japanese hospitalised patients will next be examined. To avoid complications due to the mixture of gender-biased diagnoses (e.g. war neurosis, alcohol and drug addictions, hysteria, puerperal insanity), below I shall largely concentrate on one diagnosis, namely schizophrenia.

Schizophrenia and the Social Meaning of Symptoms

Schizophrenia or dementia praecox was the most frequently employed diagnosis for pre-war hospitalised patients. In 1935, schizophrenic patients accounted for about 44.7 per cent of the admissions to about 130 mental hospitals. The condition's share of the resident population was even higher and reached 63.1 per cent, since schizophrenics were more likely to become chronic cases and to stay longer in the hospital than those suffering from other mental disorders.[18] In the post-war years, schizophrenia continued to dominate the psychiatric hospitals: in 1952, it accounted for 56.2 per cent of the resident patients, vastly exceeding manic-depressive insanity (9.0 per cent) and GPI (7.6 per cent).[19] The M/F ratio of hospitalised schizophrenics during the years between 1927 and 1931 was 1.91, meaning roughly two male patients to one female. It has continued to show male excess up to today, although the male excess has become progressively smaller – from 1.91 in the 1930s to 1.45 in 1975 and 1.30 in 1987.[20]

No historical data are available which would throw light on whether the causes of schizophrenia were differently distributed between men and women. Nevertheless, from several pieces of indirect evidence, one can reasonably assume that the respective male and female prevalence of the condition itself did not differ as greatly as the M/F ratio of hospitalised schizophrenics. The evidence concurs in suggesting that the male excess of hospitalised schizophrenics in pre-war Japan was a product of gender differences in the mechanism of committal to psychiatric institution, rather than a reflection of differences in morbidity. In other words, schizophrenic women were missing from the asylum statistics, so they must have been taken care of – or neglected – at home.

Were Asylums Men's Places?

This is most clearly shown in the discrepancy between the M/F ratio of hospital-ised schizophrenics and that of total schizophrenics, including both hospital-ised and non-hospitalised patients. Non-hospitalised schizophrenics had eluded the psychiatrists' attention until the late 1930s, when several large-scale surveys were conducted under the leadership of Yûshi Uchimura, a professor of psych-iatry at University of Tokyo from 1936 to 1958. Stimulated by this research, an even larger-scale survey was conducted in a city in Chiba Prefecture in 1946 by the newly created National Institute of Mental Hygiene. The city's rural sur-rounding region became the subject of another survey in 1953. The momentum that drove these studies culminated in 1954 in a colossal nation-wide psychiatric survey of about 23,000 individuals from 100 regions, which was acknowledged to be the largest and the most systematic of its kind ever undertaken in the world.[21] Thanks to those and other surveys, we are able to measure the M/F ratio of 'hidden' cases of mental disorders cared for at home, with which we can com-pare hospital data. Table 2 shows the number of people diagnosed as schizo-phrenic by doctors in the surveys between 1940 and 1972.[22]

Table 2 *Numbers of Schizophrenics Discovered in Psychiatric Surveys, 1940-1972*

Region	Prefecture	Year	Type of Region	Population Surveyed	Male	Female	Total	M:F Ratio
Hachijo-jima	Tokyo	1940	Island	8318	22	10	32	2.20
Muraoka-mura	Kanagawa	1941	Village	1704	4	3	7	1.33
Ikebukuro	Tokyo	1942	Large city	2712	3	3	6	1.00
Komoro-cho	Nagano	1943	Small city	5207	6	5	11	1.20
Ichikawa-shi	Chiba	1946-53	Medium-sized city	110000	109	115	224	0.95
Koshiki-jima	Kagoshima	1957	Island	6783	29	21	50	1.38
Hachijo-jima	Tokyo	1964	Island	1207	32	25	57	1.28
Henza-jima	Okinawa	1969	Island	2379	10	11	21	0.91
Oki-gun	Shimane	1972	Island	2826	12	12	24	1.00

Sources: Nakane et al., 'Prevalence Rate of Schizophrenia in Japan', 432, Table 2; *Sources of Mental Hygiene* 5 (1957), p. 4, Table 1.

The figures include both hospitalised and non-hospitalised patients, with 'un-certain cases' being excluded. M/F ratios revealed in the surveys fluctuated from one to another, from 0.91 to 2.20. However, with the exception of the survey in Hachijo-Jima Island in 1940, they do not exhibit as large a male excess as was revealed among hospitalised schizophrenics in the same time period. Statistics of the overall number of mental patients tell the same story. The nationwide sur-vey conducted in 1954 found in total 112 males and 114 females suffering from mental disorders of all kinds out of 23,000 subjects between the ages of 18 and

59 (M/F ratio = 0.98), while in 1958, 2,854 men and 1,887 women in total were discharged from mental hospitals (M/F ratio = 1.51).[23] Another set of data suggests the continuity of the same pattern in the 1970s and 1980s: while men consistently and substantially outnumbered women in the hospitalised population (M/F ratio = 1.25-1.41), female outpatients regularly outnumbered male ones (M/F ratio = 0.82-1.06).[24] All these pieces of evidence suggest that the huge male excess in the hospitalised population resulted from differential *hospitalisation*, not differential *morbidity* itself: female mental patients were under-represented in the hospitalised population, and male patients were much more likely to be treated in hospitals than at home.

Why, then, was this the case? What factors kept a greater proportion of mentally disordered women at home, and why were similar men sent to psychiatric institutions more often? I would like to argue that three inter-related factors were at work – the meanings of symptoms, the role of psychiatric institutions, and the capacity of the family to take care of its insane members. Men and women exhibited symptoms whose social meanings were different. The symptoms prioritised for hospital admission were exhibited more often by male patients, while those of female patients signalled that they could be controlled outside the walls of the asylum. The capacity of psychiatric hospitals was still small, while the Japanese family was able or even ready to bear the burden of keeping its mentally disordered member at home, without recourse to his/her institutionalisation. The balance of the capacity of institutions and that of the family thus tipped toward the latter. Under such a regime of psychiatric provision, hospitalised populations skewed towards men, and more women were treated at home. In other words, the sexual composition of the asylum population in early twentieth-century Japan resulted from the intersection of public policy over the nature and number of psychiatric institutions, and the private culture of the family.

Thus, men and women expressed different symptoms, which were construed differently by those around them, in terms of what should be done. The crucial difference lay in the pattern of dangerousness. This is most clearly seen in a study by Saburo Okuda, based on 1576 schizophrenics (873 males and 703 females) who were admitted to Matsuzawa Hospital between 1926 and 1936 and whose case records were detailed enough for retrospective analysis.[25] Table 3, only slightly modified from the original table, lists the types of what Okuda called 'anti-social acts' committed by the patients before their admission. The number and rate of patients who exhibited each type of dangerous behaviour are shown. Okuda divided his 'anti-social acts' into two categories: those which were dangerous to oneself and those dangerous to others. The two categories were further divided into 4 and 12 sub-categories, respectively. He then added up the cases that exhibited each type of dangerous act and calculated their percentages against the total numbers of male or female schizophrenics.

　　　　　　　　　　　　　　　　　Were Asylums Men's Places?

Table 3 *Anti-Social and Dangerous Behaviour among Schizophrenics Admitted to Matsuzawa Hospital, 1926-1935*

	Male		Female		Total		M:F ratio
	Number	Rate	Number	Rate	Number	Rate	
Anti-Social Behaviour	402	46.0	207	29.4	609	38.64	1.56
– Crime	56	6.4	10	1.4	66	4.19	4.51
Dangerous to Oneself							
– Suicide	109	12.5	80	11.4	189	11.99	1.10
– Disorderly behaviour	57	6.5	12	1.7	69	4.38	3.83
– Vagrancy	53	6.1	38	5.4	91	5.77	1.12
– Wandering	20	2.3	25	3.6	45	2.86	0.64
Total	239	27.4	155	22.0	394	25.00	1.24
Dangerous to Others							
– Murder	20	2.3	12	1.7	32	2.03	1.34
– Injury	30	3.4	3	0.4	33	2.09	8.05
– Abuse of Weapons	22	2.5	5	0.7	27	1.71	3.54
– Disturbance	94	10.8	39	5.5	133	8.44	1.94
– Theft	19	2.2	1	0.1	20	1.27	15.30
– Arson	30	3.4	18	2.6	48	3.05	1.34
– Litigious	30	3.4	6	0.9	36	2.28	4.03
– Lese Majesty	12	1.4	1	0.1	13	0.82	9.66
– Offence of the Order Act	6	0.7	0	0.0	6	0.38	-
– Clever crime	5	0.6	0	0.0	5	0.32	-
– Gambling	3	0.3	1	0.1	4	0.25	2.42
– Bilking	10	1.1	1	0.1	11	0.70	8.05
Total	281	32.2	87	12.4	368	23.35	2.60
Total	873	100	703	100	1576	100	

M:F ratio = Male rate / Female rate
Source: Saburo Okuda, 'Clinical and Statistical Study of Dementia Praecox', 900-901, Table 14.

The overall difference is striking: before admission, male schizophrenics were decidedly more likely to have committed acts that were, and were perceived to be, 'anti-social': 402 out of 873 men (46.0 per cent) and 207 out of 703 women (29.4 per cent). In other words, male schizophrenics admitted to Mastuzawa Hospital were 1.5 times as likely to have committed anti-social acts which were dangerous as their female counterparts. One can also assume that anti-social acts committed by women were of a less serious nature, for men had committed crimes or gravely anti-social acts about four times as often as women. Moreover, men were much more likely to be dangerous to others, while roughly the same proportion of men and women committed various types of violence against

Akihito Suzuki

themselves. All the sub-categories of dangerous acts against others exhibit massive male proportional excess, while those of dangerous acts against themselves do not show as large a male excess, apart from 'disorderly behaviour', whose inclusion into this category is somewhat questionable. Men's symptoms were more likely perceived to be seriously dangerous to others, while women's were regarded as less serious, and as directed more towards themselves.

Okuda's results are striking in showing that male and female hospitalised schizophrenics exhibited different patterns of symptoms in terms of dangerousness. His findings are, however, somewhat difficult to interpret. Do they mean that men and women tended to show different types of symptoms, due to their biological differences? Or did people employ different standards to gauge and measure men and women's disruptive behaviour? Perhaps all of these factors might have been at work. The most likely and broadly inclusive explanation is that since men and women in Japan at that time lived in separate spheres, they posited different types of danger when they suffered from schizophrenia. The male excess in dangerous acts against others was, to a considerable extent, a reflection of the fact that men were much more likely to be active in the public sphere and to be engaged in situations that had a potential of disturbance to a larger number of people. For example, the most political offences committed by schizophrenics – *lèse majesté* and offences against the Maintenance of the Public Order Act – are all infringements of norms or laws in the public sphere, which was almost exclusively a man's world in Japan at that time. It is therefore understandable that schizophrenics who had exhibited these types of dangerousness before their confinement were almost exclusively male. Public disorder and the use of violence (murder, injury, abuse of weapons) were largely a male schizophrenic's problem, since these criminal acts were largely committed by men, whether sane or insane. The only category of public dangerousness that did not show a large male excess was arson: this was understandable, for the use of fire could be widely practised by women for cooking and domestic heating. Men, who led lives in both the private and public spheres, were likely to cause a wider variety of disturbance. Their dangerous abnormality was also expressed in a manner more visible than that of women, because men normally led a more public life – taking part in politics, conducting business, etc. To sum up, the 'open' sociability of the men's world resulted in their exhibiting more visible and publicly dangerous symptoms under insanity, while the 'closed' world of women meant their schizophrenic symptoms were of a more private nature.

It should be noted that more than one-third of schizophrenics admitted to Matsuzawa Hospital exhibited tangibly 'anti-social' behaviour. Confining visibly dangerous patients was one of the major functions of the psychiatric hospital, however hard psychiatrists emphasized the role of medical cure and humanitarian care provided there. It has been a commonplace cliché of anti-psychiatric criticism that a mental hospital was more a place for social control for confining

Were Asylums Men's Places?

disturbing individuals than one in which to practise medicine, but such a characterisation is valid for pre-war psychiatric hospitals in Japan.[26] When one of the major functions of the psychiatric hospital was to confine dangerous individuals, it is quite natural that it accepted more men than women, for men were more visibly and gravely dangerous. The priority given to publicly dangerous cases for hospital admission directed more men to asylums.

One should not assume, however, a consistent social policy or ideology that assigned psychiatric hospitals the role of confining visibly dangerous individuals. Rather, it was a product of a balance between the hospital and the family. Firstly, it should be emphasized that psychiatric facilities were very small in Japan before the 1960s. Japanese psychiatrists had painfully to admit this as a sign of the 'backwardness' of their country. In 1928-29, England, Germany, Switzerland and USA had more than 250 beds per 100,000, while Japan had only 21.1, lagging behind Czechoslovakia (82.6) and Greece (30.0).[27] In 1952, the Japanese figure was still about 22.6 per 100,000, less than one-twelfth of the USA (278), and about one-fourteenth of England & Wales (313).[28] Psychiatric beds were naturally occupied by those who were severely insane and who exhibited grave symptoms, among which highly visible danger must have been given priority. Necessity, as well as social policy, dictated that confining 'hard core' patients should be a major function of psychiatric hospitals. In other words, psychiatric institutions, having only a limited number of beds, could not afford to take care of those who were 'just' insane. To enjoy the 'privilege' of being admitted to an institution, one needed to be insane in a noisy or highly visible way. The capacity of psychiatric hospitals, especially that of public ones, was too small to meet all demands, and private beds were too expensive for people with modest means to stay there for long.

On the other hand, the Japanese family at that time had a considerable capacity to take care of its insane member, due to its system of household formation. Most typically, a household consisted of two married couples and their unmarried children. Normally, the first male child continued to live with his parents after his marriage. This 'stem family' system provided a Japanese family with a large capacity for the care of its dependent member: there were normally two male breadwinners, with two adult women who contributed to the family in various ways – doing household chores, tending young children, or earning a smaller income. When one or both of the older married couple became incapacitated due to old age, the younger couple bore the burden of supporting and nursing the elderly parents. The Japanese family thus had as its built-in function a capacity to take care of its disabled members. This meant that the family had a larger capacity to cope with any crisis of mental disorder of a member than was the case for a nuclear family system. Moreover, a strong socio-cultural norm dictated that the head of the household, who was normally one of the husband-fathers, should support, manage and control other members of the family. This strong sense of patriarchal responsibility must have been a strong disincentive to refer a mental patient who was a dependent member of his family to a psychiatric hospital for long-term care. On the other hand, the incentive to send publicly dangerous patients to institutions of confinement must have been very strong, since under the Old Criminal Code of 1880, the family was liable to a heavy penalty if it let an insane family member wander around and do any harm.[29] The Japanese family could thus contain an incapacitated mentally disordered member relatively easily, though at the same time, it needed to put strict restraint upon a patient who was manifestly out of the family's control, to avoid the heavy fine. The priority given by hospitals to overtly dangerous cases was thus largely a response to the family's demand. On the other hand, families were unlikely to ask the hospital to take care of manageable patients, particularly when they had to pay for the hospitalisation. The large male excess in the asylum population thus resulted from this differential choice for different types of symptoms, which was necessitated by the balance between the family's demand and the hospital's supply, and was made possible by the large capacity of the domestic care.

The explanatory model sketched above is largely a theoretical construct. Hard and direct evidence for the applicability of this model is difficult to obtain, for one cannot demonstrate from hospital statistics the existence of 'hidden' female mental patients taken care of at home, so that this must be inferred from fragmentary or circumstantial evidence. Such evidence, however, abounds and is of three types. The first is a negative correlation between a prefecture's number of psychiatric beds and its M/F ratio: the smaller the number of psychiatric beds in a region, the larger its male excess of hospitalised patients.

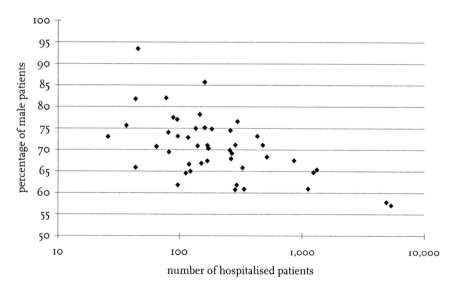

Figure 2   *Number of Hospitalised Patients and Percentages of Men, 46 Prefectures, 1940*

Were Asylums Men's Places?

Figure 2 indicates the number of hospitalised patients of 46 prefectures on the x-axis and the percentage of men against the total patients of both sexes on the y-axis in the year 1940.[30] There is clearly a negative correlation. This suggests that if a prefecture had a large institutional facility, it had more room for patients who exhibited less overtly dangerous symptoms, which led to the institutionalisation of more women. The fact that prefectures that enjoyed a larger number of psychiatric beds were urbanized ones might also have been relevant, since in urban areas, the transition to a nuclear household system was already in progress, and this shift decreased the family's capacity to take care of its insane member at home.

The second kind of evidence is qualitative and episodic. The argument above claims that in psychiatric hospitals, men outnumbered women because women were more likely to be cared for at home. The missing lynchpin of this argument, however, is hypothetical 'hidden' female patients, who were cared for at home and whose families did not knock at the door of a psychiatric hospital. As Nancy Tomes admitted in her attempt to prove 'the case of the missing female depressives', explaining the absence of hospitalisation from the records of a hospital is riddled with fundamental difficulties.[31] Nevertheless, one can frequently encounter such 'missing female schizophrenics' in case histories of the Ohji Brain Hospital (hereafter OBH), a flourishing private psychiatric hospital.[32] A.B., a 37-year-old woman married to a clerk, had been treated at home for five or six years, occasionally with doses of narcotics, before she was admitted to OBH. C.D. had been treated at home for 15 years, after a stay of two or three years at another private mental hospital. The death of her husband six months before was specified as the reason why the family asked for admission to OBH in 1928. E.F., a 46-year-old wife of a cosmetics-seller, was hospitalised at OBH twice in 1936 and 1942, each time for less than a month. During the intervening five years, she was taken care of at home. Although this type of evidence is episodic and impressionistic, it nevertheless appears in the case histories of OBH with such frequency as to make one suspect a hidden but established pattern of home care of insane women.

The third type of evidence is concerned with manic-depressive illness. The argument in this section has been so far mainly based on dementia praecox, leaving manic-depressive disorder aside, mainly because of its smaller sample size. Nevertheless, the M/F ratio of hospitalised manic-depressives is important because it brings in some further international perspectives. International comparison of the symptomatic differences of hospitalised manic-depressive illness confirms that male excess and the priority given to dangerous cases due to the small capacity of institutional provision were strongly related. As mentioned above, Japanese psychiatrists were somewhat puzzled by the statistical difference between Japanese manic-depressives and their German counterparts. While in the latter there was a clear female excess and a dominance of depressive cases, the former showed reversals in both respects – an excess in male cases and manic cases.

Table 4   *Types of Manic-Depressive Insanity*

	Manic		Depressive		Manic-Depressive	
	Male	*Female*	*Male*	*Female*	*Male*	*Female*
Matuzawa Hospital (Tokyo)	41.3%		21.7%		29.3%	
	38.7%	44.8%	26.3%	15.7%	31.8%	26%
Iwakura Hospital (Kyoto)	62%		17%		21%	
Kraepelin	14.6%		48.9%		34.5%	

Source: Hidehisa Matsumura, 'So-utsu-byo No Ippan-teki Tôkei [Some General Statistics of Manic-Depressive Illiness]', *Seishin-Shinkei-gaku Zasshi* [Journal of Psychiatry and Neurology], 41 (1937), 965-977.

In a rare attempt to explain the difference, one psychiatrist at a private asylum in Tokyo stated that the limited availability of hospital beds created the dominance of manic cases: manic and excited cases, particularly 'those trespassing into other people's houses or wandering around the Palace', must be confined, while depressive cases could be cared for and supervised at home.[33] He further enviously speculated that the excess of depressive types in Europe was due to the admission of what he regarded as 'milder' cases, because of the large institutional provision and people's readiness to refer milder cases to hospitals. This speculation grasped the core problem of the bias toward overtly dangerous cases in Japanese asylums. Indeed, several doctors were ready to admit that those who were just depressed or who harboured harmless delusions could be easily cared for at home, sometimes with the occasional help of large doses of strong sleeping pills or opium-based drugs.[34] The Japanese mental hospitals' priority for dangerous and excited patients skewed the asylum population toward men, because men were more likely to exhibit 'dangerous' manic symptoms and were therefore difficult to treat at home.

Conclusion

I have tried above to explain why the population of Japanese mental hospitals in the earlier part of the twentieth century was skewed towards men. Men might well be more exposed to causes of mental disorders than women, but such epidemiological aspects of the question have not been investigated. Rather, I have focused upon the gender asymmetry both in the meanings of symptoms and in the family's choice of institutional committal. Men and women exhibited different symptoms, which sent different messages to those around: male disorders

Were Asylums Men's Places?

were perceived to be of a more public nature and more threatening to others, while female afflictions were regarded as more private and more directed against the patient herself. This differential hermeneutics of psychiatric symptoms led, in early twentieth century Japan, to the choice of a different locus of care for male and female patients, respectively, the former committed to psychiatric institutions, the latter taken care of at home. However, the path from the contrast in the readings of symptoms to the huge male excess in hospitalised population was far from automatic. This passage was mediated by the capacity and role of psychiatric institutions on the one hand, and the capacity and readiness of the family to care for its mentally ill members on the other. When the psychiatric facility was intended for those who were dangerous to others and when its service was expensive to purchase, both for private and public clients, the precious resource was assigned to those patients who exhibited symptoms that were visibly dangerous to others. The priority for hospitalisation was thus given to male patients, who were more likely to be perceived as publicly disturbing. On the other hand, when a household had a greater capacity to take care of its incapacitated member, the family was ready to pay the human cost of caring for the patients at home, so long as their disorders could be contained within the private sphere. The option of domestic care was thus more frequently used for female patients, whose disturbing behaviour was less likely to become a public nuisance. The M/F ratio of hospitalised patients in early twentieth century Japan therefore resulted from the intersection of hospital and home, or the balance between the cost of psychiatric institutionalisation and that of domestic care. The financial cost of institutional confinement was high, while the human cost of domestic care was cheap. The large and consistent male excess in the asylum population was thus due to two factors: precious psychiatric beds were allocated to publicly dangerous cases, and the family could absorb privately troublesome cases.

Notes

*   Acknowledgements: I would like to thank those who attended the conference in Amsterdam in 2003 and Junko Kitanaka at Keio University for their helpful comments. The research on which this paper is based has been supported by the Japan Society for the Promotion of Science during 2002-2004.
1.   For a survey of the literature on the subject, see N. Tomes, 'Feminist Histories of Psychiatry', in Mark S. Micale and Roy Porter (eds), *Discovering the History of Psychiatry* (Oxford: Oxford University Press, 1994), 348-83; Jonathan Andrews and Anne Digby, 'Introduction', in Jonathan Andrews and Anne Digby (eds), *Sex and Seclusion, Class and Custody: Perspectives on Gender and Class in the History of British and Irish Psychiatry* (Amsterdam: Rodopi, 2004), 7-45.

2. Elaine Showalter, *The Female Malady: Women, Madness and English Culture, 1830-1980* (London: Virago, 1987); Mark S. Micale, *Approaching Hysteria: Disease and Its Interpretations* (Princeton: Princeton University Press, 1995).

3. See papers in Andrews and Digby, *op. cit.* (note 1).

4. Pre-WWII national statistics of mental patients and psychiatric hospitals are available in *Eisei-Kyoku Nenpô* [*Annual Report of the Bureau of Hygiene*], which was renamed *Eisei Nenpô* [*Annual Report of Hygiene*] in 1938. Both will be hereafter referred to as *ARH*. I have made extensive use of this material elsewhere. See Akihito Suzuki, 'Family, the State and the Insane in Japan 1900-1945', in Roy Porter and David Wright (eds), *The Confinement of the Insane. International Perspectives, 1800-1965* (Cambridge: Cambridge University Press, 2003), 193-225.

5. I have discussed the difference between public and private patients in Akihito Suzuki, 'A Brain Hospital in Tokyo and Its Private and Public Patients, 1926-1945', *History of Psychiatry*, 14 (2003), 337-60.

6. For early attempts at psychiatric epistemology by Esquirol and his contemporaries, see Ian Hacking, *The Taming of Chance* (Cambridge: Cambridge University Press, 1990).

7. John Charles Bucknill and Daniel H. Tuke, *A Manual of Psychological Medicine* (Philadelphia: Blanchard and Lea, 1858), 243-5.

8. Emil Kraepelin, *Psychiatry: A Textbook for Students and Physicians*, edited with an introduction by Jacques M. Queen (Canton, MA.: Science History Publication, 1990), 2 vols, vol. 1, 60. See also *Dictionary of Psychological Medicine*, edited by D.H Tuke, 2 vols. (London: J.A. Churchill, 1892, reprinted, New York: Arno Press, 1976), 1202-3.

9. Hidehisa Matsumura, 'Sô-utsu-byô No Ippan-teki Tôkei [Some General Statistics of Manic-Depressive Illness]', *Seishin-Shinkei-gaku Zasshi* [*Journal of Psychiatry and Neurology*, hereafter *JPN*], 41 (1937), 965-77.

10. See Suzuki, *op. cit.* (note 4). Waichirô Omata, *Seishin Byôin No Kigen* [*The Origins of Psychiatric Hospitals*], (Tokyo: Ota Shuppan, 1998); Kazuko Itahara and Kuwahara Haruo, 'Edo Jidai Kôki Ni Okeru Seishin Shôgaisha No Kenkyû [The Mentally Disabled in the Late Edo Period]' (1)-(4), *Shakai Mondai Kenkyû*, 48 (1998), 41-59; 49 (1999 & 2000), 93-111, 183-200; Genshirô Hiruta, *Hayari Yamai To Kitsune-tsuki* [*Epidemics and Fox Possession*] (Tokyo: Misuzu Shobô, 1985).

11. *Teikoku Gikai Kizoku-in Giji Sokkiroku* [*Parliamentary Debates in the House of Lords*] (Tokyo: University of Tokyo Press, 1979-1985), No. 12, 20 January 1900 and No. 21, 10 February 1900.

12. For more information on national mental patients' statistics, see Suzuki, *op. cit.* (note 4).

13. For a detailed account of home custody with many photographs, see Shuzô Kure and Gorô Kashida, 'Seishin-byôsha Sitaku Kanchi: Jikkyô Oyobi Sono Toukei-teki Kansatsu [Home Custody of Mental Patients: Its Situations and Its Statistical Observations]', *Tokyo Igaku-kai Zasshi* [*Journal of the Medical Society of Tokyo*], 32 (1918), 521-56, 609-49, 693-720, 762-806. This invaluable work has been reprinted in the Classics in Psychiatry series, reissued in 2000.

14. *Ibid.*, 524.

15. The mutual dependence and benefit of the public and private asylums in Tokyo are satirically described in the serialised articles in *Yomiuri Shinbun* [*Yomiuri News*].

See Yasuo Okada and Shizu Sakai (eds), *Kindai Shomin Seikatsu-Shi, vol. 20, Byôki/ Eisei [Social History of the Lives of Populace in the Modern Age, vol. 20, Disease and Hygiene]* (Tokyo: San-ichi Press, 1995), 183-223.

16.   The data for Figure I are taken from *ARH*.

17.   Yutaka Fujino, 'Shôwa Tairei To Minshû No Seikatsu To Kenko [The Showa Grand Accession Ceremony and People's Health]', in *The Records of the Showa Grand Ceremony of Accession*, 65-86; Tsuneo Matsumura et al., 'Tokyo Shinai Furôsha Oyobi Kojiki No Seishin-igaku-teki Chôsa, [Psychiatric Survey of Vagrants and Beggars in the City of Tokyo]', *JPN*, 46 (1942), 69-92.

18.   Osamu Kan, 'Honpo Ni Okeru Seishin-byôsha Narabi-ni Kore-ni Rinsetsu-seru Seishin-ijô-sha Ni Kan-suru Chôsa [A survey of the Mentally Ill and the Related Mentally Abnormal]', *JPN*, 41 (1937), 793-884, 836-43.

19.   *Seishin Eisei Shiryô [Archives of Mental Hygiene]*, 3 (1955), 13-14.

20.   Kan, *op. cit.* (note 18), 846-7; Toshiharu Fujita, 'Seishin-shikkan-kanjya-sû Ni Ttuite-no Jûgo-nen-kan No Nenji Suii [Yearly Changes in the Number of Mental Patients in the Last Fifteen Years]', *Nihon Kôshû Eisei Zashi [Japanese Journal of Public Health]*, 38 (1991), 233-45, 299-309.

21.   *Archives of Mental Hygiene*, 3 (1955), table 2.

22.   The table is based on Yoshibumi Ôta et al., 'Nihon Ni Okeru Seishin-bunretsu-byô No Hatubyô Kikenritsu [Morbidity Risk of Schizophrenia in Japan]', *Seishin Igaku*, 28 (1986), 421-6.

23.   The discharges included deaths while staying in the asylum.

24.   Fujita, *op. cit.* (note 20).

25.   Saburô Okuda, 'Sôhatsu-sei-chihô-shô No Rinshô-teki Toukei-teki Kansatsu [Clinical and Statistical Observations on Dementia Praecox]', *JPN*, 41 (1937), 885-919.

26.   This characterisation of Japanese psychiatry has been vigorously maintained by Yasuo Okada. See, e.g., his *Nihon Seishin-iryôshi [History of Japanese Psychiatry]* (Tokyo: Igaku-shoin, 2002).

27.   Nuboharu Aoki, 'Seishin-ijô-sha No Zouka To Sono Taisaku [The Increase of the Mentally Abnormal and Measures against it]', *Koshû-eisei [Public Health]*, 53 (1935), 161-8, 234-40, 304-11.

28.   *Archives of Mental Hygiene*, 1 (1953), 21.

29.   Okada, *op. cit.* (note 26), 130-1.

30.   In Figure 2 I have not used the M/F ratio, because in four prefectures there were no female patients hospitalised.

31.   Nancy Tomes, 'Women and Depression: A Historical Perspective', in Yosio Kawakita, Shizu Sakai and Yasuo Otsuka (eds), *History of Psychiatric Diagnosis: Proceedings of the 16th International Symposium on the Comparative History of Medicine* (Tokyo: Ishuyaku EuroAmerica Inc., 1997), 55-83.

32.   For Ôji Brain Hospital and its patients, see Suzuki, *op. cit.* (note 5).

33.   Matsumura, *op. cit.* (note 9).

34.   Mitsunao Koseki, 'Katei Ni Okeru Seishin-byôsha No Chiryô-kango-hô [Treatment and Nursing of Mental Patients at Home]', *Iji Kôron [Public Medical Gazette]*, no. 807 (1928), 14-15. Koseki's paper listed six drugs for excited patients, while only one for depressed patients.

CHAPTER 13

Madness in the Home

Family Care and Welfare Policies in Italy before Fascism

Patrizia Guarnieri *

Introduction

Institutions for the insane existed already in the fifteenth and sixteenth centuries, and historians of the early modern age have stressed that even then a notion existed of care, not just of confinement or segregation. But the numbers of inmates were very small. In the very long tradition of Italy,[1] Florence had 15 beds in the Pazzeria for the poor insane, founded in 1688 in S. Maria Nuova Hospital, and about 30 beds for the paying insane in S. Dorotea, opened in 1643. In the early twentieth century, there were about 1400 inmates in the two Florentine asylums.

By comparing numbers like these, historians have judged that madness – before becoming a medicalised and institutional matter – must have been mainly a family matter, as Castel and others have proposed. The family was responsible for its mad, as it was for its children, in Porter's words. But the more the process of medicalisation went on, the more families seem to disappear. In the history of the last two centuries of madness, families' attitudes are mainly described as getting rid of their insane members: by handing them over to the new professionals within special institutions or abandoning them because of the impossibility of supporting them. Increasingly, the family distanced itself. Yet the experts on mental diseases seemed to agree with such distancing: the idea of 'curability' was connected with institutionalisation, because a mentally ill person would benefit precisely from being isolated from his/her usual environment and therefore from the family.

But the asylum was neither the unique nor the ideal place for the treatment of mentally ill people. Their own family home might be better. This was the quite surprising statement that eminent psychiatrists, such as Cesare Lombroso and Augusto Tamburini, offered when the first Italian law on insanity was being drafted. In 1891, as consultants of the government, they both recommended that the law should favour the 'placement of calm and harmless [mental] patients [...] with their own or other families receiving a subsidy'. They made reference to the deliberation on the matter at the international congress on public care held in

Paris in 1889, and above all to the exemplary experiments already underway in Florence and in various other provinces.[2]

In the first year, there were 66 patients in subsidised family care in the district of Florence; the increase was continuous, and in 1911, alongside 1,452 admissions to the asylum, there were 909 welfare patients assisted at home.

The Florentine Case

Home care in Florence consisted in the official committal by the provincial administration of a certified psychiatric patient to his/her co-resident family, who received a subsidy for caring for the patient. It was important for its extent, its early beginning and long duration, and for the significance of the social, political and cultural context in which it occurred, in a city where the Chiarugi humanitarian tradition in psychiatry was still in the air. Nevertheless, it has passed unobserved by historians.

When did it start? Archival sources provided mainly by the former psychiatric hospital and the provincial administration take us back to 1866, almost 40 years before the Italian law on asylums of 1904. That beginning, in the then capital of the kingdom, is strikingly early and intriguing. It contradicts the affirmation that in the second half of the nineteenth century, families tended to delegate the caring for the most vulnerable members and to give them over to the new professionals within special institutions. It also contradicts the assumption that it was the poor in particular who got rid of their demented relatives, by locking them up in asylums, which became, in that period, completely filled. On the contrary, the evidence shows that the Florentines who officially kept their mentally ill at home were indigent.

When home care passed from being just a private solution to a system that was recognised, monitored, and funded, selective criteria had to be established that principally concerned the beneficiary. It was necessary to distinguish which patients had to stay in the asylum and which had to stay with the family.

Let's first examine those who were entitled to admission to an asylum. At the end of the nineteenth century, there were huge discrepancies with regard to admission rules among the various regions. The first post-unification law on asylums in 1904 claimed that those committed for insanity were 'people affected by insanity irrespective of the cause, when they *are* a danger to themselves and others or *are* a public scandal and *cannot be* suitably looked after or treated except within an asylum' (L.36/1904, art. 1). The dangerousness was not an intrinsic characteristic of the mental illness but a temporary and supposed condition, to be verified (the verbs in italics are, in the original Italian, deliberately in the subjunctive mood). It was intended as a restriction to limit the number of admissions.

For this purpose, specific documentation was required: a medical certificate and a sworn affidavit, attached to the relatives' request. The Regulations of 1909 indicated (sect. 39, a) that the certificate *had to state* 'the *specific facts* expressed clearly and in detail, which lead to the deduction that the individual has a clear tendency to commit violence against himself or others or offend public decency', as well as the 'necessity to admit the afflicted to an asylum'. The affidavit had to make reference again to 'the specific facts' of the danger, from 'the sworn deposition of four witnesses' who had to be knowledgeable, and above all reliable and impartial 'upright persons of trust [...] with no connection to the family of the disturbed'.

These were the intentions, but what happened? It is a fact that medical certificates and sworn affidavits were reduced to printed forms in a general, standardised and lapidary language, without providing real evidence. Moreover, even when formally respected, the spirit of the law was distorted. It foresaw that in urgent situations, hospitalisation would have to be ordered by the police. The sworn testimony of neighbours was not required for this (section 3 L.36/1904), and the danger posed by the person disturbed was invariably stated, merely to justify the urgent procedure. This was so frequently adopted that from being the exception, it passed to being the general rule until recent times, with the excuse that it was simply a short cut.

Interests and financial motives also played a role. Urgent admissions were ordered by the police and town mayors, though it was the provincial administration that paid the boarding charges of the poor admitted to an asylum. Since town councils were responsible for charity expenses in general, sending a few indigent cases to the asylum relieved them of some eventual expenses. 'If town councils were asked to contribute money for the maintenance of their insane, they would think hard about it first before so generously sending them to the asylum,' observed an administrator of the Province of Florence.[3]

Even relatives had their reasons for insisting on the danger posed by their sick, seeing that the law required it anyway for admission to a venue which was probably their only alternative, if they simply weren't able to cope anymore. To make sure that the asylum would accept the request and admit their relative, they declared ample evidence of danger and public scandal – exaggerating the risks that living with the ill relation posed. This was sometimes done in bad faith, and there were abuses of a financial nature, as well as those due to serious family conflicts. In many more cases, the emphasis made by relatives on the danger revealed the actual need for the family members themselves to be helped, at least for a period of time.

The Interests of the Sick, or the Budget?

Why was the Florentine system considered the ideal model by some Italian psychiatrists, such as the socialist Lombroso and the progressive Tamburini?[4] One of the main reasons was that it seemed to solve the big problem of over-crowding. It was necessary to avoid the asylums becoming 'a dump used not only by families but also by hospitals, by refuges and prisons'. At that stage, Lombroso and Tamburini wondered if 'instead of recovery, asylums actually contributed to incurable dementia'.[5] They recommended a model that made admissions to the asylum selective, distinguished between different types of mentally ill people, and redistributed them among the institutions in the territory but, above all, sent them back home, subsidising the families.

In reality, families were left to fend for themselves; there was either a lack of institutional care or the existing institutions were just places for chronic invalids. But Italy was already full of asylums before 1904; they continued to fill up, exceeding the worst expectations.[6] In Florence, the 'therapeutic asylum' Bonifazio – the first in Europe – which had been running under the supervision of Vincenzio Chiarugi from 1788, soon had to be enlarged; but this wasn't enough. In 1849, its director demanded new space for at least 600 beds. A country villa was purchased, where 'the chronic, calm alienated less in need of treatment' were then sent, with the remainder left in the city.[7] But this was still insufficient. In 1866, when the Province was founded in Florence (this form of local government didn't exist before the Unification of Italy in 1861) and it became directly responsible for the asylums, the provincial administration immediately changed the asylum policy and started the home custody programme.

A memo from the Prefect of Florence dated 9 February 1866 provoked astonishment among the town mayors to whom it was addressed. Making reference to unspecified norms concerning authorised private family custody of the insane, it asked for a precise prospectus of 'the maniacs [...] who have already been discharged and, at the instructions of the city council, have been placed in private custody'.[8] Many mayors knew nothing about this matter, or at least the 20 mayors whose replies still exist did not (over 40 are missing). They replied that, in their towns, all mentally insane 'were *secluded* within the Florence asylum'. Perhaps in other municipalities, especially in Florence itself, things had gone better. The prefect turned to the director of the asylum and pressed him to identify the patients who 'could be entrusted to private custody' and discharge them, if there was someone willing to take them on. The town mayors would have to prepare the families or else knock on the doors of other agencies that charged a lesser fee than the asylum.

This was a policy that, even for a small number of people, required a huge amount of work in terms of preparation and co-operation among provincial and municipal authorities, charity institutes, psychiatrists and the extended family household's components, all of whom had to agree among themselves and with the ill person. Family care was, in that phase of the project, only for those poor institutionalised patients who were discharged by the asylum after succeeding in persuading someone to come and get them. This was no easy task.

After five months, of 21 identified patients, only 6 had been received by their families. By the end of the year, however, that number had risen to 66.[9] The aim of the Province was clear: to reduce the population in the asylum and to save funds. The subsidised patients cost the Province much less at home than in the asylum: the average calculation was 0.48 lire versus 1.50 lire.[10]

But such a plan was unknowingly sabotaged by a woman named Rosa. She was a widow with three children, an indigent seamstress, living in a lane, on the ground floor where there was also a hat factory. Two of her children took home 5 lire each a week: the 16-year-old boy was an apprentice to a suitcase maker; the girl, aged 14, worked in a cigar factory. Andrea was of working age, too, but not 'suitable for any job'. He was 13 and had already entered and left Bonifazio twice, the last time being in January 1864. His mother had then decided to keep him at home. Now Rosa had learned of that subsidy – she had never received one before – and applied for it in August 1866.[11]

In these circumstances, the provincial administration had no prospect of saving money: the boy was already at home and cost nothing, except to his own relatives. Accepting Rosa's application meant authorising a new wave of candidates for public welfare, making another hole in the provincial budget. Many of those who had managed to live with their mentally sick at home would come forward, given the chance of receiving a subsidy. And so they did. Rosa's request was satisfied; the administrators couldn't reject it, because it fulfilled all the requirements. That woman's strategy interacted with the public authority strategy and made the policy of an immediate cost saving into a measure to prevent admission to the asylum.

What was the priority? If it was the budget, certain restrictive criteria were indeed necessary, as well as iron-fisted controls, not so much upon the ill, but upon the guardians, to whom the provincial administration tried to give as little as possible. The mayors had to check the economic situation of the family periodically; the municipal doctor had to certify the patient's health, and it became sufficient to declare if the mentally ill person was not getting better or worse, but still alive, so that indigent relatives would not pocket the money after his death. For patients in the asylum, it was up to the medical management to give 'prompt notice of any changes that occur in their health condition that may allow them to be placed in private home custody'.[12] Any information relating to health was of interest only in terms of cutting expenses and was in fact only required of patients maintained by the provincial administration.

The entrusting of the mentally ill to family care continued: from 66 in 1866 the number rose to 181 in 1877, and to 218 (113 men and 108 women) in 1886. An

Madness in the Home

influential politician, already a mayor of Florence, demonstrated how much more would be saved by sending some of the mentally ill to other asylums around Italy, above all to that of Pesaro, which had the merit of charging the lowest boarding rate.[13] But because the treatment was worse there, the doctors protested. Deporting the patients could not be a solution to the problem of overcrowding; the director of the Florentine asylum threatened more than once to resign over this, even if this meant losing his prestigious academic position.

When he resigned in 1885, it was his vice-director who raised the alarm,[14] and then Bini's successor, Augusto Tamburini, president of the Italian psychiatric society, concluded that Bonifazio had to be closed down, not renovated. He proposed the construction of a totally new 'building of modest proportions' for housing no more than '200 mentally ill patients [...] all acute cases'.[15] The new asylum and clinic were inaugurated in 1896 at S. Salvi; by 1900 the new admissions had reached 646, to be added to the existing patients both there and in the old Castelpulci building.[16] From that time on, the figures returned to their previous heights.

The Role of the Psychiatrists

For years, the increase in patients did not affect 'madmen, in the true sense of the word, that is people affected by clear, typical forms of psychopathy'. Information on diagnostic categories in the period from 1879 to 1891 showed that the increases were above all in the number of incurables: 'the dead wood of the asylums'. This analysis was used by psychiatrists to identify who were to be placed at home to relieve overcrowding in the asylums.[17] 'Decreasing the cost of maintaining those who are generally harmless and incurable hangs more over our province than over others,' stated the provincial council of Florence.[18]

According to Carlo Bini, discharging of patients into family care was to be carried out when 'they are recovered, but also when they are known to be harmless and calm'. And even 'when they are considered agitated and dangerous, provided that all the necessary guarantees are there, that in one case or another these insane people will be assisted and checked by whoever assumes the responsibility of custody'.[19] Custody could also be granted 'to the family as a means of experimentation, since it may be a way to hasten [...] recovery'. Experts were thinking of a type of supervised discharge, for one year, during which brief readmissions would be provided for in the event of a crisis, with a simple medical certificate, and 'the alienated would remain under a sort of supervision by the Asylum Director [...] so as to avoid a situation, as often occurs, whereby they are left to fend for themselves'.[20]

In 1909, this procedure was passed into Italian law: entrusting the alienated to the family 'by way of experiment', when he 'has reached such a level of improvement that allows him to be cared for at home' (art. 66, Regulation 1909), at the decision of the asylum director. Also, the possibility of a family that, by authorisation of the court, 'wants to host an uncured mentally ill person' would be taken into consideration, if the director did not support the provisional release that was his responsibility (art. 69, Reg. 1909). Art. 63 was given over to home custody: it was not up to the medical director to decide upon ordinary and provisional discharge, but the provincial administration. In fact, it 'may order that the family, relatives or others be entrusted with the mentally ill as provided for in section 6 (that is) the calm, chronically insane, harmless epileptics, cretins, idiots and, in general, individuals afflicted by incurable mental illnesses who are not a danger to themselves or others'.

In theory, those patients should never have been admitted to an asylum in the first place, but rather to other public and private institutions, yet the same art. 63 stated that where there were few or no alternative institutions, those categories of mentally ill had to be admitted to asylums. With this exception to the rule, which became the general rule itself, the door was opened to overcrowd asylums with chronic patients once again.

In the case of the mentally ill for whom the provincial administration could order family custody, the court and the police had to be informed, and the latter in turn had to advise the provincial administration, if the relatives or others neglected their duties of 'custody and care'. It is worth noting that although the subsidy recipients were identified by medical categories, the law did not mention the psychiatrist. Once the sick were outside the asylum, the doctor disappeared from the scene. Under the law in force until 1978, for home care a miserable subsidy could be sufficient; there was no mention of specialist medical support.

Did psychiatrists play a part in the initial experimental projects in Tuscany? The provincial deputation of Florence stated that 'in this province no subsidy is granted for home custody of the harmless demented, if the same demented persons have not been previously subjected to a visit by the Director of the Florence Mental Asylum and if he has not then explicitly acknowledged the existence of a mental illness'. It also stated that the annual confirmation was decided upon 'on the basis of certification that the recipient's condition of mental health as well as the economic circumstances of the relatives remain unchanged'.[21]

How and by whom that certificate was issued was not made clear. In practice, the system, which had started in 1866, continued for decades, during which many things changed. The Bonifazio Asylum was closed down, and the new one opened in the green area of San Salvi. The director Bini retired in 1885, and among his successors Tamburini followed everything from afar, in Reggio Emilia. In 1895 he sent the capable Eugenio Tanzi to take his place, a highly regarded professor, the founder of a prestigious journal in his specialist field and a man of fierce character, especially in his dealings with the president of the provincial administration.

Whenever the placing of the mentally ill into so-called custody (*custodia familiare*) outside the institution was concerned, Tanzi expressed an opinion that was entirely his own, and even contrary to what the administration wanted. He made no comment on the diagnostic category for those considered suitable for home care; generally, he tried to assess, case by case, the suitability of the accommodation that the administrators had procured.[22] In the autumn of 1898, at the request of the president of the provincial administration, Tanzi chose some patients deemed suitable for care in Borgo San Lorenzo, and the mayor made efforts to persuade the families to fetch them. But each attempt was in vain, and so he turned to a local charitable refuge for the elderly who were indigent and unable to work. The director of the institute agreed, setting out his conditions: the patients in question had to be male, at least five in number, all harmless and not ill, and the monthly boarding charge was 25 lire each. Yet after four months, he had no places ready. Next, the mayor started looking among farmhouses, to find an alternative there. But this did not appear realistic to Tanzi, and so nothing was done. As doctor-manager, he at least succeeded in asserting that home care was not practised merely to save money for the administration, without taking into account the interests of the mentally ill.

In October 1898, several relatives of patients turned up at San Salvi 'asking to fetch them because they had been notified by the Honorable Provincial Deputation of their receiving a subsidy for this purpose'. Tanzi had no doubt that this was true, but he was rather annoyed: 'No such information has been forwarded to me from that office, in the absence of which' he sent the relatives home and kept his patients. These documents give the impression that Tanzi was not in favour of home care. In reality, he disliked the fact that the provincial authority would decide these cases without medical advice. But when Bini retired in 1885, the number of home care cases amounted to 218, and in January 1902, the year in which Tanzi was about to leave, there were about 700.[23] This increase was faster than the rise in admissions, nor does it entirely correlate, since those never hospitalised before were included in the number of home care cases.

Even municipal medical officers played a part in the care procedures, but in a very casual manner and according to bureaucratic formulas. First, they issued a certificate of insanity at the request of the relatives (as they did for admission requests to the asylum), and then, on the annual confirmation of the subsidy, they certified 'the persisting abnormal and harmless condition of the mentally ill', if a life certificate was not good enough.[24]

Evidence shows that the mayors had a more important role.[25] It was they who had a relationship with the families of the mentally ill, both at the beginning and at the moment when custody was to be confirmed. This was especially true in the small towns, where everybody knew everyone else, and mayors acted as mediators between the poor and the distant authorities in Florence, who ordered, controlled and established sanctions, but very often took their time in sending the subsidies. Town leaders generally supported their townspeople against the provincial administration. They passed on complaints and themselves complained, almost to the point of inciting the wrath of the Province. 'I cannot understand how the payment of subsidies to these unhappy families that languish in poverty can be neglected,' wrote the mayor of Fucecchio to the president of the Deputation in 1902, 'and I cannot but agree with the measures that some of the guardians intend to adopt, that is to deliver the demented to the provincial administration whenever payment is delayed.'[26]

The subsidies were small. The difficulties involved in receiving them were many. The guardian of one demented person was old, 'helpless and cannot get to the municipal office of rates and taxes to collect the subsidy,' explained the mayor, asking the Deputation to make out the money order to the son of the invalid guardian (how that person could help the mentally ill person in the first place was not asked).[27] The 15 lire monthly subsidy received by a certain Signora Staccioli, a widow, was suspended because she had failed to take Angiola, the demented person in her charge, to the asylum for a check-up.[28] How old the two women were and in what conditions of physical health is unknown. However, it was often a big and expensive undertaking to travel as far as Florence and then to San Salvi with a mentally ill person, who was perhaps feeble or an invalid. Sometimes the deputation suspended the subsidy because the patient had not been looked after at home. The care had perhaps been inhibited 'due to the extreme poverty of the family', the mayor of Florence pointed out. The guardian needed an increase in the subsidy, but instead, they took it away and left the mentally ill person there.[29] In several other cases, the deputation simply rejected the subsidy application with the assumption that the family, already having custody of the mentally ill person, would (hopefully) keep him anyway.

We must wonder how an indigent family could possibly be expected to keep a relative with serious mental problems at home, without any psychiatric aid. It has often been said that it was in fact the poor who had filled up the asylums due to the inability of their families to look after them. However, the reason behind the decision to send a family member who required more care to an institution – be it children, the elderly, or the ill – was never only economic. Well-to-do families, in fact, owning spacious houses, kept their nervous relatives at home less and less during the nineteenth century, and preferred to leave them in paying wards in asylums or in more elegant private clinics.

Shorter explains this change in the upper classes with changing patterns of sentiment in family life and refers to his sentimental view of the modern family. In such a family, where husbands and wives married for love, mothers were more affectionate with their children, rather than indifferent, the intimacy 'of the little family's togetherness' was celebrated around the dinner table... 'Insane relatives no longer fit into the picture of bliss.'[30] The respectable families distanced themselves from those bad subjects that disturbed the idyllic portrait as described by Shorter. In truth and quite paradoxically, the close affectionate families hastened to rid themselves of their neediest members.

If a family care policy for the mentally ill failed, many times it was because the experiment 'found only enthusiastic supporters among doctors and the people, but [...] discontent among the wealthy class, who feared having contact with madmen who were given back their freedom,' as some Italian psychiatrists noted in the early twentieth century.[31] Were the poor more prone then to keep their mad with them at home? It would seem so from the relevant number of cases in Florence between the end of the 1800s and beginning of the 1900s.

The poor had difficulty surviving, but laid no claims to that kind of respectability. One might say that for this reason they may have been able to bear what those better off found to be unbecoming. For instance, they were more tolerant towards unwed mothers (it was not their idea to call their children illegitimate). The poor might also be thought of as indifferent. If they were indifferent towards newborn children – although this view has been highly criticized – it would be no wonder that they felt little affection towards their old, demented or disturbed relatives. They could have just as much abandoned them in asylums as locked them up at home without taking care of them. The choice to keep them would therefore be explained as a mere survival strategy for the family: willing to keep the mad relative at home in order to pocket the subsidies and use the money for their own needs, which were in any case primary.

Did the poor exploit their mentally ill family members whenever possible? Under what conditions did they keep them? Did they lock them up in a worse state than in the asylums? These were the questions the doctors were asking and that the administrators wanted to know. Welfare and charity require choices, criteria and controls regarding the recipients, revealing in the process much about the benefactors as well as the controllers. But what can we know about the Florentine families in question?

The archival source I came across was quite special. There were a series of printed questionnaires with the name and age of the entrusted ill person, the name of the guardian, the place of residence, and the subsidy amount granted. On the two following pages, there were 12 detailed questions about the family's circumstances, how the patients were treated and if, based on the required conditions, the subsidy was justifiable and proportionate. The answers, written in the same handwriting, are accurate and non-bureaucratic. They were signed in legible calligraphy by a woman. Even this is surprising.

Women's Care and Supervision

The woman who surprisingly turned out to be the author of those notes, Bice Cammeo, was a Jewish emancipationist of the *Unione Femminile*.[32] In 1904 she had opened an Information and Welfare Office (*Ufficio di indicazioni ed assistenza*) in Florence – like those in Milan, Turin and Rome, inspired by the Parisian model of the *Bureau Central des Oeuvres de Bienfaisance*. The final goal was 'aiding the working class in its every need', by offering small loans, helping to find a job, and above all 'supplying the most complete and accurate information' to the poor that, from the late 1860s to the 1900s (visible by default in the census), fluctuated between half and a quarter of the total population.[33] The provincial council recognised the usefulness of such a philanthropic institute and granted a financial contribution of 200 lire for the year 1906.[34] In return, it asked for a 'widespread and continuous supervision [...] over the families to whom the care [...] is being given', with a subsidy, for a demented relative. Supervision was already carried out by the local police; but some provincial deputies felt that the ladies could cope better than the policemen. And they in fact did so.[35]

In the male world of psychiatry, where all doctors and administrators were men, the women were the patients who attracted attention, even from historians, above all for hysteria. Benefactresses, philanthropists and women in search of their own as well as other women's emancipation usually devoted themselves to matters concerning maternity and children. The apparition of a woman in the harshest care for the demented reminds us that there were women in this scene: the female nurses in the asylums; at home, the wives, mothers, daughters and other female relatives, as well as neighbours. The responsibility of taking care of ill family members, even the mentally ill, almost always rested on the woman. Miss Cammeo highlighted the specific importance of the woman in the household, although the pre-printed questionnaire always made reference to the family. She always noted when a woman was lacking: that explained why the ill person appeared to be poorly looked after; there wasn't 'anybody who could wash him'.[36]

In the spring of 1906, Miss Cammeo went from home to home in Florence, visiting the mentally ill and their families. She started from the lists of subsidised mentally ill people compiled by the Municipality: these contained only names, no other personal information, not even the ages of the 'demented' or their guardian, nor their guardian's relationship to them. As for the obligatory enclosed files, the health certificate was only a pre-printed form with the generic 'visited on ... and found to be suffering from...'; the municipal medical officer then added 'harmless dementia' and that was sufficient. The Provincial Deputation wanted to evaluate if 'the harmless mentally ill person [...] is sufficiently supervised and receives the loving care his pitiful condition requires'. To various questions in the forms, there was the reply from the police office, and there was also a space for 'Observations' from Cammeo's office.

At times, when compared, the two sources disagreed. The neighbourhood police station attested that guardians had an aunt in custody who was in the hospital of S. Maria Nuova. Cammeo went to visit the woman in the hospital of San

Gallo, where she had been for months; she wanted to go back to live with her guardians – no blood ties existed – but they were unable to cope because she was too agitated and required too much assistance. Indeed, the only woman in the house already had too much to do, taking care of her father, husband and three young children, one of whom she was still breast-feeding.[37]

Stories of Families and Their Ill

Ulisse, 19 years old, appeared to be of a lucid mind and normal, even though he had spent a long time in the asylum in San Salvi. The guardian was his father, who worked as a manual labourer for the railway and received a subsidy of 12 lire a month. His mother treated him 'lovingly' and was attentive in the home. Whenever she went out, there was the landlady, who had given that family a free room out of sympathy. They lived in the Santa Croce neighbourhood and had two more children, 15 and 16 years old, who were both at school. They made a very good impression, but the subsidy they received was scant. Ulisse suffered from constant and extreme pain. The medical certificate spoke of 'mental disease after meningitis', but his bad health condition was due to tuberculosis in its last stage.

Among the patients in custody visited by Miss Cammeo, physical disabilities connected to poverty seem, in fact, to have been very frequent. Evelina, a 19-year-old, was entrusted to her 52-year-old father, a hairdresser's apprentice. She was a 'beautiful girl, young and buxom', but complained of recurrent paralysis in her right leg and was deaf and mute. Giulia, 43 years old, was entrusted to her 76-year-old father. He had retired from the railway and received a pension of 1.80 lire a day; her mother was a housewife, their other daughter was 33 years old and earned 80 cents a day as a seamstress. Giulia's family treated her 'very well', but she lived in a state of pain, her neck was swollen, she moved with great difficulty and was severely deaf, but had never been in San Salvi. They lived in a room that cost 9 lire a month. They made a very good impression, and their neighbours gave excellent references.

The observations made by Bice Cammeo followed the order of the questionnaire: what appeared to be the physical state of the ill person; their mental state; how they were treated and dressed; were they sufficiently supervised and groomed; were they left at home alone, and if so, were they in the care of another person; what was the house like, how many rooms were there, how was it furnished, and what was the cost of living in the neighbourhood; who made up the family unit, and what were the jobs and occupations of each member; impressions from the home visit; information from neighbours on the family's behaviour and morality; whether or not the ill person was able to work or do housework (gender is specified in this question); whether the afflicted person was employed outside the home, and what the earnings were?

Sometimes, the situation was obvious, and there wasn't much to report. There were painful cases, where the ill suffered and were often weakened by their age and poverty, or were afflicted by other illnesses, and the guardians sometimes needed just as much help. Emma was an idiot and needed a lot of care, but had never been in San Salvi. She lived with her mother Annetta, 61 years old, 'an unfortunate' who, in only a short time, had lost her husband and six children, mostly to tuberculosis. The family received 2 lire a week from the Jewish University and a voucher for bread.

There were many ill people who had never been admitted to asylums, especially children, and the women who took care of them were alone. Eight-year-old Umberto was entrusted to his mother, Rosamunda, a 35-year-old widow who also had another son, 10 years old and at school. Umberto was emaciated, underdeveloped, and backward due to meningitis that he had contracted ten months earlier. His family treated him with 'sufficient love', but he often remained at home alone, because his mother went out to work as a housekeeper, and his 68-year-old maternal grandmother sold sweets at the front door. The home consisted of one room with two beds and the use of a kitchen. His mother had never left him in an asylum and definitely did not keep him home for the money, because the subsidy she received was 5 lire a month.

It is enough to compare these amounts with the wages that were insufficient to live on, according to the authorities, to understand that these indigent people did not have much to gain by the payment for their ill person. The relatives did what they could, even with love and care. There are few cases in which Cammeo did not mention the family's affection, and only one case where she stated the contrary (a cobbler who locked his father up in a room full of pigeons, the only room they had). Perhaps these families had asked for a subsidy after years of caring for their ill relative when they found out about such a possibility, but the records do not specify this. There was a notable frequency of applications from workers in factories and large industries, the railways, tobacco trade, and meat markets, most likely because this type of information was better circulated where there were mutual aid societies, as well as socialist and union organisations.

Other situations were more anomalous, seen through Cammeo's own values and susceptibilities. Eleonora, aged 51, physically emaciated and entrusted to her 72-year-old widowed mother, seemed mentally normal and spoke well. She dressed in a bizarre, antique elegance. The house was untidy and did not make a good impression. The neighbours knew nothing of the two women's lifestyle. The 'demented' Eleonora said that she gave English, French and piano lessons, and the mother just nodded. So Cammeo asked where she gave lessons: to a well-known antique dealer's family. Cammeo went to visit the family and, to her surprise, not only did they confirm that Eleonora gave them lessons, but that they were extremely happy with her because, although she was a bit strange, she

Madness in the Home

was a capable and diligent instructor. Cammeo speculated that Eleonora was an 'unfortunate woman from a fallen family', therefore deserving a subsidy of 15 lire, and if she was also able to earn some money from giving lessons, her fees were ridiculously low because she posed no competition to the 'many good and balanced teachers'.

There were stories of children taken care of by their parents and vice versa; it was sometimes difficult to decipher who was supporting whom. The situation was worse in cases involving elderly invalids with only unmarried sons. There were also cases involving sisters where one was the guardian of the other, or even instances of elderly women who were old friends as was the case of Maria and Virginia. She had taken Maria into custody, but it was only Virginia's 29-year-old son, a porter, who had an income. They shared their small quarters in the centre with a couple and their two young children, but it was filthy.

These were small households, but not necessarily isolated. Cammeo testified to the strong solidarity that existed among the poor. They sometimes backed each other up to evade the inspectors. In order to get a better idea of the situation, Miss Cammeo would ask the family's neighbours about them (certainly not at the parish church). Nonetheless, she didn't always trust what they told her: 'out of a sense of solidarity, they always speak well about each other', unless they had personal rivalries.[38] Cammeo went around verifying, observing and referring. She found that all the situations were very different from one another, more so than the police reports and health certificates stated, and especially more than the periodic debates of politicians, administrators and doctors about the criteria for admission to the programme. They standardised all those having a right to family home care in the category of harmless demented, incurable, or 'only in need of custody'.

Conclusions

It is difficult to say what use was made of Bice Cammeo's observations. The doctors in the asylum probably didn't even see them. Since she was commissioned by the Provincial Deputation and made official reports, I assume that at least some of the councillors found a reason to reflect about her information. Disagreements emerged more profoundly in the Council after the questionnaire took place: some believed home care to be a dumping ground for the therapeutic and costly asylums, while on the contrary, others believed it to be a complement to asylum care. Not all the elected councillors were willing to give priority to the budget to the detriment of health and care.[39]

Although the law which contemplated subsidised home custody lasted until 1978, the ways in which it was applied changed very much. During the First World War, medical visits and biennial check-ups were suspended due to a lack of staff. During fascism, the size of subsidies diminished even more. In December 1920, based on a report by a psychiatrist from San Salvi who was responsible for visits to subsidy recipients, the Provincial Deputation unanimously voted for a 10 lire rise in subsidies across the board for the 'harmless demented'.[40] But under fascism, the head of the Province decided on draconian reductions (from 40 lire to 25 lire, from 60 lire to 30 lire, etc.), depending on the certificates.[41] The subsidy recipients were to present themselves at the asylum on days fixed in advance. They were visited by the doctor, 24 in a batch, from ten o'clock to twelve o'clock, which worked out to 5-minute visits per person.

In 1937, the director of the asylum, Paolo Amaldi, proposed another reform of the reviewing procedure: in addition to the already restrictive criteria, 'it was necessary above all to emphasize the suitability for admission to the asylum'. Since for hospitalisation 'the law does not only require the existence of some type of mental disturbance, but also that the subject be a danger', if the relatives wished to receive the subsidy, it was necessary that even the mentally ill who were capable of being entrusted to home care be declared dangerous.[42]

Rather than the harmless demented, families would have had to keep the dangerous or at least claim that they were so, the opposite of what had always been previously established. Amaldi actually expected to overturn the regulations for the benefit of the province's balance sheet. It goes without saying how little the effects of that policy benefited the lives of the more fragile mentally ill and their families, who had to carry the burden of social welfare and its inconsistencies in Italy.

Notes

*   I am grateful to Edward Shorter for his comments and editorial help.
1.   See V. Biotti and G. Magherini, *L'isola delle Stinche e i percorsi della follia a Firenze nei secoli XIV-XVIII* (Firenze: Ponte alle Grazie, 1992); L. Roscioni, *Il governo della follia* (Milano: Bruno Mondadori, 2003).
2.   See C. Lombroso, A. Tamburini, R. Ascenzi, 'Relazione a S. E. il Ministro dell'Interno sulla ispezione dei manicomi del Regno' [1891], in R. Canosa, *Storia del manicomio in Italia dall'Unità a oggi* (Feltrinelli: Milano, 1979), 199-211. About family care in Italy, see A. Tamburini, G.C. Ferrari, G. Antonini, *L'assistenza degli alienati in Italia e nelle varie nazioni* (Torino: UnioneTipografica editrice, 1918), 130-45.
3.   Quoted in Manicomio di Firenze, *Relazione della Commissione per la Riforma del regolamento* (Firenze: Galletti e Cocci, 1911), 37.
4.   See at least M. Maj and F.M. Ferro (eds), *Anthology of Italian Psychiatric Texts* (World Psychiatric Association, 2002), ad vocem; P. Guarnieri, *La storia della psichiatria. Un secolo di studi in Italia* (Firenze: Olschki, 1991), with bibliography 55-150; idem, 'The History of Psychiatry in Italy', *History of Psychiatry*, 2 (1991), 289-301.

5. Lombroso, Tamburini, Ascenzi, *op. cit.* (note 2), 201.

6. 67% of the psychiatric buildings existing in Italy in 1998 were built before 1904; 91% was in the centre or in the near suburbs of the town. See *Atlante O. P.P. in Italia*, Fondazione Benetton, 1999.

7. See F. Bini, *Schema di regolamento amministrativo e disciplinare pel Manicomio di Firenze* (Firenze: tip. Ricci, 1871), 3-9. On Bonifazio: G. Mora, 'Introduction', in his English edition of V. Chiarugi, *On Insanity and Its Classification* (Canton: Science History Publisher, 1987), xiii-cxli.

8. See Deputazione Provinciale di Firenze, *Norme pel collocamento dei mentecatti a custodia privata presso le famiglie*, circ. 9 Febr., 1866, Archive Province of Florence (APF) cat 9, cas. 1, 1865-1866, b. 18, a. 1.

9. See See Manicomio, *op. cit.* (note 3), 16.

10. APF, 1865-66, b. 18. For the financial side of the matter, see *Relazione della Commissione speciale eletta dal Consiglio provinciale di Firenze per esaminare il rapporto del prof. Augusto Tamburini sui manicomi e proporre le risoluzioni più convenienti*, but 1886, 16 ff.

11. APF cat. 9, cas. 1, 1866.

12. Archivio San Salvi, Commissione Amministratrice del Manicomio, CAM, 184, f. 22, Deputazione Provinciale di Firenze, *Mentecatti*, 28 March 1874.

13. See Manicomio, *op. cit.* (note 3), 16-7.

14. *Ibid.*, 19-20.

15. Tamburini's report is quoted *ibid.*, 9-11.

16. *La Clinica di San Salvi. Studi neurologici dedicati a Eugenio Tanzi* (Torino: tipografia Società torinese, 1926), 10.

17. Lombroso, Tamburini, Ascenzi, *op. cit.* (note 2), 201.

18. See Manicomio, *op. cit.* (note 3), 25 no. 1.

19. Art 583 in Bini, *op. cit.* (note 7), 84.

20. Lombroso, Tamburini, Ascenzi, *op. cit.* (note 2), 203.

21. APF, 1891, Firenze, 24 Oct. 1891, and 27 Oct. 1891.

22. APF, cat 9, cas. 1, 1899, b. 1959. See letters among the various provincial, municipal and medical authorities, dated 19 Sept. 1898, 7 and 17 Oct. 1898, 12, 23 and 24 Nov. 1898, 21 Febr. 1899, 22, 23, 27 and 30 March 1899.

23. APF, cat 9, cas. 1, 1899, b. 1959, cat 9, cas. 1, 1899, b. 1959, E. Tanzi's letter, 4 Oct. 1898. See APF, cat 10, cas. 2, 1902, 160, President of Deputazione Provinciale's letter, 14 Jan. 1902.

24. See APF, cat 10, cas. 2, 1902, 160, President of Deputazione Provinciale, 14 Jan. 1902.

25. APF, cat 9, cas. 1., a 46 (confirmations of subsidies) from 1900 to 1912.

26. APF, cat.9, cas. 1, 1902, 46, see Mayor of Fucecchio, 27 giugno 1902.

27. APF, cat. 9, cas. 1, 1912, 46.

28. APF, cat. 9, cas. 1, 1907.

29. APF, cat. 9, cas. 1, 1905, 233, Tanzi's request is dated 20 May 1901.

30. E. Shorter, *A History of Psychiatry* (New York: John Wiley, 1997), 50. He obviously refers to his views in *The Making of the Modern Family* (New York: Basik Books, 1975).

31.   Tamburini, Ferrari, Antonini, *op. cit.* (note 2), 571.

32.   See at least, A. Buttafuoco, *Le Mariuccine. Storia di un'istituzione laica* (Milano: Angeli, 1988). B. Cammeo, *Laura Solara Mantegazza 1813-1873* (Milano: no publisher, 1902).

33.   E. Bruno and V. Ruggero (eds), *La Donna nella beneficenza in Italia* (Torino, 1912), vol. III, 158. Cf. Comune di Firenze, *Elenco dei poveri. Relazione della Commissione* (Firenze: Barbera, 1915). Brilliant research on the poor and the early nineteenth century Florentine sources is found in S.J. Woolf, *Porca miseria* (Roma-Bari: Laterza, 1988) esp. ch. IV, original edition in *Social History*, 1 (1976). See also G. Gozzini, *Il segreto dell'elemosina*, (Firenze: Olschki, 1993).

34.   See *Atti del V Consiglio Provinciale di Firenze per l'anno amministrativo 1905-06* (Firenze: Galletti e Cocci, 1906), 113-6.

35.   APF, cat. 9, cas. I, 1907, f. 561, 2617, A. Carpi, 13 Febr. 1906; and B. Cammeo's reply, 17 Febr. 1906; letters of high esteem to Cammeo, for example, on 15 Jun. 1906, and 20 March 1908.

36.   See APF, cat. 9, cas. I, 1908, a. 2617.

37.   APF, *ibid.*, and ff., in *Dementi innocui a custodia privata. Conferme dei sussidi ai tenutari.*

38.   APF, cat. 9, cas. I, 1908, 2617.

39.   See *Atti del Consiglio Provinciale di Firenze, anno amministrativo 1916-17*, Firenze, 1920, meeting 2 Febr. 1917, 156-161, with refs. to earlier debates.

40.   APF, cat. 9, cas. I, 1920, 2591, *Protocollo Deliberazioni della Deputazione Provinciale*, 10 Dec. 1920.

41.   See, for example, the list of reduced subsidies, attached to the Delibera provinciale, 3 Sept. 1937 con *Revisione dei sussidiati. Riduzione dei sussidi*, APF, cat. 9, cas. I, 1937, 1520.

42.   Archivio San Salvi, Direzione Affari Diversi, 1938, f.n.n. *Sussidiati*, Amaldi to the Prefetto 16 June and 18 June 1937.

Psychiatric Nursing

Changing Attitudes towards 'Non-Restraint' in Dutch Psychiatric Nursing 1897-1994

Cecile aan de Stegge

Introduction

In 1907, Jacob van Deventer, founder of the Dutch teaching programme in psychiatric nursing, gave a lecture for an international audience.[1] His lecture was based on 25 years of experience with asylum reform: from 1883 until 1891, he had been chief medical officer of the Buitengasthuis in Amsterdam, and from 1892 until 1904, of the Meerenberg asylum in Bloemendaal.[2] From 1905, he was Inspector at the State Inspectorate for the Insane and the Asylums.[3] Van Deventer accentuated the great progress in psychiatry he had witnessed. Psychiatrists had – standing on the threshold of the twentieth century – finally come to realize that the focus of attention of every worker in an asylum should be directed towards the 'interests' of the insane. In earlier times, it had been supposed that merely building 'walls' around the insane was enough. Behind these walls, insane patients had often suffered the painful consequences of neglect, physical violence, and/or abuse by untrained and uninterested attendants: severe ear wounds, freezing cold, bedsores, gangrene, broken bones, mutilations, sexual perversions, the frequent use of mechanical restraint, and seclusion in isolation cells for weeks or even months.

Today, Van Deventer stated, this was history. The long struggle for 'non-restraint' had finally been won.[4] Chains and handcuffs had been replaced with vests and leather belts. These in their turn had been replaced by isolation cells, so that the freedom of bodily movement of agitated patients was hardly restricted. Ten years earlier, he would not have believed these 'cells' could ever be banned from psychiatry, unless one had replaced their use by mechanical and/ or chemical restraint.[5] Yet, psychiatry was now on its way to replace the 'isolation cell' by a 'single room', of which the door could remain open. He concluded: 'The "principle of non-restraint" is entirely "ratified".'[6] While former inspectors had maintained that only 'mechanical' restraint could stop certain patients from uncontrolled behaviour such as masturbating or smearing faeces, from 1870, 'non-restraint' had been adopted as a desirable method.[7] Each category of patient was to be allowed as much freedom as possible; each individual patient was to receive individual attention. A modern 'hospital for the insane' would offer bed treatment, hydrotherapy, physiotherapy, and occupational therapy.[8]

The growing diversity of treatments was, he said, due to development of 'the art of caring for sick people'.[9] Once the insight had grown that the insane were 'sick', psychiatrists had acknowledged that their overcoming of neglect as well as of restraint depended on the degree into which they could trust the personalities of their 'caring' personnel.[10] They had to be enabled to offer more humane and adequate care.[11] Educating 'attendants' to 'nurses' by explaining the reason why the insane could show strange, irritating or even aggressive behaviour would motivate them to refrain from using force or mechanical restraint.[12]

The Dutch Society for Psychiatry & Neurology had designed a three-year course in nursing the insane.[13] Van Deventer said that this was best offered to both male and female attendants, preferably in mixed groups.[14] Both genders had their own specific talents and qualities and could complement each other well in psychiatric nursing. While 'caring' was an excellent task for the female nurse, 'supervising labour-therapy' was a task for males.[15] Meanwhile, one shouldn't think that every 'lady from the bourgeoisie' was suitable to nurse on all wards. In departments for men of the lower classes, some 'upper class ladies' tended to assume an air of superiority that was not accepted by their patients.[16] On such wards, as well as on the units for dangerous or immoral male patients (referring to those with a tendency for nude exhibition or masturbation), male nurses would probably do a better job.[17]

The Dutch course was based on the premise that the psychiatric hospital – this term was actually used by Van Deventer – itself embodied the proper school for psychiatric nurses. Only such hospitals employed doctors with enough working experience to teach student nurses. A qualified psychiatric nurse should be able to deal with *all* psychiatric patients: the quiet, the semi-agitated and the agitated, but also the 'sick' insane who were both mentally and physically ill. Therefore, the student had to gain working experience in departments for *all* these categories, which could only be found in psychiatric hospitals.[18] During the first year, lessons improved the students' general education in reading, writing, arithmetic, history, geography and the like. This was a necessary check on their learning capacity, while also guaranteeing that they would be able to understand the rest of the programme and be capable of social intercourse with patients of all classes. During the second year, the course offered lessons on anatomy and physiology of the human body, nursing the sick, hygiene and pathology. On the wards, the students could develop technical skills in the use of instruments, binding of wounds, etc. The third year concentrated on knowledge needed to nurse the insane: psychiatry, caring for the insane, and knowledge of the second Dutch Insanity Law of 1884. Nurses had to know what documents this law required before a patient could be admitted, as well as what means of restraint asylums were supposed to register.[19]

The registration form of the State Inspectorate mentioned eight means of mechanical restraint: binding the hands, restraining gloves (either loose or attached to a belt), the straitjacket or strait suit, binding the feet, foot chains, binding to a chair, and a strait chair.[20] There were also different possibilities for secluding patients: the 'isolation room' or 'single room' (in Dutch *afzonderings-kamer*, situated near a common room, furnished and containing a large window); the 'isolation cell' (in Dutch *isoleercel*; 'isolated' from other rooms, with a 'peephole' instead of a window, a heavy door with padlocks, fixed furniture or no furniture at all), and the closed box bed (in Dutch *dekselbed*). The register should contain the name of the patient involved, the doctor who had ordered its use, the reason for using mechanical restraint or seclusion, the judgement of this measure by the doctor, and that of the inspector.[21] Neither nurses nor the role of nurses in registration were mentioned on the form.

Van Deventer stressed that Dutch psychiatry had witnessed a rapid decrease of mechanical restraint and seclusion since most psychiatric hospitals had organised courses in 'nursing the insane' and held examinations. He had recorded a significant reduction in the use of isolation cells at Meerenberg after he had started educating nurses and introduced female nurses on to male wards.[22] This proved that psychiatric nurses could restrict their use of mechanical restraint and seclusion to cases where these devices were the only means of preventing a complete upheaval, suicide or serious harm.

Almost a century has passed since Van Deventer expressed this opinion. Between 1892 and 1997, Dutch psychiatric hospitals trained more than 55,500 Dutch nurses, 34 per cent male and 66 per cent female. It is unclear, however, whether all these nurses practised according to his standards of 'non-restraint' and even how long his standards of 'non-restraint' survived him.[23] This chapter hopes to shed some light on changes in Dutch attitudes towards 'non-restraint' during the twentieth century. One source is the successive textbooks that psychiatric nurses have used to prepare themselves for their final examination. Another is the requirements of the State Inspectorate for nurses' use of restraint.

The Textbooks and Requirements of the State Inspectorate

Between 1897 and 1938, ten Dutch asylum doctors published nine different textbooks with the purpose of preparing students for the final examination leading to qualification as a psychiatric nurse. These authors were: J. van Deventer (1897, 1 edition), B. van Delden (1897, 1 edition), D. Schermers (1898, 11 editions), J.C.Th. Scheffer (1906, 5 editions), P.H.M. Travaglino (1910, 1 edition), J.G. Schnitzler (1915, 4 editions), W.H. Cox (1927 and 1929, 1 edition), H.J. Schim van der Loeff & J.A.J. Barnhoorn (1930, 4 editions), and finally A.P. Timmer (1938, 5 editions).[24] With their reprints, these textbooks add up to a total of 34 editions, published between 1897 and 1964. Up to the mid-1960s, these textbooks were compulsory reading for psychiatric nurses. The authors were doctors in large psychiatric hospitals when they published their books. Their textbooks can therefore be considered a reflection of the standards of care in psychiatric nursing at the time they were written.[25] On the other hand, they were also the means to set 'standards' in psychiatric nursing. They provide a useful source for historical research into the use of restraint and seclusion.

With regard to the Dutch phenomenon of 'pillarisation': the authors of these textbooks worked in psychiatric institutions that were either non-denominational or belonged to two different denominations. Though it is indeed possible to distinguish a non-denominational, a Calvinistic, and a Roman Catholic 'trend' in their books, the authors also greatly influenced each other and were – throughout this period – largely of one mind with regard to the subject of restraint.[26] On the basis of changes that can be observed in the textbooks, three periods can be distinguished. First, a period (1897-1925) during which all authors expressed their sympathy with the principle of 'non-restraint' that had been introduced in the mid-nineteenth century by the English psychiatrist John Conolly. Second, a period (1926-1955) after the publications of Dr. W.M. van der Scheer, who was inspired by the German psychiatrist Hermann Simon. Van der Scheer wanted nurses to value the principle of 'responsibility' above that of 'non-restraint'. The third period (1956-1964) started after the introduction of psycho-active drugs in 1953. The principles of 'non-restraint' and 'responsibility' then became combined in a new approach.

From 1960 onwards, many textbooks were produced by nurses themselves and by psychologists, psychotherapists as well as by psychiatrists. This great quantity makes it hard to determine which nurse read which book for his/her final examination. Therefore, for this period, only the best-known textbooks written by psychiatric nurses were studied: P. Stevens, J. Pepping & A.P. Lammens (1960, 1961), B. Verdel (1965), F. Kramer (1968, 1974), C.J.M. Nieland, L. van der Laan and P.F. Rooyackers (1969, 1970), G. Roodhart (1975, 1977) and A. Bos & van R.R. Leeuwen (1994).[27] In successive books, the principle of 'individualised nursing care' gained increasing emphasis. This resulted in a diminishing tolerance for 'standard routines' in the use of mechanical restraint and seclusion: the most recent textbook contained explicit instructions on the use of these measures.

The State Inspectorate also issued specific regulations for nurses with regard to mechanical restraint and/or seclusion, not only requiring registration but also – from 1924 – prescribing what technical skills psychiatric nurses ought to possess. Here it is necessary to explain something about the educational system for nurses in the Netherlands. In 1920, when the Law on Protection of the Nursing Diploma was prepared for discussion in Parliament, nine of 11 professional organisations who were consulted thought that the Dutch psychiatric institution-based course in 'nursing the insane and the nervously ill' had become worthy of a diploma in its own right.[28] The Parliament accepted this 'two diploma sys-tem'.[29] *Two* vocational training routes were acknowledged as 'basic learning routes for nurses'.[30] A general route (general hospital-based) gave access to Diploma A. The psychiatric route (psychiatric institution-based) gave access to Diploma B. Each required three years of combined theoretical training and practical working experience. Both general hospitals and psychiatric institutions that wanted to go on training nurses had to obtain a permit from the State Inspectorate. In return for this, the Inspectorates would prescribe what the nurses had to learn, check their final examinations, and register those who were qualified with Diploma A or B.[31] The law stipulated a fine for anyone who advertised themselves as 'nurses' without possessing one of these diplomas.

The first requirements of the Inspectorate about the content of courses in 'general nursing' and 'nursing the insane' were published in December 1923.[32] To be admitted to the final examination in B-nursing, candidates were expected to be at least 22 years old and had to produce a testimonial, signed by the chief medical officer of their institution, stating that they had satisfactorily worked for three years on a variety of wards. They also had to hand in a Practical Experience and Report Book (PE&R). The exam took two hours: one to assess theoretical knowledge, one to demonstrate technical skills.

Originally, the State Inspectorate had intended to revise the PE&R book every five years, to keep pace with changes in actual psychiatric practice. The book was indeed changed in 1929 and 1933. Then, the Inspectorate announced that the economic depression made it impossible to continue the labour-intensive practice of changing the booklet every five years. From 1970, however, the PE&R book was changed several times, until it had to give way to a modern, reflective learning style.

1897-1925: Medical Abhorrence of Mechanical Restraint

The authors of the first well-known Dutch textbooks on nursing the insane – Van Deventer (1897), Van Delden (1897), Schermers (1898) and Scheffer (1906) – were impressed with John Conolly's ideology and method of 'non-restraint'.[33] His first principle was 'to exclude all hurtful excitement from a brain already disposed to excitement', and he therefore objected to the use of mechanical restraint.[34] Such means would irritate patients and make them feel animal-like. Conolly's view on 'asylum management' was that the total climate should indicate respect for patients' comfort in the smallest details: food, clothing, bedding, tasteful surroundings, friendliness, respect, etc. The dedication that attendants felt for looking after these 'details' (a job, according to Conolly, that consisted of endless 'fatiguing, depressing and often repulsive tasks') would be a decisive factor in the success of non-restraint.[35] If attendants were able to live up to these high standards, Conolly was convinced they would only have to resort to a few minutes of 'manual restraint' to 'hold' an agitated patient experiencing a sudden impulse of aggression. He preferred this brief 'manual restraint' to any means of mechanical restraint, and also favoured 'temporary seclusion'.[36] For the latter, he had created different facilities. When confronted by troublesome behaviour, his attendants had a choice between 'single rooms' (for short-term seclusion or retreat), 'padded cells' (for very agitated patients prone to injure themselves by head-banging) and 'non-padded cells' with fixed furniture and built-in toilet, high, bare walls, and a heavy door with a peephole (for very agitated patients who were a risk to other patients).[37]

Dutch textbook authors knew that in the Netherlands also, nurses were the most important agents in turning the non-restraint method into a success. Therefore, they began with a sketch of the 'inhuman' and violent history of nursing the insane.[38] This was illustrated with pictures of obsolete means of restraint, such as the strait suit, strait gloves, coffin beds, shackles, etc.[39] This sketch was followed by an appealing description of Conolly's non-restraint and the statement that since then many patients had proved they were capable of being awarded greater freedom.[40] As well as the atmosphere in the former 'asylums', buildings had changed for the better. [41]

Following Conolly, the authors of this period experienced a dilemma with regard to the question of whether they should write about means of mechanical restraint. On the one hand, they were confronted with regulations from the Second Insanity Law (1884) and the State Inspectorate for the Insane and the Asylums. The fact that seclusion and mechanical restraint had to be registered made it necessary to describe both measures, but they considered the list of methods to be fairly long and feared that publishing it would create the impression that 'mechanical restraint' was a frequent practice in Dutch asylums.[42] Probably, they also believed that giving practical instructions on how to *use* these means would entail an 'open invitation' to psychiatric nurses to go on using them, instead of using their own physical presence ('manual restraint'). Most authors tried to overcome the dilemma either by not writing about means of mechanical restraint at all or by depicting them as 'relics of old times'.[43] Van Deventer only mentioned them in his chapter on 'admission': nurses might be confronted with some means of restraint when patients entered the asylum for the first time.[44] In that case, they should remove these devices as soon as possible, while taking care not to run any risk of personal harm. This was achieved by having enough staff to be able to 'hold' the agitated patient.[45] Meanwhile, showing 'tact' was more important than showing 'courage'.[46]

B. van Delden, a doctor at the non-denominational Medical Asylum for the Insane in Utrecht, considered mechanical restraint one of the most important hindrances to the public's acceptance of the asylum as a 'psychiatric hospital', though he did not deny its existence. His motto was: 'Openness instead of secrecy'.[47] He published the registration form in his textbook.[48] He warned not to infer from this list that these means were used frequently.[49] Van Delden stated that in the Utrecht asylum of 1896, he had known only one imbecile patient on a ward of a 150 who had to be treated with mechanical restraint. He included no 'instructions' on the practical use of such means.

When he wrote his book, D. Schermers was chief medical officer of a large Calvinistic asylum in Loosduinen. He gave instructions on the use of gentle, brief 'manual restraint', but the first means to combat 'agitation' was to show understanding. Agitation could be a consequence of illness, but also be justified anger about the behaviour of fellow patients or nurses. Nursing staff had to ask themselves: did I do anything that brought this about? If this did not help, the patient was to be calmed down through 'speech'. If that failed, they could try 'holding on to' the patient (with enough colleagues, preferably by the clothes and always without pinching).[50] Only when the patient started to embody physical danger to fellow patients or staff, was he to be put in 'isolation'.[51] In such cases, the doctor had to be asked for advice; only in cases of absolute emergency were nurses permitted to decide themselves.[52] The only means of mechanical restraint Schermers described in his textbook was the straitjacket.[53] While explaining that the use of this device had a dangerous side, Schermers pointed out that the jacket was much smaller, allowing the patient more freedom to move his limbs, than the strait suit had been.

The fourth author, J.C.Th. Scheffer, was chief medical officer of a non-denominational asylum as well as of an adjacent sanatorium for nervous sufferers near Leyden. He gave very little information on mechanical restraint, but his statements on the straitjacket were ambivalent. Though stating that this means of restraint could only be found 'in the attics of asylums or in museums', he mentioned that it was still used from time to time for the transport of a dangerous insane patient.[54] The third edition of his textbook was compatible with Conolly's method of non-restraint: if an agitated patient could only be kept in bed or a bath by means of 'mechanical' or 'manual' restraint, 'temporary seclusion' was to be preferred.[55] Another method in such situations was to administer barbiturates, but these could only be given by order of the doctor.

The subject of seclusion was treated entirely differently. All authors agreed that in psychiatry, one simply couldn't do without it. Already in 1897, both Van Deventer and Van Delden discriminated between two different facilities: a 'single room' was meant for patients who created 'unrest' on their ward, e.g. by screaming. However, an 'isolation cell' was to seclude dangerous patients against their will; it needed to be stripped of all comforts, as well as of objects that could be used to injure oneself.[56] Its sole goal was to protect patients from bodily harm. The decision to put someone in such a cell, particularly when a longer period was foreseen, was to be taken by the doctor.

Suicidal patients, though, were not to be secluded in either kind of room. If guarding them could not be achieved without seclusion, they had to be permanently watched there.[57] If a disturbed patient had to be taken to an isolation cell, this had to be done by at least three nurses. Most authors wrote only about male nurses in this regard; only Van Deventer also mentioned female ones. During the period of seclusion, the patient had to be observed constantly, and after one hour, staff had to assess whether the patient was approachable again. At regular intervals, attempts should be made to see if the patient had calmed down sufficiently to be taken out of the cell. No patient was allowed to stay in a cell for longer than 12 hours in succession. Both patient and cell had to be washed every 12 hours.

Analysing the first editions and the next ones (in particular those of Schermers and Scheffer) brings to light that an important architectural change has taken place in psychiatric institutions. 'Seclusion departments', a long way from the rest of the wards and consisting solely of isolation cells, gave way to a variety of 'isolation rooms', sometimes in combination with 'single rooms', *within* the pavilions. The textbooks make clear that after this architectural shift had taken place, so that the act of 'seclusion' could take place within a ward itself, doctors no longer considered their former objections ('dehumanization' or 'reducing patients to the status of an animal') as so very relevant.

The textbooks also reveal that so-called 'humane' medical treatments like 'methodical bedside nursing', 'prolonged bath therapy', and 'wet packs' were used for the same categories of patients who formerly would have been treated with mechanical restraint or seclusion. As early as 1897, Van Delden wrote that 'the frequent seclusion of patients in isolation cells' had greatly decreased as a result of 'methodical bedside nursing'.[58] According to Schermers, the straitjacket had become superfluous by 1921: by then, agitation was looked upon as a result of illness, so that doctors would want to treat it medically, including the use of drugs.[59]

As mentioned above, the State Inspectorate issued the first regulations on the final exam in psychiatric nursing in December 1923. A nurse should have gained experience with at least 20 diseases and have mastered at least 50 technical nursing skills. Among these latter were making a report on a patient whose admission was legally certified, 'holding an agitated patient', giving a 'cold (wet) pack', putting patients in an isolation cell, and either 'keeping' or 'guarding' dangerous patients (to prevent suicide or aggressive outbursts).[60]

Combining the textbooks and the regulations of this period, one can conclude that during the years between 1897 and 1925, 'non-restraint' had grown more popular. In 1892, when Van Deventer and his colleagues had organised the first final examination in 'nursing the insane', questions had still been asked like: 'Are you permitted to use means of mechanical restraint, and if so, what means under what circumstances?' and 'What aspects does a nurse have to be alert of when taking care of the interior of a single room or an isolation cell?'[61] By 1925, however, neither the State Inspectorate nor the authors of textbooks expected nurses to master a skill in the use of *any* of the means of 'mechanical restraint', mentioned on the Inspectorate's registration form, while alternative techniques such as 'manual restraint' and 'giving a wet pack' were not mentioned on the registration form.[62] Doctors underlined the fact that the 'modern' straitjacket was *smaller* than the nineteenth-century strait suit, so that freedom of movement was evidently considered very important. With regard to seclusion, nurses were advised to use the utmost caution. Whenever possible, they should prefer a 'single room' to the isolation cell. All in all, as a consequence of the general acceptance of the non-restraint policy expected of nurses, during this period modern medical treatment methods by (more or less) trained nurses may for a large part have indeed *replaced* former means of mechanical restraint.

1926-1955: Restraint as an 'Educational Means' for Psychiatric Nurses

The second period starts with a publication by the psychiatrist W.M. van der Scheer, general director of the provincial psychiatric hospital near Santpoort, in a magazine for nurses.[63] Here, he stated that regular contemporary responses to agitation – 'nursing methods' like 'methodical bedside nursing' – were in fact disguised means of restraint, because these were means of control, without improving the patients' condition.[64] Their use had resulted in 'fool's liberty', while patients were allowed to regress further and further.[65] Consequently, special wards for the most troublesome and agitated patients were needed, to apply more serious means of mechanical restraint or forced treatment.[66] On such 'closed wards', situations occurred that one would rather conceal from the outside world.[67] Therefore, it was time tc replace Conolly's method of 'non-restraint' with the method of 'active therapy', as introduced by Simon of Gütersloh.

The basic principle was that one should desist from considering patients 'not responsible'; agitated behaviour was not caused by illness but was the consequence of environmental neglect. Therefore, psychiatric nursing had to be reorganised radically, first of all on wards for agitated patients. All patients had to be given 'fitting' work.[68] For a start, a patient could work within the 'community' of the pavilion or ward. Later, they could work elsewhere: in a central hall for occupational therapy, within a live-in ward without supervision by nurses, or even within normal society. Psychiatric nurses should supervise their patients' work with an attitude of friendship and equality, but also watch for progress, so that any patient ready for the next step was promoted at once. Even the most troublesome insane patient should be considered 'a social creature' and receive a negative reaction from the people in his surroundings in response to 'irritating behaviour'. It was a matter of permanent observation and education.[69]

Nurses were allowed to use 'educational measures' such as reward and punishment, which had to be awarded as a direct response to positive or negative behaviour.[70] Each reward or punishment had to consist of stimuli that would really 'affect' the patient in question. A reward could be a sweet or tobacco, a little more freedom, a walk, a day off etc.; punishment would be the opposite. Uniformity in the type or quantity of reward and punishment had to be avoided. None should be 'favoured'. If 'soft' educational measures did not have the expected effect, the first tough 'educational' measure involved a few minutes of segregation in an ordinary but not very cosy room. If the agitation was not effectively subdued, a five-minute seclusion in the 'single room' followed, and if need be, after that half an hour of seclusion in a 'seclusion cell'.[71] After that, if necessary, a lukewarm bath (one to one and a half hours) and only as a very last resort could the doctor be asked to prescribe a narcotic. As this method had to be applied in a consistent manner, much depended on its correct interpretation by the nursing staff. For each measure taken – whether light or severe – the nurses had to supply a written report, including their motivation and the effects. To become good pedagogues, nurses were invited to reflect upon their own behaviour and reactions. Van der Scheer insisted that psychiatrists should organise 'talk sessions' for the nursing staff on their ward, in order to exchange experiences with them and supervise them.[72]

All in all: Van der Scheer opposed Conolly by returning to the same ideas that Conolly had valued. He also strove after a style of hospital management in which the nurses and occupational therapy would be of crucial importance, while emphasizing the importance of a civilised atmosphere and respect for patients. Like Conolly he stressed 'details': chronic female patients should be provided with a brassiere, and chronic male patients should not have too short a pair of trousers.[73] He detested 'wet packs' and did not mention any means of mechanical restraint. Yet there was an important difference between him and Conolly. Van der Scheer delegated more responsibility to the nurses than Conolly had done a century earlier, because they were supposed to educate their patients. He also insisted that nurses' motivation in using seclusion had to be considered when judging the appropriateness of this measure. If nurses could prove that they had done all they could to prevent seclusion and give sound arguments why they had finally resorted to this measure – to 'teach' the patient that he was 'a nuisance to the community' – then it was legitimate.

All medical authors of nursing textbooks that were edited or written after 1926 (Scheffer 1929; Hamer & Haverkate 1932, 1938, 1946, 1950; Cox 1927 and 1929; Van der Loeff & Barnhoorn 1930, 1932, 1936, 1947; Timmer 1938, 1942, 1947, 1952, 1957) stressed the impact of Van der Scheers's campaign to replace 'wrongfully applied nursing methods' by educating patients through a variety of occupational therapies.[74] As A.H. Oort wrote in 1929: 'the "active therapy" made Dutch "asylums" break with their efforts to imitate the general hospital.' Instead, a modern 'psychiatric institution' should resemble a 'small community' where 'the ill and the underprivileged' lived together as well as possible.[75]

Changing Attitudes

To implement such communities, authors sought to stimulate nurses' interest in individual patients. W.H. Cox, for instance, tried to persuade his student nurses to 'listen' to themselves as well as to their patients, so that they would eventually be able to see the resemblance between the normal and abnormal. He also underlined the necessity of a 'broad general education' for psychiatric nurses. Since nobody could undergo all human experiences himself, anyone wanting to be successful in dealing, as a nurse, with 'unusual people' should read a lot of novels and listen to other people's stories. Patients were not just 'passive recipients of care'; they would perhaps not always venture to express their complaints but would not forgive the nurses if their feelings were ignored.[76]

The other authors of this period also accentuated the importance of 'mutual trust' between nurses and patients. Nurses should study the arts of observation and conversation, to get acquainted with the personal reactions of individual patients. They should avoid 'standard nursing methods' but be able to pinpoint the 'weak' or 'strong' points that could be stimulated for punishment or reward. This would make their 'educational nursing task' easier, because patients would accept fair and 'tailor-made' authority.[77]

For the avoidance of mechanical restraint, the most important measures mentioned were 'manual restraint' or the prolonged bath. Visual material was used to show how nurses should 'hold' agitated patients. Scheffer (fifth edition, 1929) was the first to publish two drawings on the matter.[78] Schim van der Loeff & Barnhoorn (1930) and A.P. Timmer used photographs.[79] Most authors hardly mentioned the use of traditional means of restraint like the straitjacket.[80] A 'modern' method, however, emerged in the form of the 'strait sheet'.[81] This device was said to allow patients more room to move their limbs and breathe than the 'wet pack'. It was, therefore, considered a rather 'humane' device and recommended as an 'educational measure' in case patients 'needed' a lesson in self-restraint.[82] Though 'medical' methods were considered the responsibility of the doctor, by discussing the dose of certain drugs and more especially by describing some of these as possible 'means of punishment', the authors may have created an impression that nurses could administer these also as an 'educational method'.[83]

Over time, the authors gave their 'educational guideline' two different uses: one for the curable and one for the incurable patient.[84] Curable insane patients, whose agitation was caused by their illness, had to be 'educated' under the direction of the doctor, so that they could eventually return to society. Slightly less curable patients were also 'educated' to be able to return to a less restricted community, e.g. a nursing home or care in their own home.[85] The doctor was also important here. Incurable patients, however, whose agitation was more likely to be caused by 'fool's liberty' would remain in 'the small asylum community'.[86] For them, nurses could use a bath or a strait sheet as an 'educational measure', as long as they were able to give a sound reason for doing so. After Van der Scheer, all nursing measures were dominated by the concept of 'education', but for incurable patients, this was a responsibility that rested almost solely in the hands of nurses. Over time, the authors also created a distinction between different types of seclusion. They did not allow long-term seclusion and tried to prevent it.[87] Short-term seclusion, as a response to the 'primary agitation' of a curable patient, needed supervision by a doctor or head nurse. But short-term seclusion, applied as an 'educational measure' for 'secondary agitation', was an educational measure that nurses were allowed to administer independently.[88]

The State Inspectorate supported this 'educational and individualising trend' wholeheartedly. In 1929, they changed their regulations for the final exam in psychiatric nursing. This reflected the growing demands on nursing skills in communication, observation and writing reports. In the final practical exam, candidates were expected to have a conversation of half an hour with a patient they had never met before, in front of an examination board which consisted of five doctors.[89] They then had to give a report of what was the matter with this patient, leaving only half an hour for a demonstration of technical skills. The Inspectorate also changed its regulations with regard to the PE&R book: from 1929, this contained two extra skills with regard to restraint: nurses were now expected to administer medicines to patients, on the basis of doctors' prescriptions, and to feed patients who refused to eat, provided they would never forcibly tube-feed.[90]

In 1930, the Inspectorate edited – for the first time since 1884 – new regulations on the registration of mechanical restraint and seclusion. The diverse 'means of mechanical restraint' were no longer exactly defined: all measures that caused the patient to be restricted in the movement of more than one of his limbs had to be registered, including the 'wet pack'.[91] 'Seclusion' was defined as 'in a room destined for this use', and this also had to be registered, while the difference between 'isolation cells' and 'single rooms' disappeared.

In 1933, the State Inspectorate published a fresh version of the PE&R book. Certain psychiatric hospitals were said to use less restraint because they offered more active therapy, and so the importance of skill in 'active therapy' was stressed.[92] Candidates had to master 85 practical nursing skills. Among these at least 45 were considered 'typical' for psychiatry and 40 'general' nursing skills. The 'psychiatric skills' included 19 varieties of occupational therapy and 4 spare-time activities: party games; music, dance or drama activities; gymnastics; and outdoor sports. Nurses were supposed to have a considerable amount of recorded skills in both kinds of activities.

Three years later, another new registration form was introduced. This time 'seclusion' had to be registered only when it was during the daytime and had lasted for more than two hours. Therefore, all nocturnal and 'short term seclusions' fell outside the registration policy. The regulations of the Inspectorate clearly resembled the attitude towards restraint that was expected of psychiatric

Changing Attitudes

nurses by textbook authors. On the other hand, the requirement that nurses should be skilled in the use of a strait sheet was now part of the examination. So, after forty years *without* reference to 'mechanical restraint', such a skill suddenly belonged to the final test in psychiatric nursing, while also experience in 'holding an agitated patient' still needed to be recorded. Maybe the Inspectors hoped that the 'smaller' and less hampering strait sheet would replace the wet pack.

The Inspectorate took its controlling task with seclusion less seriously than before. 'Educational isolation' for chronic patients had come solely under the authority of the psychiatric hospitals and their staff, perhaps because it was very frequent.[93] All in all, it seems that between 1926 and 1955 the attitude towards non-restraint had changed fundamentally, from 'non-restraint' towards a rather severe 'educational nursing regimen', condoning the use of a strait sheet and/or short-term seclusion. This severe nursing regimen, however, was only for the chronically ill.[94]

1956-1964: Restraint as an Impediment to Self-Realization

The principles that had dominated the two previous periods ('non-restraint' and 'returning "responsibility" to the individual patient') became radicalized by a new generation of doctors in the *Algemeen Leerboek voor het verplegen van geestes- en zenuwzieken*.[95] This was published in 1956, re-printed in 1960 and 1964, and it was the first 'oecumenical' and social-psychiatric nursing textbook.[96] J.H. van der Drift, director of the Calvinist psychiatric hospital at Wolfheze, showed the importance of nursing by joining the earlier paragraphs on 'nursing sufferers of mental and nervous disorders' and those on 'specific medical treatment methods' into one text. 'Nursing' thereby became an integral element of medical treatment.

Van der Drift relied heavily on Van der Scheer's book of 1933. He acknowledged that psychopharmacology had contributed significantly to a change of climate in psychiatric institutions. Yet, the 'real revolution' in Dutch psychiatry should be ascribed to the broadly accepted principle of giving patients 'responsibility'.[97] 'Medical treatment' in psychiatry was described as 're-education of the patient'. Both psychiatrists and nurses could exert a beneficial influence, provided they undertook all kinds of activities with their patients (work, play, cultural activities, conversation) while being aware of their own behaviour towards them.[98] Since the quality of medical treatment depended on the quality of the nursing staff, he stressed the importance of training for nurses, especially by revitalising the need for self-reflection that had been stated earlier.[99] A psychiatric hospital should be more than just an institution supplying care; it should also socialise its professional personnel, especially the nurses, through 'sound teaching' and 'team discussions'.[100] Student nurses should be offered a chance to 'practice' newly learned skills – on one another or on dolls – before applying them on real patients. They should be able to become member of professional nursing organisations and attend conferences.[101]

These measures in the sphere of 'human resources management' were not only necessary to recruit more personnel but had a sound 'medically motivated' basis.[102] If the psychiatric hospital took good care of its employees, the outcome of medical treatment (including skilful nursing) could become more successful. Van der Drift expected that as many as 70 or 80 per cent of the patients would eventually be re-integrated into society, though some with a small 'social defect'. (In the previous period, this percentage was said to have been 50 per cent.)[103]

Re-education of patients for the benefit of the community was no longer proposed; the highest goal of treatment was not in 'adaptation'.[104] Inspired both by psychoanalysis and Jaspers' phenomenology, Van der Drift proposed allowing each patient to develop his/her personality to the full.[105] To achieve this, doctors and nurses should closely follow the patient's perceptions and study what this individual recounted of his/her experiences. Since each patient possessed a capacity for responsibility and freedom, he/she should participate in conversation and be treated as an autonomous person. Since this philosophy was largely incompatible with a frequent use of restraint, the 1956 textbook embodied a return to 'non-restraint' *via* 'nurses' responsibility for good communication'. A nurse would use the utmost caution before applying any means of mechanical restraint and needed to be able to adapt his/her use of a 'seclusion room' to a variety of purposes, for instance try to use an open door or negotiate with the patient over the times for visiting.

During the short period in which (among others) this textbook was compulsory material for the final exam, the Inspectorate did not change any of its regulations.[106] As a result, the old PE&R book became incompatible with the attitude towards restraint that was now expected. The nurses therefore organised themselves in order to bridge this gap. In 1958, a group of head nurses started meeting to revise the teaching programme.[107] Consequently, from 1962 onwards, the text of a 'modern' concept PE&R book was printed *within* the official book of the Inspectorate.[108] In this new 'draft-text', all earlier skills with regard to restraint were revised. Skills in 'mechanical' restraint were not mentioned, and those in 'manual' restraint were replaced by others that presupposed an interpersonal relationship with the patient. For example: 'guarding a dangerous patient' was replaced by 'taking action in relation to an aggressive patient'. 'Isolation' was renamed 'segregation' (in Dutch: *separeren*), while 'modern' nursing tasks, e.g. 'taking care of a group of patients' and 'supporting individual patients to operate more independently' had gained a much more prominent place.[109]

In 1962, the Inspectorate permitted psychiatric hospitals to let candidates pass their final exam if they had recorded some of the skills from this new part of the book.[110] Thus, psychiatric hospitals had a chance to develop their own profile with regard to the theoretical ideas and technical skills they wanted to teach their nurses on restraint. Therefore, 'non-restraint' seemed to have regained some strength, as in the period between 1892 and 1925, when it was a guiding principle for the attitude of psychiatric nurses towards patients.

1960-1994: Restraint and Seclusion as a 'Nursing Responsibility'

Between 1960 and 1966, five Roman Catholic religious brothers (all head nurses and/or teachers) became the first psychiatric nurses to write their own point of view.[111] Their text fed the already lively discussion at that time, defining nursing as: 'the science that delivers general and understandable knowledge, necessary to care with responsibility for a sick human being, in order to relieve his suffering and to restore his health'.[112] The word 'science' and the fact that nursing was portrayed as 'a responsible and goal-directed activity' were the key elements that expressed a break with tradition. In the earlier nursing textbooks 'doctors knew best'; they bore the final responsibility for all tasks, including tasks that nurses performed.[113] In the end it was always the psychiatrist who was responsible.

In opposition to this, the Brothers prepared their aspirant readers for a 're-sponsible job'.[114] The fundamental rule was that every individual patient, regardless of his/her behaviour, was a 'human being who thinks, loves and hates and is capable of sharp and quick apprehension'.[115] The necessity to learn to tune into every individual patient in the way this particular patient could approve of was precisely what made nurses' work so attractive. For because every individual patient had his/her own preferences, the nurses' task would never become 'routine'. A nurse should be able to adapt his/her own attitude towards each of them. All patients being 'sensitive but defenceless human beings' needed to have the right atmosphere to regain their health. Creating this atmosphere within a ward was considered a *nursing* responsibility. Therefore, all nurses were to gain 'educational authority' by being a trustworthy educator, though adults who had 're-gressed into a stage of childhood by their illness needed 'correction' and sometimes even 'punishment'.[116] However, neither a 'general rule' on this, nor a mandate from the head nurse would do. Every ward nurse should always be able to give a sound, personally motivated reason for his/her reactions towards individual patients.

Here, echoes of the earlier medical authors and their arguments for 'individualisation' of treatment and nursing methods can be heard. Yet, the Brothers added a new element, translating Van der Drift's principle that all people had a right to 'realize' their own personality to the shop floor of psychiatric nursing. An unprejudiced contact with every individual patient was necessary to evade the pitfall of dealing with problems this person caused *others*, instead of those he/she experienced. Nurses should prevent 'lack of care' by mastering the 'basic forms of human contact' to assist even the least approachable patient, as well as by supporting them in a variety of practical matters.[117] The Roman Catholic brochure of 1966 was the most explicit text for such thoughts; its title was 'Guarding becomes coaching'. It condemned all repressive nursing regimens that patients in traditional psychiatric hospitals had endured.[118]

The Brothers avoided commenting on existing means of mechanical restraint and gave no instructions about their application.[119] Yet, the Brothers did change the general attitude towards restraint, establishing the principle that there could be no 'rules' or 'routines' any longer.[120] It should, for example, not be 'routine' to seclude patients after their legally certified admission on an acute ward. 'Routine practices' were considered 'bad nursing'. Nurses were not supposed to 'persuade' the psychiatrist involved to seclude these patients, and if necessary, they should even contest his decision to seclude.

F. Kramer, a leading male nurse at the psychiatric institution of Franeker, who published a textbook in 1968, did mention 'restraint' but simply mentioned the correct procedure for using a seclusion room. He did not mention any means of mechanical restraint and appeared to accept the use of seclusion as an 'educational measure'. Not surprisingly, he even called his paragraph on seclusion: 'Corrective measures'.[121]

The next textbook – first published in 1975 – by G. Roodhart, another male nursing author, working as a tutor in the Central School in Goes, showed greater openness than the Brothers and Kramer.[122] Roodhart even named one of his chapters 'The use of means of restraint'.[123] Both means of mechanical restraint and seclusion were mentioned, and he was the first author to mention explicitly 'strait belts' (to contain agitated patients) as well as the use of the strait sheet.[124] In doing this, Roodhart acknowledged that ward nurses had an ever-growing responsibility in the use of restraint and he offered the technical instructions they needed. He warned that devices of mechanical restraint were dangerous and that practising their correct application was indispensable.

The last textbook during this period, again written by male nurses (Bos & Van Leeuwen, 1994), contained evidence that between 1975 and 1994, psychiatric nurses had reconsidered their role with 'Means and Measures' such as mechanical restraint and seclusion.[125] This had resulted in describing in detail when, where and how such means were to be used.[126] It emphasized the need for 'reflection' on the ways in which they could use (and abuse) 'power' over their patients: the power of rules, the power of ethical norms, the power of sanctions, the power of professional knowledge, the power to manipulate and the power of means of restraint. This book also contained information on patients' rights, as well as the last version of the registration form on mechanical restraint and seclusion produced by the State Inspectorate.

Between 1960 and 1994, all regulations of the Inspectorate about the registration of restraint and expected nursing skills were changed regularly. The

Dutch Law on the Nursing Diploma of 1921 was changed in 1970.[127] This change was enforced by a group of assertive student nurses who declared the official PE&R book for their final exam 'nonsensical and outdated'.[128] They refused to work as 'attendants' and demanded a psychological and sociological emphasis, as well as a say in their training programme. The Inspectorate actively supported this: a new Law and a new Chief Inspector created the preconditions for emancipation.[129] The Chief Inspector advised the Minister of Health to introduce the requirement for psychiatric nurses to write at least one reflective essay about their way of relating to one or more patients during their training. This was done in 1970.[130] A fundamental change in the teaching programme was also advised. A first revision, in 1973, made the subject of 'psychiatric nursing' a 'theoretical subject' to be examined by both psychiatrists and nursing teachers in the final examination, instead of merely a 'practice' to be demonstrated to psychiatrists. This presupposed 'evidence-based psychiatric nursing knowledge'. A second revision, in 1975, restyled the teaching programme with about twice as many theoretical lessons as before, including psycho-social sciences, medical sciences and 'general cultural development'. Meanwhile, the former PE&R book had been restyled into a personal 'portfolio', to be used in monitoring one's own personal learning process. The Inspectorate expected nurses to have practised and reflected on their use of mechanical restraint and segregation of patients.[131] Thus, psychiatric nursing students were now actively studying 'psychiatric nursing' instead of 'consuming' the knowledge of doctors. Experienced ward nurses had to be a 'model' and critical 'coach' for their younger colleagues. In 1986, this emphasis on nursing responsibilities was strengthened.

A comparable delegation of responsibility to ward nurses is mirrored in the changes of regulations on the *registration* of restraint. In 1979, the Inspectorate was forced to re-introduce a register on restraint as a result of pressure from patients, their advocates and the Parliament.[132] From now on, it was expected that psychiatric nurses should also play a role in this. Unfortunately, this new register did not become successful, because the definition of 'restraint' was widened too far. However, a new system was published in 1985.[133] Since then, nurses have had to register separation, segregation, mechanical restraint and the involuntary administration of medication and/or food (if combined with separation, segregation or fixation). A new addition was *'protective measures'*: 'all nursing measures meant to *protect* severely invalid and/or dependent patients from the risk of severe personal injury' (often a strait belt).[134] In 1990 this system was replaced by a new procedure for 'Untenable Situations in Psychiatric Hospitals'.[135] This time the Inspectorate tried to define not only the 'Means and Measures', but also the context in which these were used, with a number of qualitative requirements.

Thus, from 1960, textbooks encouraged ward nurses to be cautious and to reflect critically on their use of restraint. Meanwhile, the Inspectorate's regulations kept on requiring them to be skilled in *using* Means and Measures correctly. The emphasis on the nurses' attitudes, however, coinciding with a growing movement for patients' rights and investment that led to smaller wards and many more qualified nursing staff led to conflicts between student nurses and experienced ward nurses about means of restraint and seclusion. Most likely, the students tried to diminish the use of restraint, because they had been taught to be more critical of it.[136] For many of them, it may have been confusing that they also were expected to 'practise' with the use of restraint, in order to acquire the required skill.

Conclusion

It may be concluded that from Van Deventer's time until 1926, Dutch psychiatry had a special interpretation of 'non-restraint', which differed in its use of mechanical restraint and seclusion. Since any use of *mechanical restraint* was rejected until 1930, psychiatric nurses were not even trained in the correct appliance of these means. Instead, they were supposed to master skills in the use of *other* techniques, such as 'manual restraint' and 'modern nursing methods', e.g. bed rest, wet packs or prolonged bath therapy. Such 'modern nursing methods' did not have to be registered. With the exception of the period between 1926 and 1962, when the Inspectorate required *all* psychiatric nurses to have skills in using a strait sheet or wet pack, this Dutch attitude stayed fairly constant. Both textbook authors and Inspectors felt uneasy with mechanical measures that hampered the freedom of bodily movement. Instead of the strait *suit*, psychiatrists preferred the strait *jacket*; after the '*wet pack'* came the strait *sheet*, and after that came the strait *belt*. However, a remarkable detour from this general attitude occurred in 1985, when the Inspectorate decided to describe certain means of mechanical restraint as '*protective measures'*. This detour, however, did not last beyond 1994.

The Dutch attitude towards 'seclusion', however, is another story. Even in Van Deventer's time, certain forms of seclusion were considered less serious than mechanical restraint. An important reason for this was that three strong arguments against putting patients in an isolation cell were no longer considered relevant (it makes them feel animal-like, it 'invites' nurses to neglect them, and it puts them at risk of going mad because of their extreme isolation) after the geographically isolated 'cell blocks' in the asylum grounds had given way to isolation rooms *within* the pavilions where the patients lived. Still, the forced removal of a patient to such a cell to protect him from the *danger* of hurting himself or others was considered a very serious measure, only for untenable situations. No one doubted, however, that seclusion cells were a necessary facility, not only to protect patients, but also to protect nurses. The removal of a patient who merely *disturbed* others to a 'single room', if possible with an open door, was not considered so bad. Some patients might even appreciate this, since it would provide privacy, protection and extra nursing attention.

The Dutch attitude towards seclusion changed fundamentally between 1926 and 1955, when psychiatry adopted the principle that its patients were to be looked at as 'responsible people'. During these years, putting patients in short-term seclusion, preferably in a single room, was considered 'appropriate' if it had an 'educational' goal. Some patients simply had to learn that their behaviour was a nuisance to the community. With chronic patients, short-term seclusion could even be imposed by nurses themselves, when they chose to use the isolation cell. The Inspectorate agreed to this change of attitude.

After World War 11, largely as a consequence of the introduction of psychotropic drugs, substantial investment in facilities, a strong movement for patients' rights, and the emancipation of nurses in their practice, the Dutch attitude towards seclusion was influenced by the principle of 'non-restraint' again, though used in a modern way. It came to serve not as a *guideline*, but as a 'guiding *principle*' in modelling nurses' attitudes. The acceptability of 'educational seclusion' gradually gave way to the demand that nurses should merely take care of problems patients experienced *themselves*. Confronted with the fear that many patients experienced during seclusion, authors underlined that nurses should take cautious and responsible decisions about it. A generally diminishing tolerance for unnecessary restriction in patients' freedom was translated into greater expectations of nurses' capability to negotiate with patients and to monitor symptoms of oncoming unrest or aggression. The nursing textbook of 1994 was the first to contain a detailed discussion of arguments nurses could use in considering the use of seclusion. Thus: the Dutch attitude towards non-restraint was finally translated into a clearly circumscribed need for reflective and professional nurses. The fact that since 1997 nurses have to be able to defend their personal choices on seclusion before disciplinary law may lead to the overall conclusion that the national attitude towards seclusion has finally arrived at a stage that Van Deventer could have only dreamed of.

Notes

1.   J. van Deventer, 'L'éducation, les droits et les devoirs des gardes-malades attachés aux hospitaux pour maladies mentales', in G.A.M. van Wayenburg (ed.), *1er Congrès International de Psychiatrie, de Neurologie, de Psychologie et de l'Assistance des Aliénés, Amsterdam, 2-7 Septembre 1907* of *Rapport van het Internationaal Congres voor Psychiatrie, neurologie psychologie en Krankzinnigenverpleging*, Amsterdam 2-7 September 1907 (Amsterdam: J.H. de Bussy, 1908), 660-96: 662-3.
2.   The Buitengasthuis was an annexe of the general hospital of Amsterdam where only insane, contagious, incurable or terminal patients were admitted; Meerenberg was one of the largest, but certainly the most innovative asylums of the Netherlands.

It was opened in 1849 and had been mentioned by John Conolly himself as 'the only continental asylum of Europe' in which doctors had tried to work on the basis of non-restraint. See: J. Conolly, *The Ttreatment of the Insane without Mechanical Restraint* (London: Smits, Elder & Co, 1856), 345.

3.   The State Inspectorate for the Insane and the Asylums was part of the Ministry for Internal Affairs, Department of Poor Relief; the State Inspectorate for Health Care was part of another Ministry. This lasted until 1948.

4.   Later in his lecture he would refer explicitly to the work of Pinel and Conolly. Van Deventer, *op. cit.* (note 1), 665.

5.   J. van Deventer, 'Isoleeren of niet isoleeren?', *Psychiatrisch Bladen*, 1 (1896), 19-23: 21.

6.   Van Deventer, *op. cit.* (note 1), 662. He probably referred to the fact that on the basis of the First Insanity Law (1841), most former Dutch asylums had been either closed or transformed into 'hospitals for the insane' where diverse categories of insane patients – after segregation of the sexes, social classes, violent and quiet patients – were housed and treated in specific wards, based on a rational classification of their behaviour.

7.   The Second Insanity Law (1884) obliged asylums to register their use of restraint, with the intention to restrict it. Inspector J.N. Ramaer (in 1871 the founder of the Dutch Society of Psychiatry) had – on the basis of a broad general acceptance of non-restraint – succeeded to get this registration policy incorporated in the Second Insanity Law. See: J. Vijselaar, 'Zeden, zelfbeheersing en genezing (1849-1884)', in J. Vijselaar (ed.), *Gesticht in de duinen. De geschiedenis van de provinciale psychiatrische ziekenhuizen van Noord-Holland* (Hilversum: Verloren, 1997), 41-73: 65.

8.   Van Deventer preferred the use of the term 'hospital' for the asylum. So did almost all other authors of textbooks for nurses.

9.   Van Deventer, *op. cit.* (note 1), 671.

10.   *Ibid.*, 672. On page 673 he mentions necessary qualities for psychiatric nurses such as: being civilised/refined, intelligent, enterprising, punctual, methodical, vigilant, trustworthy, being able to work on one's own. He does *not* mention terms as 'obedient' or 'subservient'.

11.   *Ibid.*, 661.

12.   *Ibid.*, 674. In 1892, the first examinations in psychiatric nursing were held.

13.   The Dutch Society for Psychiatry (NVP) had been founded in 1871 as a platform for the exchange of scientific knowledge as well as practical experience. The term 'Neurology' was added in 1897; since then the Society has been named the Dutch Society for Psychiatry and Neurology (NVPN). In 1890 the NVP had asked Van Deventer and two colleagues to design a nursing course, in order to raise the quality of the 'attendants' (men and women) in the asylums by educating them into 'nurses'. Their design was accepted, and in 1892 the first examinations were held.

14.   This did not apply to subjects with a relation to intimate parts of the human body. See Van Deventer, *op. cit.* (note 1), 678.

15.   *Ibid.*, 675. Van Deventer stated that among both sexes he had encountered an equal capacity for 'dedication' to work with the insane. He had merely witnessed other 'qualities'. Van Deventer acknowledged 'caring capacities in the female nurse'

with respect to the general atmosphere in a ward and with respect to the care for food, clothes, sleep, hygiene and direction of the household. He acknowledged 'caring capacities in the male nurse' with regard to guiding the labour as well as the dangerous and/or immoral behaviour of (male) patients.

16.   *Ibid.*, 685. It is important to realize that in the Dutch psychiatric hospitals of these days, the majority of the patients came from the lower classes. See also M. Gijswijt-Hofstra in this volume.

17.   Van Deventer, *op. cit.* (note 1), 668-9, 676 and 685.

18.   *Ibid.*, 677.

19.   Vijselaar, *op. cit.* (note 7), 65.

20.   The form did *not* mention 'medication' (scopolamine or hyoscine), 'forced feeding' (such as tube feeding) or the 'wet pack'. Apparently, the Dutch State Inspectorate did not see the need to control the use of such means.

21.   Besluit van 3 juni 1884, tot vaststelling van modelregisters voor de gestichten voor krankzinnigen, in gevolge het bepaalde in het zesde lid van artikel 4 der wet van 27 april 1884 (Staatsblad 96), artikel Staatsblad 110 ('s-Gravenhage, 1884), nr 110-112: 63.

22.   Van Deventer told his audience that the number of secluded cases in Meerenberg in the last ten years had gone down from 679 (of 1489 ill patients) in 1893 (= 45.6 per cent) to 282 (of 1589 ill patients) in 1903 (= 17.7 per cent). This meant that the practice of secluding patients in Meerenberg was more than halved over the last ten years.

23.   Valid or comparable empirical data on the actual *use* of seclusion and mechanical restraint by psychiatric nurses between 1897 and 1997 are lacking: in 1915 the State Inspectorate concluded that the registration of 'mechanical restraint' and seclusion had come to an end in 1914. See: C.J. van de Klippe, *Dwangtoepassing na onvrijwillige psychiatrische opname, een juridische beschouwing* (Nijmegen: Ars Aequi Libri, 1997), 37. Between 1936 and 1974 the State Inspectorate issued no annual reports on the state of affairs in psychiatric institutions. See: Staatstoezicht op de Volksgezondheid, *Verslag over de jaren 1969-1974 van de Geneeskundige Hoofdinspectie voor de Geestelijke Volksgezondheid* ('s-Gravenhage: Staatsuitgeverij, 1976), o (foreword). During the 1980s the Dutch Parliament enforced the State Inspectorate to re-introduce an adequate registration policy and to intensify its control. See: Onze redacteuren, 'Kamer stemt in met regeling inzagerecht in medische dossiers', NRC *Handelsblad* 21-4-1982; 3; Jet Bruinsma, 'Psychiatrische ziekenhuizen: Isoleren van patiënt overal toegepast', *Volkskrant* 27-5-1982, 3; Hoofdredactie, 'Ten geleide: Isoleren', *Volkskrant* 28-5-1982, 3. In all later reports of the State Inspectorate, the Inspectors complain that their data on seclusion and restraint are incomplete.

24.   J. van Deventer, *Handboek der Krankzinnigenverpleging* (Amsterdam: J.H. & G. van Heteren, 1897); B. van Delden, *Onze krankzinnigen en hunne verpleging* (Utrecht: C.H.E. Breijer, 1897); D. Schermers, *Handleiding bij het verplegen van krankzinnigen* (Leiden: D. Donner, 1898); J.C.Th. Scheffer, *Voorlezingen over zenuwzieken en krankzinnigen en hunne verpleging* (Haarlem: De Erven F. Bohn, 1906); P.H.M. Travaglino, *Leiddraad bij de voorbereiding tot het examen in krankzinnigenverpleging* (Amsterdam: F.van Rossen, 1910); J.G. Schnitzler, *Krankzinnigen en hun ver-*

pleging (Amsterdam: J.H. de Bussy, 1915); W.H. Cox, *Handleiding voor den cursus in de verpleging van zielszieken* I & II (Amsterdam: J.H. de Bussy, 1927 and 1929); H.J. Schim van der Loeff & J.A.J. Barnhoorn, *Zielszieken en hunne verpleging* (Roermond/ Maaseik: Romen en Zonen, 1930); A.P. Timmer, *Leerboek voor verplegenden van zenuwzieken en krankzinnigen*, (Haarlem: De Erven F. Bohn, 1938).

25.   The authors on many occasions explicitly referred to 'acts' by nurses (nowadays we would call these 'nursing interventions') they had witnessed in practice and considered to be sensible and useful.

26.   Five textbooks were reprinted and/or revised many times: Scheffer was reprinted five times (*non-denominational*, 1906-1929), Schnitzler four times (*non-denominational*, 1915-1930), Timmer five times (*non-denominational*, 1938-1957), Schermers eleven times (*orthodox Calvinistic*, 1898-1964; from the fifth edition of 1932 until the eighth in 1950 his book was revised by the two doctors B.Ch. Hamer and J.H. Haverkate; from 1956 by the doctors B.Ch. Hamer and F.J. Tolsma), Schim van der Loeff & Barnhoorn four times (*Roman Catholic*, 1930-1947).

27.   P. Stevens, J. Pepping and A.P. Lammens, *Psychiatrische Verpleegkunde* I-III (Heiloo: Stichting St. Willibrord, 1960); Brother Bosco Verdel, *Handleiding Psychiatrische verpleegkunde* (Boekel: Huize Padua, 1963); W.A. van den Hurk, *Bewaken wordt begeleiden, Moderne psychiatrische verpleging* (Amsterdam: IVIO, 1966); F. Kramer, *Psychiatrische verpleegkunde* (Lochem: De Tijdstroom, 1968, 1970 and 1974); C.J.M. Nieland, L. van der Laan, P.F. Rooyackers, *Verpleegkundige lessen voor de opleiding tot het diploma B* (Leiden: Spruyt, Van Mantgem en De Does, 1969 en 1970); G. Roodhart, *Basis psychiatrische verpleegkunde* (Amsterdam & Brussel: Elsevier, 1975, 1977); A. Bos en R.R. van Leeuwen, *Psychiatrische verpleegkunde. Het verplegen van patiënten met een verstoord functioneren* (Leiden: Spruyt, Van Mantgem & De Does, 1994).

28.   See C. aan de Stegge, work in progress.

29.   Handelingen der Staten-Generaal, 1920-1921, 64th meeting, 16 March 1921: 1831-40.

30.   *Staatsblad* no. 702, 2 May 1921. The Dutch Law on Protection of Nursing Diplomas was accepted in 1921, and became effective in 1924.

31.   The State Inspectorate for Health Care (a part of the Health Department of the Ministry of Labour) controlled the final examinations for the A-diploma and registered the sicknurses; the State Inspectorate for the Insane and the Asylums (belonging to the Department of Poor Relief of the Ministry of Internal Affairs) controlled the final examinations for the B-diploma and registered the psychiatric nurses.

32.   *Nederlandsche Staatscourant*, 31 December 1923, no. 252.

33.   John Conolly (1794-1866) was an English asylum doctor and chief medical officer of Hanwell, a public asylum near London. Conolly pleaded for 'moral treatment' as a new way of 'asylum management'. The climate within an asylum should be based on the director's authority, a regular daily routine, allocating patients places on wards according to the nature of their behaviour (quiet, agitated, semi-agitated, ill). Other factors constituted occupational therapy, religious exercise, good nourishing food, various material amenities and the offering of a general degree of physical comfort. As far as he was concerned, the use of mechanical restraint had a counterproductive effect, because it equalled neglect. If restraint was needed, he preferred a

Changing Attitudes

few minutes of 'manual restraint' or 'temporary seclusion', exerted by a group of three or four trained and gently operating 'attendants'. See J. Conolly, *op. cit.* (note 2), 41 and 46. See also: Nancy Tomes, 'The great restraint controversy: A comparative perspective on Anglo-American psychiatry in the nineteenth century', in W.F. Bynum, Roy Porter and Michael Shepherd (eds), *The Anatomy of Madness. Essays in the History of Psychiatry.* III. *The Asylum and its Psychiatry* (London and New York: Routledge, 1988), 190-1 and 196-202.

34. Conolly, *op. cit.* (note 2), 101.
35. *Ibid.*, 103.
36. Gunnel Svedberg, Carl-Magnus Stolt and Gunilla Bjerén, 'Prolonged Bath as Treatment, Care and Restraint. Ideology and Practice in Swedish Psychiatric Care during the First Half of the Twentieth Century', in Gunnel Svedberg, *Omvårdnad-straditioner inom svensk psykiatrisk vård under 1900-talets första hälft,* (Stockholm: Karolinksa Institutet, 2002), V: 1-27: 5.
37. Vijselaar (ed.), *op. cit.* (note 7), 51.
38. Van Delden, *op. cit.* (note 24), 75-85; Schermers, *op. cit.* (note 24), 180-91; Scheffer, *op. cit.* (note 24), 221-4.
39. Schermers, *op. cit.* (note 24), 1911, et seq.; Scheffer, *op. cit.* (note 24) 1914, et seq.
40. Van Delden, *op. cit.* (note 24), 76-7; Schermers, *op. cit.* (note 24), 188.
41. Schermers, *op. cit.* (note 24), 188.
42. Van Delden, who published the registration form in his book, explicitly expressed this fear. Van Delden, *op. cit.* (note 24), 196.
43. Scheffer, *op. cit.* (note 24), 223.
44. Van Deventer, *op. cit.* (note 24), 1.
45. *Ibid.*, 1 and 11 (holding at times of forced feeding), 20-1 (taking care in the isolation cell), 101-2 (holding during transport).
46. *Ibid.*, 102.
47. Van Delden, *op. cit.* (note 24), 85.
48. *Ibid.*, 195.
49. *Ibid.*, 196.
50. Schermers, *op. cit.* (note 24), 205.
51. Like in Van Delden's approach, suicidal patients should not be left on their own at any time.
52. Schermers, *op. cit.* (note 24), 206.
53. *Ibid.*, 209.
54. Scheffer, *op. cit.* (note 24), 222-3 and 236.
55. *Ibid.*, third edition 1919: 338. This edition was revised by A.H. Oort.
56. Van Deventer, *op. cit.* (note 24), 17-9 and 20-2; Van Delden, *op. cit.* (note 24), 151-3; The other two authors seem to have become acquainted with this difference much later. Schermers, *op. cit.* (note 24, edition 1921), 365; Scheffer, *op. cit.* (note 24, third edition, 1919), 328.
57. Viz. Van Deventer, *op. cit.* (note 24), 58; Van Delden, *op. cit.* (note 24), 153; Schermers, *op. cit.* (note 24), 190 and 245.
58. Van Delden, *op. cit.* (note 24), 196.
59. Schermers, *op. cit.* (note 24, fourth edition, 1921), 367.

60.   The terms 'keeping' and 'guarding' refer to the necessity of continuous alertness on closed wards.

61.   See: J. Van Deventer, W.P. Ruysch and A.O.H. Tellegen, 'Rapport van de Examencommissie', *Psychiatrische Bladen*, 11 (1894), 11-6: 15-6.

62.   In England the 'wet pack' was considered as a means of restraint and needed to be registered. See: Tomes, *op. cit.* (note 33), 198. This was not the case in the Netherlands during this period.

63.   W.M. van der Scheer, 'De verpleging van onrustige krankzinnigen in nieuwe banen', *Nosokómos* (1926): exact pages unknown because I used a copy that was edited independently. See also *idem*, 'De nieuwere inzichten in de behandeling van geesteszieken en de in ons Ziekenhuis bereikte resultaten', *Psychiatrische en Neurologische Bladen*, 32 (1928), 101-5. Van der Scheer further enlarged on his ideas in a book: *Nieuwe inzichten in de behandeling van geesteszieken* (Groningen: J.B. Wolters, 1933).

64.   Van der Scheer developed these thoughts more and more. In his book of 1933, *op. cit.* (note 63), he denounced the whole concept of a special ward for the agitated, bringing all agitated patients together in one place, as a mistake in itself (132); in this book he also supplied examples of mistakes in his own management, which had led to agitation in a patient (124-5) and comparable thoughtless actions by nurses (126).

65.   *Ibid.*, 12-9.

66.   Van der Scheer never worried about exact definitions: enforced bed rest, prolonged bathing, (wet) packs, medication, mechanical restraint, all this was captured by the word restraint. He wrote from his own experience: colourful and direct. He did not beautify the reality of practice and also wrote about very ordinary things.

67.   Van der Scheer, *op. cit.* (note 63: 1933), 50-1.

68.   Van der Scheer meant work of a level of complexity that corresponded to the patient's capability.

69.   Van der Scheer, *op. cit.* (note 63: 1926), 14.

70.   The teaching of conditioned reflexes is meant here, the 'training' that teaches people to associate good behaviour with a reward (pleasure) and bad behaviour with punishment (pain), derived from Pavlov.

71.   Van der Scheer did not give exact definitions of these terms. His 'seclusion room' probably was a 'single room' and the seclusion cell, the modern 'seclusion cell' within the pavilion. Van der Scheer, *op. cit.* (note 63: 1926), 10.

72.   *Ibid.*, 14.

73.   Van der Scheer, *op. cit.* (note 63: 1933), 136-7.

74.   As mentioned in note 26, B.Ch. Hamer & J.H. Haverkate took care of the revisions of Schermers' textbook from 1932 onwards. They renamed this book as *Schermers' Leerboek bij het verplegen van krankzinnigen en zenuwzieken* (Leiden: Gebr. Van der Hoek, 1932). H.J. Schim van der Loeff & J.A.J. Barnhoorn also stressed that it was very likely that in the near future ever more open wards would be created, where patients were allowed to be hospitalised exclusively on medical grounds, without legal certification. They expected this to have a very positive influence on the climate in psychiatric hospitals. See: Schim van der Loeff and Barnhoorn, *op. cit.* (note 24, second edition: 1932), 6.

75.   Scheffer, *op. cit.* (note 24: fourth edition, 1929), 335-6.
76.   Cox, *op. cit.* (note 24: 1927), part 1, 87.
77.   Schim van der Loeff & Barnhoorn, *op. cit.* (note 24), 276.
78.   Scheffer, *op. cit.* (note 24: fifth edition, 1929), 329-30.
79.   Schim van der Loeff & Barnhoorn, *op. cit.* (note 24), 287-91. They used these photographs until the fourth edition of 1947, 368-72. A.P. Timmer, *op. cit.* (note 24: first edition 1938), 251-2; second edition (1942), 250-1; third edition (1946) 249-50, fifth edition (1957) no pictures anymore. Apparently by this time he thought manual restraint wasn't necessary anymore.
80.   W.H. Cox differed between psychiatric hospitals in this regard: modern, well operating hospitals did not use mechanical restraint, bad hospitals did, he seemed to imply. See Cox, *op. cit.* (note 24: 1927), 67.
81.   Schim van der Loeff & Barnhoorn, *op. cit.* (note 24: first edition, 1930), 279. These Roman Catholic doctors were the first to mention the term 'fixation-material' and the first to mention the strait sheet.
82.   Hamer & Haverkate, *op. cit.* (note 74: seventh edition 1946), 311.
83.   M. Louter has interviewed a diversity of patients who complain about a frequent disciplinary use of an emetic. See M. Louter, work in progress. See also T. Pieters and S. Snelders in this book. My own interviews with nurses do not assert the impression that nurses felt free to decide on medication by themselves. They were merely entitled to prepare medication according to doctors' prescriptions.
84.   With 'over time' is meant that the editions of nursing textbooks that were published during the 1920s make less distinction between curable and incurable patients than the editions of nursing textbooks that were published during the 1940s or the 1950s.
85.   In the Netherlands, community nursing started as early as in 1917, in Amsterdam; in 1937 a special extra course in 'pre- and aftercare' was organised, to be followed by experienced and qualified B-nurses who worked in the community.
86.   Hamer & Haverkate, *op. cit.* (note 74: sixth edition, 1938), 390.
87.   Long-term seclusion they did not allow.
88.   Van der Scheer, *op. cit.* (note 63: 1933), 125.
89.   This way of taking (part of) the practical exam lasted in the Netherlands until 1973.
90.   This probably was a consequence of the fact that a specific teaching book had been published on the use of physics and chemistry in nursing. This made the nurse more responsible for preparing the right dosis per patient (following prescriptions) out of a liter bottle with medication. See: A. Schoondermark: *Natuur en scheikunde voor de leerling krankzinnigenverpleegster* (Amsterdam: H.J. Paris, 1925).
91.   See: Van der Klippe, *op. cit.* (note 23), 41; see also Tomes, *op. cit.* (note 33), 198.
92.   C. aan de Stegge, work in progress.
93.   Van der Klippe, *op. cit.* (note 23), 41.
94.   Albeit completely unintended by the most important ideologist of the epoch, for Van der Scheer was thoroughly aware that his nursing method of 'education' demanded a lot of nursing staff; he often expressed his frustration about the fact that the number of nursing staff was too low. See Catharina Th. Bakker & Leonie de Goei,

Een bron van zorg en goede werken. Geschiedenis van de geestelijke gezondheidszorg in Noord-Holland-Noord (Amsterdam: SUN, 2002), 207.

95.   B. Chr. Hamer & F. J. Tolsma, *Algemeen Leerboek voor het verplegen van geestes- en zenuwzieken* (Leiden: Spruyt, Van Mantgem & De Does, 1956), 438-9. It was the ninth revision of the textbook that was originally written by Schermers (1898), *op. cit.* (note 24).

96.   The editorial board consisted of authors from all denominations including non-religious persons. Also, one of the authors of this edition did not work in an asylum, but in an outpatient service. It was a quite remarkable break with tradition that these last services, formerly considered as pre- or aftercare, had grown important enough to be invited to have their say in the basic training for psychiatric nurses. The book contained 50 pages on social psychiatric nursing.

97.   Hamer & Tolsma, *op. cit.* (note 95), 438.

98.   *Ibid.*, 440-5.

99.   *Ibid.*, 463.

100.   Van der Drift explicitly stated he preferred the term 'psychiatric hospital'. See: Hamer & Tolsma, *op. cit.* (note 95), 439.

101.   *Ibid.*, 463.

102.   'Human resources management' is not the term Van der Drift used. It certainly is what he had in mind.

103.   Hamer & Haverkate, *op. cit.* (note 74: fifth edition, 1932), 294; Hamer & Haverkate, *op. cit.* (note 74: eighth edition, 1950), 388.

104.   See: Hamer & Tolsma, *op. cit.* (note 95), 472.

105.   The way a patient dressed, for example, was now interpreted as 'self-expression'; education by the nurses in this matter should no longer benefit the reputation of the institution, but the patient's own need for self-expression.

106.   The only other nursing textbook still in use was the one by Timmer, *op. cit.* (note 24), who edited a fifth revision of his textbook in 1957.

107.   Cecile aan de Stegge, 'Verpleegkundigen opleiden voor de psychiatrie', *Maandblad Geestelijke Volksgezondheid*, 56 (2001), 691-708: 701.

108.   The examination committees of neutral as well as of the Roman Catholic and Calvinist hospitals had co-operated with the organised head nurses to edit this text.

109.   See all PE&R books in B-nursing, edited between 1962 and 1970 (Zeist: Uitgeversbureau Van Lonkhuyzen), that can still be found in the houses of former psychiatric nurses.

110.   See Aktiekrant Aktiegroep Willem of 5-2-1970, Verslag van een aktie-bezoek aan Psychiatrisch Centrum Heiloo; to be found in Internationaal Instituut voor Sociale Geschiedenis, Nieuw Dennendal (1965-1969-1974 (989), no. 38, Stukken betreffende Aktie Willem.

111.   See Stevens, Pepping and Lammens, *op. cit.* (note 27: part 1), 1. Verdel, *op. cit.* (note 27); Van den Hurk, *op. cit.* (note 27).

112.   See Stevens, Pepping and Lammens *op. cit.*, (note 27: part 1), 1. In other texts the Roman Catholic brothers often explicitly wrote that they considered nursing to be an 'art'; it was not solely a technique but a technique that should be fulfilled with love and attention. They also did not consider nursing to be an *intellectual* or a mainly

verbal activity. They thought it much more important to coach and guide or support patients in their practical matters than to talk.

113.　See also: Catharina Th. Bakker, 'De broeders en de nieuwe tijd (1950-1970)', in Bakker & De Goei, *op. cit.* (note 94), 199-238: 228.

114.　The text of the first trio is composed in the form of short lectures, followed by a large number of questions that should be answered by the nurse. The text is composed like a Catholic Catechism but *without* prescribed answers.

115.　Stevens, Pepping and Lammens, *op. cit.* (note 27), 2.

116.　*Ibid.*, 19.

117.　In a text of 1978, Stevens explicitly described these 'basic forms of human contact' like caring for people, animals, plants and objects together; playing games; being able to organise or participate in a feast; going out together; working together; eating together and talking in a group. See P. Stevens, *Basis psychiatrische verpleegkunde, opleiding tot verpleegkundige 1e leerjaar* (Heiloo, July 1978, internal publication), 7.

118.　See Van den Hurk, *op. cit.* (note 27), 5.

119.　See the three mentioned texts in note 112 as well as Nieland, Van der Laan, Rooyackers, *op. cit.* (note 27).

120.　And – thus – most likely also the use of restraint.

121.　In the last edition of his textbook Kramer mentioned that the two State Inspectorates (on General Health Care and on Mental Health Care) had agreed that the Dutch word '*isoleerkamer*' in future could only point to such a room in a general hospital, where one hoped to prevent contagion; the former '*isoleerkamer*' in psychiatry would in future be called '*separeerkamer*'. See: F. Kramer, *op. cit.* (note 27: 1974), 67.

122.　From the beginning of the 1970s, so-called Central Schools were set up in the Netherlands; in such schools, raised by general hospitals in co-operation with psychiatric institutions to lower costs (this was necessary because also other learning routes for nurses were created), teachers took care of the theoretical part of schooling (A- and B-) nurses; the hospitals and institutions would take care of offering working experience and coaching.

123.　Roodhart, *op. cit.* (note 27), 133-5.

124.　Until today it has – despite all efforts – been impossible to trace the exact moment in time that this strong canvas belt – closed with a metal lock – was introduced in the Netherlands. On the basis of my interviews with nurses I am convinced it must have been towards the end of the 1950s that the strait sheet in many cases was replaced by this belt. In the Netherlands the restraining belt is called 'the Swedish belt'. This probably stems from the fact that in Sweden these belts were already used from the 1930s.

125.　Bos & Van Leeuwen, *op. cit.* (note 27), 116-22.

126.　'Means and Measures' was the term for a diversity of means of restraint as used by the State Inspectorate from 1985 onwards. See: Hanneke van de Klippe, *Dwangtoepassing in de psychiatrie, Een kritisch literatuuronderzoek naar de rechtsontwikkeling inzake dwang na opname* (Utrecht: NcGv, 1992), 59.

127.　*Nederlandse Staatscourant*, 31 July 1970, no. 145: 4 and 5.

128.   This was 'Action group Willem', a group of students in psychiatric nursing in the psychiatric hospital Willem Arntsz Hoeve in Den Dolder. Within six weeks, this group managed to enforce a breakthrough with regard to the training programme in psychiatric nursing. C. aan de Stegge, work in progress.

129.   From 1968 onwards, the Exceptional Medical Expenses Act (AWBZ) brought an end to the link between mental health care and poor relief. See Marijke Gijswijt-Hofstra in this volume. In 1969 a new Chief Inspector was installed: Prof. P.A.H. Baan. Baan protected Action group Willem. See: C. aan de Stegge, work in progress.

130.   In later revisions, the number of expected written essays was enlarged significantly.

131.   *Nederlandse Staatscourant*, 13 June 1975, no. 111.

132.   See: Van der Klippe, *op. cit.* (note 23) 47.

133.   Geneeskundige Inspectie voor de Geestelijke volksgezondheid, *Referentiekader Middelen en Maatregelen*, October 1984, 2nd version. See: Van de Klippe, *op. cit.* (note 126), Bijlage 10. The publication of 1984 became effective in 1985. The Inspector explained that the terms to be used in this system had to match with the terms of the Psychiatric Hospitals Compulsory Admissions Act that was prepared for introduction. (This new Law became effective in 1994.)

134.   *Ibid.*, Appendix 10, 7.

135.   Geneeskundige Inspectie voor de Geestelijke Volksgezondheid, *Referentiekader Noodtoestanden bij patiënten in psychiatrische ziekenhuizen* (Den Haag: Centrale Directie Voorlichting, Documentatie en Bibliotheek van het Ministerie van Welzijn, Volksgezondheid en Cultuur, 1990).

136.   J.P.M. Hendriks, 'Publicatie van besluit van 30 mei 1975 tot Algehele Wijziging regeling opleiding diploma B Ziekenverpleging', *Nederlandse Staatscourant*, 13 June 1975, no. 111.

CHAPTER 15

Nurses in Swedish Psychiatric Care

Gunnel Svedberg

The history of psychiatric nursing in different European countries varies, although there are of course also conspicuous similarities. From the middle of the nineteenth century and throughout the twentieth, staff within Swedish psychiatric care have looked towards Germany, the Netherlands and the UK for inspiration. In spite of this, the Swedish model of nursing has in some important respects come to differ from that in these countries. One of the most obvious differences is that in some countries, psychiatric nursing was established as a separate branche with its own staff systems and separate recruitment and training of students, in close association with asylums. During the first half of the twentieth century, leading Swedish nurses were in agreement with their American counterparts, who forcefully asserted that 'there is no such thing as mental nursing apart from general nursing or general nursing apart from mental nursing'.[1] All Swedish nurses received general training and supplementary training in one field of nursing. Thus, in Sweden, psychiatric care has been one of several fields of nursing open to general nurses.

In this paper, I wish to outline Swedish developments in psychiatric nursing, with a focus on professionalisation and professional identity during the first half of the twentieth century. Gender and class perspectives are inevitable in this context. A tentative explanation of the background to developments in Sweden is also offered.

Psychiatric Care in the Eyes of Foreign Visitors

Travel reports from asylums abroad can provide a view of contemporary values and give impetus to analyses and comparative studies from today's perspective. In the 1880s, two foreign travellers visited Swedish asylums and left accounts in book form. They were G.A. Tucker, an Australian psychiatrist,[2] and the American industrialist and philanthropist William P. Letchworth.[3] At the turn of the twentieth century, the Hungarian psychiatrist Kárlmán Pándy arrived.[4] All three had undertaken study trips to many countries and made comparisons between them. They held up English and especially Scottish psychiatry as exemplary, in particular the openness and lack of coercion and the friendly, home-like care environments. At the end of the nineteenth century, Scandinavian travellers nevertheless regarded the German Alt-Scherbitz asylum with its lack of surrounding fences and well-developed allotment programme, as a model of coercion-free care.[5]

Swedish asylums seemed poorly equipped to the foreign travellers. But cleanliness was conspicuous, and there were flowers on the tables. Most critical was the American, who was distressed by what he regarded as a harsh and forbidding attitude. His overall impression of the Scandinavian countries was that they were more interested in protecting society than caring for the patients. The visitors recorded the restraints they saw being used and the number of patients in isolation. It would appear that these visitors regarded a coercion-free and home-like environment as the primary criterion of good psychiatric care and that this was predicated upon careful recruitment and thorough training of suitable personnel.[6] Foreign visitors commented with amazement and appreciation on the fact that young Swedish women from middle-class homes would train as nurses in order to earn a living, and had found working in psychiatric care a dignified alternative to life as a wife or daughter at home. The fact that individual women had worked among male asylum patients in the eighteenth and nineteenth centuries was not unique to Sweden. On the other hand, the extent and focus of Swedish women's work among male asylum patients were less common at the turn of the twentieth century and beyond, since gender segregation in asylums had gradually become more rigidly implemented, including the staff.

At the turn of the twentieth century, there were complaints in Swedish asylums about problems with personnel. In 1904, the psychiatrist Herman Lundborg paid a month-long study visit to 'Holland, a country where psychiatric care is at a high level'.[7] The overall theme of his travelogue was training of personnel. According to Lundborg, Swedish asylums had to make do with persons who were not up to their difficult task, and the turnover of male and female attendants was rapid, with many having to be dismissed for carelessness, drunkenness or violence against patients. An asylum nurse had to have specific character traits: conduct herself with dignity and calm, without showing fear; have patience, tact and true humanity, without being squeamish, he declared.[8] Lundborg gave a detailed account of the three-year training of women from cultured homes at the Meerenberg asylum in Holland. Women there acted as supervisors and were in charge of male wards. They were assisted by male personnel to carry out bathing and heavier tasks. In his view, the Dutch were surely on the right track, and there was much to learn from them. Corresponding principles with female nurses as supervisors on male and female wards[9] were adopted in Sweden, except that the nurses in Sweden were recruited via the nursing colleges where probationers received about three years' training in general nursing, including training in psychiatric care at certain asylums. However, the majority of

Nurses in Swedish Psychiatric Care

the nursing staff at the asylums consisted of both male and female attendants[10] who were recruited and trained at asylum-based schools. The attendants were subordinate to nurses, regardless of their length of service and personal qualifications, though they were nevertheless found in supervisory positions in wards where there were no nurses.

The fact that Lundborg and other psychiatrists chose to focus so completely on the merits of women in this context correlates well with the perception of gender characteristics at the time, where women were deemed to have a given mandate as moral agents and caregivers within conventionally feminine areas of activity.[11] Psychiatrists could state with authority that it was an incontestible fact that women are better suited to nursing care than men,[12] a standpoint which was seized upon by early nurses.[13]

Compared to many other European countries, Sweden had a fairly uniform system. It had a 'strong' centralised government administration with central agencies for education and health care, where representatives of the professions had a great deal of influence, and anything that could be linked to science and education was highly esteemed. Although the Lutheran national church, despite early and extensive secularisation, in principle encompassed the entire population until the year 2000, it had no real influence on societal issues. It is noteworthy that Swedish psychiatrists on study trips to Holland and elsewhere avoided asylums operated by religious orders, or commented briefly that the influence of doctors was limited to 'purely medical matters' at asylums run by religious orders, which offered 'nothing of interest'.[14]

Pioneers in the Training of Swedish Nurses

Swedish nurses have considered psychiatric care the domain of trained nurses ever since formal training was established in the middle of the nineteenth century. Asylums soon came to be seen as one of several alternative fields of activity for trained nurses. Deaconess Marie Cederschiöld is regarded as the first Swedish woman formally trained as a nurse. She studied at Kaiserswerth in Germany in 1850, at the same time as her British counterpart, Florence Nightingale.[15] Marie Cederschiöld also visited the Emden Irrenanstalt, an asylum in Hannover. On her return home, she started a training programme for nurses at the Ersta deaconess house, Sweden's first school of nursing. As of 1860, there are references to deaconesses working in asylums.[16]

The first secularised training programme for nurses was started in 1868 by Emmy Rappe, who trained at Florence Nightingale's school at St. Thomas Hospital in London. She had been well received at the school and given an audience with Miss Nightingale. However, she was critical of the training, especially its theoretical component, which she found inadequate. Emmy Rappe made several study visits to various specialised hospitals, one of them the Colney Hatch Asylum in London. She reported home that she found this institution very interesting. After one year of training there, she became matron at the Department of Surgery at the Uppsala Academic Hospital and principal of the nurse-training school founded by the Red Cross. Several nurses from the school started by her eventually served in psychiatric care. After working for many years as matron and in nurses' training, Emmy Rappe concluded her professional career with nine years' service as supervisor at Uppsala Asylum. At this time – the turn of the twentieth century – local schools for female and male attendants were started in Uppsala and at a few other asylums, thus separate from nursing training.[17]

Deaconesses trained in the Kaiserswerth model and female nurses trained at nursing colleges inspired by the Nightingale model were consequently the first trained members of the nursing staff at the asylums, and their training gave them a natural authority as supervisors and nurse tutors. In Sweden, the secular Nightingale model of nursing came to be the dominating model for all nursing training, including psychiatric nursing as one of the specialisations for general nurses.

Although the Nightingale model is English, psychiatric nursing in Britain was seen as a special branch of nursing, followed a different path of development, registered separately, and there were tensions between general nurses and psychiatric nurses.[18]

My conclusion is that the great interest in psychiatric care shown by the pioneers of Swedish nurses' training contributed to making work in asylums one of several alternatives for general nurses trained at nursing colleges, which at this time only accepted female students.

The Nightingale Legacy

It is uncertain how much the Swedish protagonists of the Nightingale model of nursing really knew about Miss Nightingale's intentions and changing standpoints over time.[19] It is clear, however, that Swedish nurses' training embraced principles which also are found in Nightingale's extensive writings and correspondence. Florence Nightingale's book *Notes of Nursing: What it is and what it is not*, was published in 1859. It appeared in a Swedish translation only a year later and, remarkably, in a second translation the following year.[20]

In 1884, the Sophiahemmet school of nursing was established, with its own board of directors and organised theoretical training provided by female tutors. This was the programme which most closely adhered to the Nightingale model. Sophiahemmet's first principal was Alfhild Ehrenborg, who had studied the Nightingale system at its source.[21]

Nurses in Swedish Psychiatric Care

According to the Nightingale model, the school should be a separate unit independent of the hospital, managed by women and with its own board of directors, where the training of students was prioritised.[22] Several nurse-historians have stated that in the U K, this was not realised in practice, and that students came to be exploited as inexpensive labour.[23] Although similar assertions can be made with respect to Sweden, nursing colleges were nevertheless able to maintain a degree of autonomy vis-à-vis the hospital management, as well as more control over the training than in the asylum-based schools for attendants. Principals and tutors at the nursing colleges were nurses. Although mostly attached to general hospitals, the colleges were formally independent. Doctors, pharmacists, dieticians and other professionals were appointed to teach relevant subjects, while the nurse tutors taught nursing. In the selection of students, emphasis was placed on personal characteristics such as maturity and sense of responsibility, with character-building considered part of the training.

Florence Nightingale wanted training to be governed by a secular board, in which religious orders had no formal influence. She nevertheless believed that the ethical foundation should be based on Christian values: that nurses should be religious and devoted and must have respect for their calling.[24] Florence Nightingale has been described as a 'radical theologian'.[25] A radical liberal theology with relations to the feminist movement also existed in Sweden in the middle of the nineteenth century. The debate concerning expansion of the role of women into traditionally male domains of public service saw the emergence of a new exegetical approach to misogynistic Biblical passages that legitimised the subordination of women. Elements in Luther's vision of freedom and calling that supported emancipation were emphasized.[26] An ethic based on Christian traditions and values continued to characterise the education and lifestyle within the training of nurses; nursing ethics was considered the main subject in nursing education.[27]

Florence Nightingale collaborated well with men and made sure that those with influence in medicine and society were well represented on the board responsible for nurses' training. This has been interpreted as a strategy to gain legitimacy for her projects and adapt realistically to existing conditions.[28] A similarly pragmatic and collaborative attitude, where open conflict was avoided, was also prominent among leaders of Swedish nursing.[29] As an ethical guideline, early Swedish nurses repeatedly cited Florence Nightingale's standpoint in their writings that the nurse's work is different from the doctor's, but no less important, although subordinate to his in medical matters.[30] Investigators of the relationship between nurses and doctors maintain that leading nurses in the Nordic countries did not act obsequiously.[31]

Professionalisation Strategies

At the turn of the twentieth century, both the science and practice of psychiatry were exposed to intra-disciplinary critical review, as well as public distrust, in Sweden and other countries. There was a great need for renewal, and impulses for change came primarily from Germany. Bed rest came to be associated with a humane, scientifically based form of psychiatric care, which offered alternatives to confinement in cells and mechanical restraints. Prolonged baths were to be administered to the most severely disturbed, violent or untidy patients. Wards should resemble those in somatic hospitals, while at the same time providing a home-like and appealing environment. Middle-class women with health care training would fit in well with this vision.[32] These endeavours have been interpreted as part of the professionalisation strategies of psychiatrists, who wanted to raise the status of their cadre by association with more successful somatic medicine.

In early twentieth-century Sweden, some nursing colleges were sending students to asylums for three months of theoretical and practical training, which qualified them as headnurses at asylums. Nurses were appointed to this position on both female and male wards in a few asylums. The trend towards the increasing employment of nurses in the asylums was supported by professors of psychiatry and appears to have been appreciated by the nursing profession, which saw participation in reform work as appealing. But not all psychiatrists were satisfied. The educational level of many nurses was lower than expected; some were not even capable of applying a fomenting bandage or giving an enema. Psychiatrists found that nurses were more interested in surgical procedures than in psychiatric care.[33] Furthermore, some medical directors were hesitant to recruit nurses because it led to conflicts with the attendants.

Attendants had to complete a one-year traineeship, extended to two years in 1931. A nurse provided 15 hours' teaching of nursing theory with practical exercises, and doctors provided 30 hours of training in pathology. There was also an advanced 50-hour theory course which could open the door to supervisory positions.[34] Training at a general hospital was not included in their curriculum, and nursing colleges were closed to men.

Attendants formed local trade unions modelled on the labour movement in the early decades of the twentieth century and challenged the sovereign right of medical directors to decide on the recruitment, advancement and dismissal of personnel. Male attendants were periodically subject to sharp and collective criticism by medical directors. Attendants claimed that union activists were especially exposed to censure and that medical directors had decided to 'get rid of all socialists' and replace them with female workers.[35]

The attendants' trade union, *Svenska Hospitalspersonalens förbund* ('The Union') was open to both male and female attendants, but relatively few women were union members. The Union fought in the traditional way with collective demands such as regulated working hours, better working conditions and better wages. They wanted a just system of advancement, where supervisors would be trained and appointed from the cadres of attendants based on years of service and merit. This would require improved training that could be considered equivalent to or even better than the nurses' training. 'The merging of personnel in a common trade union' comprising all health care workers at the asylums and solid support for the trade unions were seen as prerequisites for pushing through demands and wishes. The Union distanced itself clearly from the notion of female supervisors for male attendants. There was a feeling within it that the 'women system' and 'management in skirts' had expanded alarmingly on male wards in the asylums.

Despite the large proportion of female attendants at the asylums, this category has not been subject to historical analysis. A probable explanation is the relative lack of sources, since there is little information about them in medical archives, and the union literature contains few specific references to this group.

Nurses working in psychiatric care have, like other nurses, belonged to Sweden's only nursing association, the *Swedish Society of Nursing*, established in 1910 as a professional association with middle-class, bourgeois leanings and considered to have an elitist character. At the time, many of the poorly trained general nurses were not admitted.[36] Improving the training of nurses was a prominent element in the professionalisation effort. This Society has supported and participated in issues concerning nurses in psychiatric care. Several nurses active in psychiatric care have held positions of trust within it, one serving as chair for many years.

Nurses were recruited to positions as matron and headnurse in the asylums. Their principal task was to supervise care on the wards and implement improvements. Nurses wrote nursing notes. They participated in medical treatments. Nurses' tasks included instruction at the local schools for attendants. In the first half of the twentieth century, a nurse might manage the pharmacy, work in the laboratory or on the surgical ward at the asylum.

In psychiatric care, nurses worked with doctors in an alliance of mutual loyalty and interdependence, which can be described as a 'gender contract'. Nurses assumed extensive administrative tasks and management responsibilities for large wards. In return, they were supported in their professional endeavours and claims to high positions in the care-giving hierarchy which *inter alia* included the subordination of attendants.

In 1912, the 18 Swedish asylums employed 66 (female) nurses, 22 of whom served on units for male patients. At the same time, there were 682 male attendants, all for male patients, and 774 female attendants, including 50 who served on male wards.[37] Over time, the proportion of nurses increased, as did the proportion of female attendants on male wards.

Nordic Collaboration

Nursing associations in the Nordic countries – Denmark, Finland, Iceland, Norway and Sweden – established the federation *The Northern Nurses' Federation* (*NNF*) in 1920. Solidarity in their collective work was emphasized, and the five nursing associations referred to the federation as 'five flying swans in a flock' to outwardly indicate unity of their development direction.[38] Their congresses included presentations on psychiatric care for all nurses, as well as a section for members active in this field. Meeting protocols suggest a high degree of unity within the federation in terms of what had to be done, both to improve conditions in the asylums and to give all nurses theoretical and practical training in psychiatric care; this would enable nurses in all fields to provide good nursing care and promote preventative care in society. A greater emphasis on basic psychological-ethical training was thought desirable throughout the curriculum. Recruitment of nurses to asylums in the different Nordic countries was a regular topic for several reasons. Generally trained nurses were few at the time, and work at asylums did not seem to be the preferred choice for many of them. Furthermore, there was resistance to generally trained nurses at asylums from attendants, who claimed to be mental nurses, and also ambivalent attitudes to general nurses from some doctors, who preferred to recruit attendants to the superior posts at the asylums.

Nurses referenced their own experiences from study visits to the USA and reports from other countries. The mental hygiene movement in the 1930s was discussed on the basis of examples from Yale University in New Haven and hospitals in Washington.[39] Discussions within NNF in many ways parallel discussions among US nurses working in psychiatric care.[40]

One of the leading nurses within the federation was the Swedish-speaking Finn Karin Neuman-Rahn, author of the first Swedish textbook on psychiatric care, which was published in 1924.[41] The book was devoted to nursing ethics and aspects of care; inspiration for it came partly from studies in both Germany and Sweden.[42] The book also appeared in a German translation.[43]

Despite certain differences between the Nordic countries, they are ideologically closely related. To a varying degree in the different countries (female general) nurses, trained at nursing colleges, were engaged on male and female wards at the asylums as head nurses.[44] Denmark led the way in this.[45] Iceland's first asylum was established in 1907 and from the outset employed female head nurses, initially trained as general nurses in Scotland or Denmark.[46] In Finland, secular training of nurses started in 1889 – twenty years later than in Sweden – and here again the Nightingale model was used.[47] Swedish conditions differ from those in other Nordic countries in that Sweden from an early stage has had a fairly large cadre of well-trained and professionally well-organised female and male attendants, who performed most of the nursing work. The proportion of

Nurses in Swedish Psychiatric Care

nurses within psychiatric care still remains small today.[48] There was a small number of male, health care-trained deacons in the Nordic countries[49] where, generally speaking, the nursing profession remained in the hands of women until the 1950s.

Increased Female Personnel

Around 1920, the benefits and disadvantages of increasing the use of female staff on male wards and generally trained nurses as supervisors of attendants were topics of debate within psychiatry in many Western countries.[50] In Sweden, asylums in Denmark were held up as models from which positive experiences were being reported and where violence by patients against staff was a rarity: 'Agitated patients who are ready to fight with any man who approaches them and wants to order them about will often listen to a woman and become calmer and easier to treat when they hear friendly words.'[51] But what type of female staff should be recruited: female attendants or nurses? The question had become more pointed in the wake of a number of strikes carried out by women in the 1920s. Swedish government-employed telephone operators had participated in a well-publicised strike which resulted in serious clashes and police action. Some 2,000 telephone operators had gone on strike, supported by the labour movement. Other operators, with links to the middle-class white-collar movement, remained on duty and kept operations going with the aid of extra personnel called in by the employer.[52] In that same spring of 1922, a strike took place in a British asylum where female nurses locked themselves in with patients and resorted to fisticuffs when they were forcibly removed by the police.[53] This event is unlikely to have passed unnoticed within Swedish psychiatry.

Resumption of the debate about employment of nurses in Swedish asylums should probably be seen against the background of these strikes, associated with the labour movement. It seems likely that medical directors and asylum boards wanted to be sure of having staff that were loyal to the employer, which in this case implied a category of women without links to the labour movement. The situation must also be seen against the political state of the nation, where a combative and growing labour movement was set against a conservative, middle-class power structure. At this time, the collective consciousness also included memories of the Finnish civil war and Russian revolutions, where antagonism between socialists of every hue and groups representing middle-class values had led to armed conflict and bloodshed. These events had also left traces in Sweden in the form of open demonstrations of class differences, mutual distrust and fear of violent clashes.

In conjunction with the proposed adoption of the law of an eight-hour working day by Parliament in 1921, the Society of Nursing had lobbied for the exclusion of nurses from regulated working hours. The nurses' intentions have been interpreted as an attempt to find differentiating circumstances and define a clear border, relative to subordinate personnel and, in particular, to labourers, with whom they did not want to be compared.[54] The result was that all nursing personnel at health care institutions were excluded from the eight-hour legislation.[55] In 1938, an eight-hour working day was introduced at asylums, but even in the late 1940s, nurses in practice worked unregulated hours.[56] The tenacious efforts by nurses to adapt working hours and performance to the needs of the job were probably motivated by several factors, all pointing in the same direction. On the one hand, asylum patients probably had a genuine need for the presence of staff at all times, considering how the care was organised at the time with many patients forced to spend a long period in the asylum, having sporadic or no contact with family and friends. On the other hand, the nurses' efforts reflected a need for life content among women who had elected to work in health care, thereby relinquishing their option of starting a family. But the motive was probably also a more or less conscious way of obtaining competitive advantages vis-à-vis other categories of staff. Nurses portrayed an image of co-operation and devotion to duty. Their working hours were planned so that they could be present at ward rounds and medical procedures. This allowed them to maintain control over the medical aspects of patient care and collaboration with the psychiatrists. As a consequence, attendants were denied contact with medical treatment, which they saw as a gateway to higher positions.

Inevitably, a class and gender conflict ensued within psychiatric care which was carried on at different levels and by various means: by professional strategies at the group level, and by subtle negotiation at the individual level. It is relevant that the class identity of nurses appears to have been shaped by the colleges of nursing and the positioning of the Swedish Society of Nursing, rather than by family background (which was generally lower middle-class).

Against the background of these obvious tensions between different categories of staff, it is bewildering and contradictory to find numerous accounts of positive collaboration between all staff categories and hear descriptions in interviews of the good family-like spirit that characterised the secluded environment where personnel of all types both worked and lived. My belief is that this is not simply the reflection of an idyllic retrospective construction; the conflicts were kept under wraps. Perhaps this was an expression of professionalisation strategies, since a more confrontational approach appeared to be unproductive. Research in other areas of the civil service has demonstrated the existence of similar, hidden conflicts behind a facade of cosy co-operation both among Post Office workers and primary school teachers, who were also involved in class and gender conflicts.[57]

During the period of economic depression in the early 1930s, there was unemployment in many areas of society. Nurses looked for work in the asylums

Nurses in Swedish Psychiatric Care

to a greater extent than before. When the economic depression abated and the construction of new general hospitals was under way, the proportion of nurses dropped in the asylums. Contributory reasons probably included uncertainty about the future development of the personnel organisation as well as the periodic resurgence of conflicts between nurses and attendants. In 1940, about half the supervisory positions in asylums were held by nurses (300), while the rest were held by female (123) or male (195) attendants.[58] Nurses also served as head nurses in the general hospital psychiatric units, which started to appear in the 1930s. Lower positions at the asylums and the psychiatric units were held by both female and male attendants. For male patients, there were still wards staffed only by women. Female wards remained the exclusive domain of female staff well into the 1960s, when wards with both male and female staff started to appear. Extramural community work in Sweden was attached to the asylums and to the general hospital psychiatric units until the 1970s, but was available to a small extent.

Reformed Training Programmes

How to resolve the training of different categories of mental health care personnel came to be a complicated matter that extended over several decades. It is clear that this was not because of curriculum issues of a technical nature, but because of a power struggle that touched on controversial matters and emotionally charged spheres.

Numerous training proposals appeared in the 1930s and 1940s. Extensive investigations were made, ministers were petitioned, and union journals became involved.[59] Attendants fought for uniform training for all mental health care personnel and access to advanced positions. The path to this goal seemed to go via more extensive training, with an increasingly medical approach for attendants. England had an organisation with separate recruitment and a specific training programme for personnel within psychiatric care; this was held up as a model for desirable development and described as 'infinitely superior' by the attendants. Training as nurse-tutor was open to male nurses as well. The notion of a 'hospital nurse', i.e. someone trained at a nursing college, being competent to work in psychiatric care following minor supplementary training, was seen as unthinkable in England. Frustrated male attendants pointed out that only male personnel worked on male wards in most other European countries.[60]

However, the Board of Health in Sweden wanted leading positions staffed by medically well-trained personnel. The formal reason why nurses were in demand at asylums was their medical training; a trend that increased in the 1940s with the advent of various somatic treatments. From 1955, the nursing college curriculum included two months' training in psychiatric nursing for all nurses, with the option of a further six months of specialist training within the framework of the three-year nurses' programme.

However, it was more difficult to reach agreement with regard to the attendants' reformed training programme. One proposal followed the next, only to be rejected by the other party. It took until 1956 for a two-year basic training to be initiated for attendants, comprising extensive practical and theoretical training, including four months' experience at a general hospital. The planned path to advanced positions was nevertheless via a training programme at nursing colleges, which were at the same time opened to male students.

It was the representatives from the nursing and medical professions to the 1949 Royal Training Commission who achieved acceptance of the demands for an extensive training programme for attendants, but still with the requirement of nursing college training for access to leading positions.

The title of nurse was protected in 1958, when state registration of the profession was initiated. Protection of the title came late in Sweden, probably because both the Royal Medical Board and the Swedish Society of Nursing wanted to prevent a development similar to certain other nations that had a separate asylum training system and register for psychiatric nurses. It took time and effort to enforce generic training for all nurses, including psychiatric care, and develop a single register. For a position as nurse in psychiatric care, a nursing college education was consequently required. Working as an attendant required no education beyond compulsory school, although asylum-based training for attendants had been available since 1905 and a two-year – now three-year – training had been offered at the upper secondary school level since the 1970s.

During my research interviews, many older nurses have touched on the consequences of the new training system for attendants.[61] Attendants trained under the old system were excluded from the further training they had asked for. Furthermore, their opportunities for advancement to senior positions diminished with the growing availability of nurses who wanted to work in asylums. Their younger colleagues, who had graduated from the new training programme for attendants, had much better theoretical knowledge than what had been provided by the old training and a somewhat different outlook on care content, which occasionally led to conflict among the attendants.

Men as Nurses

Male nurses who were former attendants have described problems in relation to attendants who wanted to continue demanding a different training system, and regarded nurse-trained former attendants as traitors. Male nurses became involved in conflicts if they distanced themselves from a collective masculinity of attendants, which they found destructive. The attendant's identity was contrasted with that of the nurse, giving rise to a search for alternative modes of conduct between caregivers and patients and a gender identity with a new repertoire. Under the influence of the politically radical ideologies of the 1960s, the nursing profession could be associated with a gender-conscious, forceful masculinity concentrated on solidarity. A masculine identity emerged, with a focus on male emancipation, in the footsteps of the growth of feminism and reinforced by the gay rights movement, both of which were critical to male hegemony. However, as a result of the introduction of a government equality project in the late 1970s, the number of men recruited fell sharply, at the same time as the ambition to strengthen the link between masculinity and the caring practices increased.[62]

In the 1960s and subsequently, there was discussion about the feminine professional title of 'nurse' and its effect on recruiting men to the profession. Several different designations were proposed, following various government enquiries. In the 1970s, the alternative masculinised variant of 'sjukskötare' appeared and was intended as a gender-neutral designation. This attempt to change the professional title was fiercely resisted by the Swedish Society of Nursing, which refused to yield to normative male ideals. Instead, the Swedish Society of Nursing launched the feminine variant 'sjuksköterska' as a gender-neutral professional title. Over time, this has gained support within an increasingly gender-conscious public policy and the purportedly gender-neutral, masculinised term was relegated to history.

Numerous studies show that male nurses are satisfied with their profession and see their minority position as an advantage, which among other things shows up in their career development. They work to a large extent in technologically advanced and high-status positions.[63] In the 1980s, the proportion of men in the nursing profession was approximately 11 per cent.[64] In 2004, 14 per cent of students in the nursing programme and 27 per cent in the specialised training programme in psychiatric care at the *Department of Nursing, Karolinska Institutet* are men.

Psychiatric Nurses' Identity

It can be deduced from both the written and verbal accounts of nurses from the first half of the twentieth century that they saw themselves as agents of reform within psychiatric care with a mission to work for development and change. This may have contributed to their relatively high self-esteem and disinclination to accept personal blame for shortcomings in the care system or criticism relating to asylum conditions.

A work ethic with elements of a Lutheran sense of duty emphasized work as a source of joy, which was primarily self-rewarding.[65] The meaning of the concept a 'calling' in relation to the nursing profession has varied over time.[66] Nurses who worked in psychiatric care in the 1940s do not refer to religious belief as a fundamental tenet for their work.[67]

Nurses from that period describe a struggle to give psychiatric patients more humane conditions and a reasonable quality of life. The lack of equipment and inflexible routines were seen as near insurmountable obstacles in their work. The fact that representatives of other personnel categories fought for the same issues does not diminish the impression that nurses saw this as their specific duty.

Nurses' narratives present the perception that violence against nurses was rare and that the common notion of mental patients as violent and dangerous was exaggerated. The professional identity of nurses appears to be linked to the ability to control fear, which was seen as a prerequisite for being able to ward off violence from the patient. When violence is mentioned in the narratives, it is linked to specific situations that were stressful for the patient, inappropriate treatment routines or professional shortcomings.[68]

After the Second World War, Swedish psychiatry was influenced primarily by the USA and Great Britain. As a result, the previously very negative attitude to psychodynamic psychotherapy in Swedish psychiatry could no longer be maintained. Nurses within psychiatric care who had already looked to the USA for inspiration were being influenced by Hildegard Peplau and other authors focusing on interpersonal relationships in nursing, based on psychodynamic theory and practice. From the middle of the twentieth century, training in psychiatric care, for instance in the Stockholm region, acquired a psychodynamic focus.[69] Ideological differences between nurse tutors and proponents of more 'traditionally medical-biological' practical training placed student nurses in an awkward position for a few decades. Since the 1970s, psychotherapy training is open to nurses in multi-professional programmes.

In 1977, nursing education at academic level was initiated, with the expressed objective that the training should have a scientific basis, and that nursing should be evidence based. What this means in terms of nurse identity remains to be seen.[70]

Concluding Discussion

The professionalisation strategies of nurses in the field of psychiatry included the recognition of psychiatric care as an area of activity for women trained as general nurses in nursing colleges. Ever since the training of nurses began, definition of the area of activity in medical terms has been linked to femininity, a caring ideology associated with ethics, and training with elements of personality moulding. In this context, there are a number of factors which in different ways may have contributed to the fairly successful professionalisation result.

Nurses in Swedish Psychiatric Care

Sweden has generally had a stable government, a 'strong' centralised administration, as well as a central agency for public health and health care issues in which medical experts have had a major influence. During the twentieth century, health care has been a public responsibility in Sweden, financed primarily through taxes. Overall, this has allowed the government to drive development forcefully, as well as taking a major responsibility for psychiatric care, even in cases where decisions have been questioned by one or other personnel category or by the public. These circumstances worked to the advantage of nurses, since they were supported by the medical authorities. Why the attendants failed to drive home their demands via their union remains an unanswered question, particularly when there was a close relationship between the trade unions and the Social Democrats, the party which has formed most governments since the 1930s.

Sweden is probably one of the most profoundly secularised societies in the Western world and became so fairly early. Religious orders have been active in psychiatric care to an extremely limited extent. Individual priests on the boards of asylums or who served at the asylums had very little influence on care. A national church which places relatively little emphasis on gender segregation and female subordination, and with no real influence on societal and medical issues, appears in this case not to have slowed the development.

The lingering tradition since the eighteenth century of women occasionally working in asylums with male patients made it impossible to paint a scenario of violence against female personnel, since there was a continuum of contradictory examples. From the turn of the twentieth century, there have been a few asylums which employed female general nurses as headnurses on every ward at all times. In other words, there was already an established system for reference purposes. The critics of this system were primarily attendants, especially men whose opportunities for advancement to senior positions were curtailed, while they were at the same time denied access to the nursing colleges, which prior to 1950 only accepted female students. Concern that the labour movement, with links to the attendants' union, would develop a heightened class struggle appears to have worked against them. The nurses' links to the middle-class women's rights movement, which employers generally found preferable in view of their greater willingness to co-operate, worked to the advantage of the nurses.

Notes

1.   H.E. Peplau, 'Historical Development of Psychiatric Nursing: A Preliminary Statement of Some Facts and Trends', in S.A. Smoyak and S. Rouslin (eds), *A Collection of Classics in Psychiatric Nursing Literature* (Thorofare: Slack, 1982), 10-46: 19.
2.   G.A. Tucker, *Lunacy in Many Lands* (Sydney: Charles Potter, Government printer, 1887).

3.   W.P. Letchworth, *The Insane in Foreign Countries* (New York and London: G.P. Putnam's sons, 1889).

4.   K. Pándy, *Die Irrenfürsorge in Europa – Eine vergleichende Studie* (Berlin: Reimer, 1908).

5.   G. Schuldheis, 'En ny anstalt för sinnessjuka', *Hygiea*, 1 (1905), 209-40. 11 (1905), 332-53. S.A. Skålevåg, 'Constructing curative instruments: psychiatric architecture in Norway, 1820-1920', *History of Psychiatry*, 13: 49 (2002), 51-68.

6.   G. Svedberg, 'Utländska besökare på hospital vid sekelskiftet 1900', *Psyche*, 1 (2000), 10-15.

7.   H. Lundborg, 'Om sinnessjukvård', *Allmänna Svenska Läkartidningen*, 37 (1904), 657-65: 659.

8.   *Ibid.*

9.   G. Boschma, *Creating Nursing Care for the Mentally Ill: Mental Health Nursing in Dutch Asylums, 1890-1920* (Pennsylvania: UMI Dissertation Services, 1997); *idem*, 'High Ideals Versus Harsh Reality: A Historical Analysis of Mental Health Nursing in Dutch Asylums, 1890-1920', *Nursing History Review*, 7 (1999), 127-51; *idem*, *The Rise of Mental Health Nursing: The Rise of Psychiatric Care in Dutch Asylums, 1890-1920* (Amsterdam: Amsterdam University Press, 2003).

10.   Various designations have been used in Swedish as well as English translations: Swedish: skötare, sinnessjuksköterska/sinnessjukskötare, mentalsjuksköterska/mentalsjukskötare, mentalskötare or skötare inom psykiatrisk vård. English: attendant, mental nurses, assistant psychiatric nurse, psychiatric nursing auxiliary or second level nurse in psychiatric care.

11.   L. Bland, *Banishing the Beast: Sexuality and the Early Feminists* (New York: the New York Press, 1995); C. Lindén, *Om kärlek: litteratur, sexualitet och politik hos Ellen Key* (Stockholm: Symposion, 2002); U. Manns, *Den sanna frigörelsen: Fredrika-Bremer-förbundet 1884-1921* (Stockholm: Symposion, 1997).

12.   B. Gadelius, *Sinnessjukdomar och deras behandling förr och nu: En populär framställning* (Stockholm: Hugo Gebers Förlag, 1913), 122.

13.   A. Meyerson, *En blick på utvecklingen af Sveriges sjukvård och sjuksköterskeväsende* (Stockholm: Svensk Sjukskötersketidnings Förlag, 1918), 66.

14.   'Berättelse rörande studier i vissa sinnessjukvårdsfrågor – särskilt arbetsterapi och hjälpverksamhet – I Danmark, Tyskland, Holland och Schweiz avgiven av 1928 års studiedelegation för vissa hospitalsbyggnadsfrågor m.m.', SOU [Swedish Official Government Reports Series], 7 (1929), 50.

15.   R. Christianson-Rykling and M-L. Norrman, 'Två samtida banbrytare i sjuksköterskeyrkets framväxt', *Vårdfacket*, 5 (2000), 48-51; Y. Iverson, *Tro verksam i kärlek: En bok om Ersta* (Stockholm: Verbum, 1988).

16.   Marie Cederschiöld Diary 1848-1851 (Stockholm: *Ersta Diakonimuseum*), 52; G. Svedberg, *Omvårdnadstraditioner inom svensk psykiatrisk vård under 1900-talets första hälft* [Nursing traditions in Swedish psychiatric care during the first half of the twentieth century. Summary in English.] (Stockholm: Department of Neuroscience, Karolinska Institutet, 2002), 90.

17.   E. Dillner, *Sjuksköterskeutbildningen inom Svenska Röda Korset åren 1866-1904* (Stockholm: Bonnier, 1934); *idem, Åtta decennier och en del år därtill: Några data och*

Nurses in Swedish Psychiatric Care

fakta kring sjuksköterskeutbildningen i Sverige (Stockholm: Svensk Sjuksköterskeförenings förlag, 1962); Emmy Rappe, *Letters to Sophie Adlersparre 1866-1869* (Stockholm: *Kungliga Biblioteket*, Ia7a:3, 924-5); Svedberg, *op. cit.* (note 16).

18.   M. Arton, *The professionalisation of mental nursing in Great Britain, 1850-1950* (London: University College London, 1998); M. Carpenter, *Working for Health: The History of the Confederation of Health Service Employees* (London: Lawrence and Wishart, 1988); C. Chatterton, 'Women in Mental Health Nursing: Angels or Custodians?', *International History of Nursing Journal*, 5: 2 (2000), 11-19; P.A. Nolan, *A History of Mental Health Nursing* (London: Chapman & Hall, 1993).

19.   M.E. Baly, *Florence Nightingale and the Nursing Legacy* (London: Croom Helm, 1986).

20.   E. Dillner, 'Förord till den svenska översättningen', in Florence Nightingale, *Anteckningar om sjukvård ... ur vårt tidsperspektiv* (Stockholm: SHSTF, FOU report 31, 1989).

21.   Meyerson, *op. cit.* (note 13), 58.

22.   Baly, *op. cit.* (note 19); R. van der Peet, *The Nightingale Model of Nursing* (Edinburgh: Campion Press, 1995).

23.   O.M. Church, 'Nightingalism: Its Use and Abuse in Lunacy, Reform and the Development of Nursing in Psychiatric Care at the Turn of the Century', in V. Bullough, B. Bullough and M.P. Stanton (eds), *Florence Nightingale and her era: A Collection of New Scholarship* (New York: Garland Publishing, 1990), 229-44; Van der Peet, *op. cit.* (note 22); M. Tallberg, *Den sekulära sjuksköterskan i Finland från 1700-talet till den enhetliga utbildningens början 1930: Vården och utbildningen speglade mot förhållandena i övriga länder* (Kuopio: Publications of the University of Kuopio, 1991), 114.

24.   Baly, *op. cit.* (note 19); Tallberg, *op. cit.* (note 23), 94-6.

25.   V. Webb, *Florence Nightingale: The Making of a Radical Theologian* (St. Louis: Chalice Press, 2002).

26.   I. Hammar, *Emancipation och religion: Den svenska kvinnorörelsens pionjärer i debatt om kvinnans kallelse ca 1860-1900* (Stockholm: Carlssons, 1999).

27.   Tallberg, *op. cit.* (note 23). Svedberg, *op. cit.* (note 16).

28.   Baly, *op. cit.* (note 19), 187-204; B-M.R. Sommer, *Vilka skäl kan Florence Nightingale ha haft till att förankra sjuksköterskorna i ett etiskt lydnadsråd till läkarns?: En litteraturstudie i hermeneutisk fördjupning* (Stockholm: Enheten för vårdpedagogik, Institutionen för pedagogik, Lärarhögskolan i Stockholm, 1996); Tallberg, *op. cit.* (note 23).

29.   S. Nicklasson, *Sophiasystern som blev politiker Bertha Wellin Pionjär för moderat politik* (Stockholm: Carlsson Bokförlag, 1995).

30.   E. Rodhe, *Ur sjukvårdens etik* (Stockholm: Svensk sjukskötersketidnings förlag, Third Edition, 1927 [first edition 1912]).

31.   Nicklasson, *op. cit.* (note 29). Tallberg, *op. cit.* (note 23), 59.

32.   Svedberg, *op. cit.* (note 16).

33.   G. Wretmark, 'Svenska psykiatriska föreningen 75 år', in L. Ljungberg and G. Wretmark (eds), *Svenska psykiatriska föreningen – en återblick* (Stockholm: Liber, 1980), 7-17: 11.

34.   G. Zetterström, 'Utbildning av sinnessjukvårdspersonal', *Nordisk Psykiatrisk Medlemsblad*, Festskrift (1956), 80-6; 'Sjukvårdspersonalens utbildningsfråga', *Humanitet*, 9 (1946), 149.

35.   H. Truedsson, *Svenska sinnessjukvårdspersonalens förbund Minnesskrift 1908-1933* (Lund: Svenska sinnessjukvårdspersonalens förbund, 1933), 60.

36.   A. Emanuelsson, *Pionjärer i vitt: Professionella och fackliga strategier bland svenska sjuksköterskor och sjukvårdsbiträden, 1851-1939* (Stockholm: SHSTF, FOU 1990: 34, 1990).

37.   'Årsberättelser från hospital 1912' (Stockholm: *Riksarkivet*, Medicinalstyrelsens arkiv Hospitalsbyrån; E 5 F: 12).

38.   Sjuksköterskors samarbete i Norden (SSN). Svensk sjuksköterskeförening/ SSF. Handlingar rörande nordiskt samarbete (Stockholm: Tjänstemannarörelsens arkiv och museum TAM, SSN-kongresser 1920-1950, F7a: vol. 1-4); N.B. Wingender, *Fem svanor i flok: Sygeplejerskers Samarbejde i Norden 1920-1995* (Copenhagen: Sygeplejerskers Samarbejde i Norden, 1995).

39.   Sjuksköterskors samarbete i Norden (SSN), *ibid.*

40.   O.M. Church, *That Noble Reform: Emergence of Psychiatric Nursing in the United States, 1882-1963* (Chicago: University of Illinois, 1982).

41.   K. Neuman-Rahn, *Den psykiskt sjuka människan och hennes vård* (Stockholm: AB Nordiska Bokhandeln, 1924); D. Matilainen, *Idémönster i Karin Neuman – Rahns livsgärning och författarskap – en idéhistorisk-biografisk studie i psykiatrisk vård i Finland under 1900-talets första hälft* (Åbo: Åbo Akademi University Press, 1997).

42.   Matilainen, *op. cit.* (note 41).

43.   K. Neuman-Rahn, *Der seelisch kranke Mensch und seine Pflege* (Jena: Gustav Fischers Verlag, 1924).

44.   Å. Fause and A. Micaelsen, *Et fag i kamp for livet: Sykepleiens historie i Norge* (Bergen: Fagbokforlaget, 2002); K. Ludvigsen, *Kunnskap og politikk i norsk sinnssykevesen 1820–1920* (Bergen: Institutt for administrasjon og organisasjonsvitenskap, Universitet i Bergen, Rapport nr. 63, 1998); M. Lysnes, *Behandlere – voktere? Psykiatrisk sykepleies historie i Norge* (Oslo: Universitetsforlaget, 1982); K. Melby, *Kall og kamp: Norsk Sykepleierforbunds historie* (Oslo: JW Cappelens Forlag, 1990); idem, *Kvinnelighetens strategier: Norges Husmorsforbund 1915-1940 og Norges Laererinneforbund 1912-1940* Skriftserie 4/97 (Trondheim: Senter for kvinneforskning, Universitetet i Trondheim, 1995); idem, *Professionalisation and Gender: Nurses in Norway* (Trondheim: Senter for kvinneforskning, Arbeidsnotat, Skriftserie 5, 1993); Skålevåg, *op. cit.* (note 5); G. Svedberg, 'En historia om psykiatri utan bälten: Berättelser från Island', *Psyche*, 2 (1997), 6-8; Svedberg, *op. cit.* (note 16); G. Sjöblom, 'Den gamla Grelsbyandan', in K. Eriksson and D. Matilainen (eds), *Vårdandets och vårdvetenskapens idéhistoria – Strövtåg i spårandet av 'caritas originalis'* (Vasa: Åbo Akademi, Vårdforskning, Institutionen för vårdvetenskap 8, 2002), 173-91; S. Vatne, *Korrigere og anerkjenne: Sykepleiers rasjonale for grensesetting i en akuttpsykiatrisk behandlingspost* (Oslo: Det samfunnsvitenskapelige fakultet, Institutt for sykepleievitenskap, 2003), 21-2.

45.   B. Burhe, 'PM angående kvinnlig sjukvårdspersonal å mansavdelningar vid ett par danska hospital respektive användningen av skolade sjuksköterskor å dessas båda könsavdelning', (Stockholm: *Kungl. Medicinalstyrelsen*, 1927, Stencil, Bil. 2, 7-8.

46.　Svedberg (1997), *op. cit.* (note 44).

47.　Tallberg, *op. cit.* (note 23), 6.

48.　'Psykiatri i Norden – ett jämförande perspektiv: Delbetänkande av psykiatriutredningen', sou [Swedish Official Government Reports Series], *Socialdepartementet*, 4 (1992).

49.　Lysnes, *op. cit.* (note 44); Meyerson, *op. cit.* (note 13).

50.　Svedberg, *op. cit.* (note 16).

51.　Burhe, *op. cit.* (note 45).

52.　B. Nilsson, 'Telefoniststrejken 1922. Tio dagar som skakade Stockholm', in C. Florin, L. Sommestad and U. Wikander (eds), *Kvinnor mot kvinnor: Om systerskapets svårigheter* (Stockholm: Norstedts, 1999), 45-74.

53.　Carpenter, *op. cit.* (note 18), 65-70; Chatterton, *op. cit.* (note 18).

54.　Emanuelsson, *op. cit.* (note 36), 68, 112-21.

55.　E. Bohm, *Okänd, godkänd, legitimerad: Svensk sjuksköterskeförenings första femti år* (Stockholm: Svensk sjuksköterskeförenings förlag, 1961), 128-9, 250-4; Emanuelsson, *op. cit.* (note 36), 68, 112-21; Nicklasson, *op. cit.* (note 29), 265-302.

56.　Informant 14. Born 1897. Nurse 1925. Private Nurs 1925-27. Psychiatric nurse at Sandbyhov, Norrköping 1928-32. Head Nurse at Beckomberga Mental Hospital until 1957.

57.　C. Florin, *Kampen om katedern: Feminiserings- och professionaliseringsprocessen inom den svenska folkskolans lärarkår 1860-1906* (Umeå: Almqvist & Wiksell International, 1987); B. Lundgren, *Allmänhetens tjänare Kvinnlighet och yrkeskultur i det svenska postverket* (Stockholm: Carlsson, 1990).

58.　'Betänkande angående utbildning av sinnessjukvårdspersonal – 1949 års kommitté för sinnessjukvårdspersonalens utbildning' (Stockholm: *Inrikesdepartementet*, 1951), 90.

59.　*Ibid.*; P. Björck, 'Behörighetsvillkoren för översköterskor', *Social-Medicinsk Tidskrift*, 10 (1936), 181-6; J. Emers, 'Utbildning av sjuksköterskor och övrig mentalsjukvårdspersonal', in G. Holmberg, L. Ljungberg and C. Åmark (eds), *Modern svensk psykiatri* (Stockholm: Almqvist & Wiksell, 1968), 378-83; Truedsson, *op. cit.* (note 35), 94, 107, 178; Zetterström, *op. cit.* (note 34), 149; 'Sinnessjukvårdspersonalens utbildningsproblem', *Humanitet*, no. 10 (1946), 169-70; 'Statens sjukhusutredning av år 1943, betänkande iv: Synpunkter och förslag rörande sinnessjukvården', sou 1948:37, (Stockholm: *Inrikesdepartementet*, 1948); M. Söderström, 'Förslag till riktlinjer för utbildning av personal vid statens sinnessjukhus', *Humanitet*, October (1933), 187-8.

60.　A.N., 'Glimtar från tjänstgöring på engelska sinnessjukhus', *Humanitet*, no. 6-7 (1950), 132; I. Larsson, 'Glimtar från engelska sinnessjukhus iii', *Humanitet*, no. 12 (1950), 255 8; Truedsson, *op. cit.* (note 35), 127.

61.　Svedberg, *op. cit.* (note 16).

62.　H. Eriksson, *Den diplomatiska punkten – maskulinitet som kroppsligt identitetsskapande projekt i svensk sjuksköterskeutbildning* [Abstract: The Diplomatic Point – Masculinity as an Embodied Identity Project in Swedish Nursing Education. Summary in English.] (Göteborg: Acta Universitatis Gothoburgensis, Göteborg studies in educational sciences 172, 2002).

63. *Ibid.*; H. Robertsson, *Maskulinitetskonstruktion, yrkesidentitet, könssegregering och jämställdhet* (Stockholm: Arbetslivsinstitutet, Arbetsliv i omvandling 2003: 13, 2003).

64. E. Pilhammar Andersson, *Det är vi som är dom: Sjuksköterskestuderandes föreställningar och perspektiv under utbildningstiden* [Abstract: Now we are them! Registered Nurse Students' Perceptions and Perspectives during the Nurse Training Programme.] (Göteborg: Göteborg studies in educational sciences 83, 1991), 97.

65. Svedberg, *op. cit.* (note 16).

66. Å. Andersson, *Ett högt och ädelt kall: Kalltankens betydelse för sjuksköterskeyrkets formering 1850–1930* (Umeå: Institutionen för historiska studier, Umeå universitet, 2002).

67. Svedberg, *op. cit.* (note 16).

68. G. Svedberg, 'Berättelser om rädsla inom psykiatrisk vård' [Abstract: Narratives on fear within psychiatric care], *Svensk Medicinhistorisk tidskrift*, 3: 1 (1999), 83 101; Svedberg, *op. cit.* (note 16), Study 11; Gunnel Svedberg and Gunilla Bjerén, 'Violence against Nurses in Swedish Psychiatric Care – Narratives on a gendered culture from the first half of the twentieth century'; G. Svedberg, 'Sjuksköterskors berättelser om rädsla inom psykiatrisk vård före moderna psykofarmaka', *Social Vetenskaplig Tidskrift*, 8: 1-2 (2001), 20-39.

69. A. Engquist, *Psykiatrisjuksköterskan: Ideal eller verklighet? Utvärdering av hälso- och sjukvårdslinjens inriktning mot psykiatrisk vård* (Stockholm: Högskolekansliet Utbildningsförvaltningen FoU report 1988, 2), 61.

70. Although there were also re-organisations of the nursing programme during the second half of the twentieth century, the basic structures since the 1850 pioneers remains in current nursing training: one general training programme for all nurses, which is intended to provide a qualification for nursing posts, including that of nurse in psychiatric care. At the Nursing Department, Karolinska Institutet, three years of study (180 ECTS credits) leads to a Bachelor of Science in Nursing, and nurse registration by the Swedish National Board of Health and Welfare. Reg. nurses can specialise in psychiatric care (60 ECTS credits), or eight other nursing specialisations or in midwifery science.

Psychotropic Drugs

CHAPTER 16

Mental Ills and the 'Hidden History' of Drug Treatment Practices

Toine Pieters and Stephen Snelders

Hyoscyamine, 1879: 'We may make a desert and call it peace'.[1]

Largactil, 1961: 'The patient can do extremely well at first sight but he experiences the world as empty, cold and theatre-like [...] sometimes he becomes more handicapped than by taking a simple sedative...'[2]

Psychopharmacology and Historiography

There can be no history of psychiatry without a history of psychopharmacology. Whether on medical prescription or as self-medication, whether to sedate or to cure, whether promoted by pharmaceutical companies or clamoured for by an anxious population, the consumption of psychoactive drugs has been an integral part of the politics of mental health.

Psychotropic drugs have been and still are important, although recurrently controversial, intervention tools in the treatment of mental ills. The administration of psychoactive substances has remained an underlying variation in mental health care, regardless of changes in therapeutic fashion. Psychiatrists, as trained doctors, have continued to prescribe psychotropic drugs, while at the same time there has been a steady consumer demand for these substances, whether in the form of patent medicines, prescription medicines, or natural remedies. Even in the 1970s, the period of anti-psychiatric revolt and critique of psychopharmacology, chemical 'liberation' with the help of *other* drugs such as LSD was an alternative for chemical 'straitjackets' leading to mental liberation and de-conditioning.[3]

In the second half of the nineteenth century, the production, marketing and consumption of therapeutic drugs such as morphine and other opiates, hyoscyamine, hyoscine (scopolamine), potassium bromide and chloral hydrate became an integral part of the cure and care of mental ills, both inside and outside the walls of the asylums.[4] In the 1950s, the celebrated 'psychopharmacological revolution' introduced new drugs: neuroleptics or major tranquillizers such as chlorpromazine (Largactil, Thorazine) and reserpine (Serpasil) for the psychotics, minor tranquillizers such as meprobamate (Miltown), chlordiazep-oxide (Librium) and diazepam (Valium) to handle anxiety and tension, stimulants such as methylphenidate (Ritalin) for the depressed, hallucinogens such as lysergic acid diethylamide or LSD (Delysid) for neurotics and alcoholics.

The historiography of psychiatry has paid relatively little attention to the use of psychotropic drugs or other somatic treatments in mental health care. Ten years after Andrew Scull drew attention to this omission, there have been not sufficient systematic efforts to open up this field of research.[5] For instance, recent reviews of the history of psychiatry and mental health care in the Netherlands hardly refer to any studies specifically devoted to the use of psychotropic drugs.[6] Of course, the use and even the importance of drug therapies in treating psychiatric problems have been credited. But the specifics and contexts of drug use have hardly been explored.[7]

A basic problem in the integration of the history of psychopharmacology in the history of psychiatry is the tendency to take a perspective based on the dichotomy between a 'biological' and a 'psycho-social' psychiatry.[8] It is our hypothesis that this perspective hides the far more complex and versatile roles that psychotropic drugs play and have played in treating mental ills. Our own research suggests developments and transformations that do not necessarily concur with the constructions of either a biological or a psycho-social psychiatry, or with theses of the 'first' and 'second' biological revolution in psychiatry. Anything more than a superficial awareness of the historical continuities that have shaped the careers of psychotropic drugs is missing in most accounts.

We therefore propose a different position, which focuses on the evolution of psychotropic drugs within various practices and cultures, inside and outside the 'Bedlams' of the world.[9] In order to deepen our understanding of continuities as well as discontinuities with regard to the use and meaning of psychotropic drugs, we need accounts that go beyond descriptions of the scientific, medical or social development of a drug. In their conception, making, marketing and uses, therapeutic drugs show that they are far more than just medical commodities. They also reflect developments and transformations in the science and art of healing as a cultural process. Moreover, pill-making and pill-taking are part of the medical market, which is essentially cyclical in nature and subject to supply and demand interactions. We will explore these kinds of dynamics in two rather different case studies. While differing widely in time period, geographical location and method of research, it is especially noteworthy that both studies suggest similar conclusions regarding the continuities of psychotropic drug use within the context of asylum psychiatry.

First, we discuss the European career paths of the new psychotropic drug hyoscine (alternatively named scopolamine) at the end of the nineteenth century on the basis of a primary and secondary literature review around the nightshade alkaloids. We argue that interpretations of a new 'alkaloid period' of asylum treatment, or of a paradigm shift from romantic to scientific medicine around 1850, do not suffice to explain the increasing use of hyoscine and other nightshade alkaloids in treating mental ills. Here, drug treatment practices show much greater continuity with earlier centuries than a focus on nineteenth-century asylum psychiatry allows for.

Second, we explore the career paths of chlorpromazine in the 1950s and the 1960s, primarily in the Netherlands, on the basis of sampling and analysing Dutch scientific, clinical and popular writings as well as interviews with expert witnesses. Historians generally agree that the introduction of chlorpromazine, marketed either as Thorazine or Largactil, marked the start of a new era of drug treatment in psychiatry.[10] But to what extent are we dealing with a paradigmatic turn in the history of psychopharmacology? Was there indeed such a thing as a revolution if we examine chlorpromazine treatment practices as part of a less straightforward history of the long run of psychotropic remedies?

A comparison of these two case studies shows, with all due acknowledgement of the different historical contexts and the different nature of the historical source materials, that the developments and transformations show more continuities between the end of the 19th century and the 1950s than is accounted for to date.

From Nightshade to Hyoscine[11]

The use of plants from the family of nightshades (*Solanaceae*) has a long documented tradition of medical investigation and use since antiquity. Extracts from *Atropa belladonna, Datura stramonium, Hyoscyamus niger* (black henbane) and other nightshades were used as pharmacotherapeutic remedies for all kinds of physical and mental illnesses. Henbane was used in antiquity, for instance, in cases of problems with sexual potency. We find the herb as an ingredient in Paracelsus's sedative arcana and in the Pharmacopoeia Amstelredamensis of 1636. Apart from medical uses, the herb also had widespread application in religion, magic and recreation; indeed, it is not always possible to differentiate between these. In the Netherlands, the flavouring of tobacco and beer with henbane, which has hallucinogenic side-effects, was popular until well into the seventeenth century.[12] The nightshades were included as standard prescriptions in the *materia medica*. Around 1830, nightshade extracts were in use as sedatives in cases of mental disorders (mania, nervous disorders) and neuralgia.[13]

Pharmaceutical research into alkaloids, starting with Sertürner's (1805) discovery of 'Morphium' or morphine, a salt-forming 'alkaline' substance obtained from opium, led to the isolation of the nightshade or tropane alkaloids. In 1833, *hyoscyamine* was isolated from *Hyoscyamus* by the German pharmacists P.L. Geiger and L. Hesse. Their German colleague Emanuel Merck followed up on this finding and developed a procedure for the mass-production of the new alkaloid. In the process, a link was forged between the alkaloid firm of Merck and academic science. Merck's hyoscyamine was investigated by the Viennese pharmacologist Carl Ritter von Schroff in the 1850s. On the basis of mainly physiological examination, Von Schroff concluded that the drug had sedative and hypnotic properties. In 1875, the British alienist Robert Lawson reported on the administration of hyoscyamine to his patients in the West Riding Pauper Lunatic Asylum in Yorkshire. At this time, the medical staff there was very keen on experimenting with drug therapies, using chloral hydrate, nitrous oxide, ether, ergot, opium and other substances.[14] Lawson reported exceptionally good results from the administration of hyoscyamine in cases of 'recurrent, acute, and sub-acute mania, monomania of suspicion, and the excitement of senile dementia', even reporting *cures* of patients with chronic mania and often with chronic alcoholism. Hyoscyamine worked where bromide of potassium or tincture of cannabis had failed.[15] Following Lawson's study, hyoscyamine was increasingly used as a sedative and hypnotic in asylums in different countries.[16] We also find a number of new studies in the German and British medical and pharmacological literature in the years 1875-1880 about the properties and effects of hyoscyamine.[17]

In the 1880s, hyoscine (later named scopolamine) was isolated from hyoscyamine. The company Merck produced its own hyoscine in 1882. Robert Kobert, then professor at the world's first pharmacological university laboratory at Dorpat (in Russian Estonia), played a central role in the testing and development of hyoscine as a psychiatric drug.[18] In 1886, Kobert received samples of the drug from Merck, with the request to investigate its properties. Kobert delegated the research to his pupil August Sohrt, whose dissertation was summarized in Kobert's subsequent article on the properties of hyoscine.[19] Kobert included the results of preceding research on the nightshades. He was not only familiar with the work of Lawson and others on hyoscyamine, but also with the fact that researchers at the end of the 18th century, such as the Viennese physician Anton Störck, already knew about the therapeutic effects of henbane extracts. The study of Kobert and Sohrt was followed by the introduction of hyoscine into asylums. For several reasons, the Merck company became the leading producer of hyoscine. First, it had earned itself a reputation for chemical purity and high quality with its hyoscyamine and other alkaloid products (guaranteed by the company). Second, Merck had close ties to academic pharmacology and related fields, and maintained a close relationship with the medical community. Third, Merck had gained respectability among doctors by projecting a scientific image in the marketing of pharmaceuticals.[20]

Hyoscine was found to be of better use in sedating patients than hyoscyamine. Having a standardized measurement of the dose eliminated the problems of under- or overdosing.[21] Because it could be injected subcutaneously, it was deemed especially suitable in the treatment of the severely disturbed insane.[22]

There was some discussion about hyoscine's range of indications. Kraepelin considered it a very 'energetic' substance and recommended caution.[23] The Dutch psychiatrist M. Ruland reported having only satisfactory experiences with the administration of this drug.[24] The discussions in medical journals seem to point to an increasing interest in the use of hyoscine, as do references in the Merck reports of medical investigations and uses.[25] Around 1895 hyoscine, by then renamed scopolamine, had become increasingly incorporated in the treatment of manic patients. It retained its status as an essential part of the armoury of sedative and hypnotic drugs beyond the Second World War.[26] In the 1950s, scopolamine was still in use in Dutch mental hospitals. Routinely, an injection of 10 mg morphine in combination with 0.25 mg scopolamine was used (the so-called 'ten M and a quarter') to calm the agitation of patients with mania and psychosis, and in severe cases to produce drastic sedation (*platspuiten*).[27]

In the older historiography, the transformation in the materia medica from botanical extracts to standardized compounds with extensive use in clinical practice has been presented as linear and generally unproblematic, a product of autonomous knowledge production.[28] In his history of psychiatry, Edward T. Shorter calls the second half of the nineteenth century the 'alkaloid period of asylum treatment'.[29] Matthias Weber suggests that nineteenth-century psychopharmacology experienced a paradigm shift, or as Fleck has called it, a *Wandlung in Denkstil*. Weber sees around 1850 a 'scientific' medicine (*naturwissenschaftliche Medizin*) taking the place of 'romantic' medicine. According to Shorter, romantic psychiatry placed, for instance, distress within the category of morals and passions.[30] In Germany and elsewhere this approach disappeared in favour of a focus on chemical-physiological studies.[31]

There are some problems in understanding the psychiatric use of hyoscyamine and hyoscine from this perspective. We know that already at the end of the eighteenth century, henbane extracts were applied by doctors to calm down patients with 'maniacal deliria'.[32] Störck, for instance, tested the therapeutic use of henbane on animals, himself, and his patients.[33] As Andreas-Holger Maehle has convincingly argued, experimental pharmacology and the use of a case history method in establishing the therapeutic benefits of a drug was essentially an eighteenth-century innovation. Starting from this thesis, we can seriously question historical approaches that relate the uses of new alkaloid drug therapies in the *treatment* of insane patients with a shift towards scientific medicine.[34] The medical use of henbane-extracts in the second half of the nineteenth century was basically not much different from that in the sixteenth century, whatever the difference in the theoretical explanations of the effects might have been. In the sixteenth century, for instance, doctors recommended the internal use of belladonna (which as we now know contains the same alkaloids as henbane) to *cool down* in the case of mental disorders and disturbances. After going out of fashion in the seventeenth century, the use of belladonna was again generally accepted at the end of the eighteenth. Simultaneously, it also acquired a high status in homeopathic medicine.[35] Was there, then, a paradigm or conceptual shift in the introduction of hyoscyamine, hyoscine or scopolamine in psychiatric *practice* in the second half of the nineteenth century?

From a practical perspective, it is difficult to speak about Lawson's observations with hyoscyamine either in terms of a 'discovery' or a 're-discovery'. Hyoscyamine extracts are mentioned again and again in pharmacopeia and textbooks during the *whole* of the nineteenth century. An example from Germany is the psychiatrist Alexander Haindorf, who described the use of belladonna and *hyoscyamus* in 1811 as successful interventions in cases of mental disorders. He might, as Weber comments, not have been specific in his recommendations, but his contemporary Johann Heinroth was: he wrote about the use of nightshade extracts to dampen nervous excitation in 1818. Even Karl Wilhelm Ideler, for historians a figurehead of romantic psychiatry, used belladonna as a sedative. And they were psychiatrists who, according to Weber, relegated the primacy in mental disorders to the psyche, not the soma.[36]

Experimental research into the therapeutic use of nightshade extracts was carried out by J.-J. Moreau de Tours in France in the 1840s and by Carl Ritter von Schroff at the University of Vienna in the 1850s, at least 20 years before Lawson's research.[37] Moreau differentiated between the effects of belladonna and other medicines on both acute and chronic psychiatric patients: in the first case, according to him, they were therapeutically successful, in the second they were not. The rationalizations might have differed, but this hardly affected the everyday practice of testing and using therapeutic drugs. The nightshade extracts or alkaloids were applied to sedate patients and depress their psychic functions with the aim of producing momentary relief of symptoms. Moreau hoped that this momentary relief might extend into a cure of the patient.

To proceed from medical practice to rationalizations of this practice, there is no discontinuity in the arguments in favour of or against the use of nightshade extracts before and after 1850. Doctors tested the new standardized Merck preparations of hyoscyamine and then hyoscine from at least 1855 (Von Schroff) onwards, on animals, patients and themselves, without a fundamental change in the nature, direction and standards of testing. However similar the clinical testing procedure, the therapeutic setting underwent significant changes: the rapid growth of the asylum population created a demand for hypnotic and sedative substances to help in nursing the increasing numbers of insane patients there. As Shorter points out, the great majority of patients around 1900 received diagnoses like 'hysterical madness' that in retrospect are not transparent, but might nowadays be considered as some form of psychosis, with attendant violent behaviour.[38] In the treatment and care of these patients, standardized medicines such as hyoscine were in demand. Merck offered the medical profession the standardized medicine suitable for treating large number of patients on a regular basis. In an effort to determine what conditions could be improved by hyoscyamine and subsequently hyoscine or scopolamine, doctors tested the industrial preparations on a wide variety of psychiatric conditions like mania, melancholia, chorea and general paralysis.[39] Kobert, for example, considered hyoscine to be a suitable medication for patients with varying diagnoses, such as 'dementia after primary madness', periodical mania, paranoia, melancholia, puerperal mania, paralysis and 'secondary dementia'. This resulted in hyoscine being recommended in most therapeutic reports as an adequate means of calming down severely agitated patients with mania, who previously could only be prevented from causing trouble to staff and other patients by physical isolation.[40] In our view, the subjective experiences of the patients were neglected in this appropriation of hyoscine by the nineteenth-century asylum psychiatry and pharmacology. It seems never to have been taken into account that hyoscine might provide patients with a remarkable and disturbing dream life, in a similar way as the hyoscine-containing so-called 'witch ointments' had done before.[41] Of course, side-effects were noticed, including visual and auditory hallucinations, even prolonged depression and what we would now call psychosis, but these were never seen as a decisive argument against drug treatment.[42]

There was no sense of effecting 'new cures' through the use of hyoscine at the end of the nineteenth century. What we do find, however, is that the use of these drugs in the context of the growing asylums sometimes led to a critique that sounds familiar to us: the patients were not cured, but instead kept sedated to the extent of turning them into spiritless creatures or 'living dead'. An editor of *The Journal of Mental Science* wrote in 1879 that 'We may make a desert and call it peace'.[43] In 1902, a Dutch psychiatrist voiced the same criticism: the drug might bring peace and quiet to the asylums, but (echoing Schiller's *Don Carlos*) it was the peace of a graveyard.[44] This criticism regarding chemical forms of restraint not only applied to the use of hyoscine or scopolamine, but was part of a continuous debate about the pros and cons of using hypnotics and sedatives in psychiatric practice as a means to establish peace and quiet and make patients amenable to 'reason'. The dynamic balance of positive and negative sentiments was typical of the career of most psychotropic drugs.

In 1912, the German psychiatrist Max Seige pointed to the repetitious quality of the reports on psychotropic drugs in medical journals. In his view, they always started with very optimistic reports about promising therapeutic results, soon followed by communications about the occurrence of side-effects or therapeutic claims that failed to materialise, gradually resulting in a reduction of the range of indications and uses.[45] Whether we focus on the introduction and use of hyoscine, the bromides and chloral at the end of the nineteenth century or the introduction and use of barbiturates like Veronal (barbital) and Luminal (phenobarbitone) at the beginning of the twentieth century, a 'Seige cycle' of therapeutic optimism and disappointment manifests itself that corresponds with a cycle of subsiding and growing criticism within the field of psychiatry.[46] Regardless of what preoccupations prevailed among psychiatrists, the question of whether the application of sedatives and hypnotics itself was justified did not seem to be up for discussion, as these were frequently regarded as a necessary evil.[47] An extensive armoury of sedatives, tonics, stimulants and anti-epileptics helped doctors, nurses, patients and the general public to cope with the daily discomforts of mental ills and other nervous problems, both inside and outside the walls of the asylums.[48] As we will show, the arrival of the psychotropic drug chlorpromazine in 1953 did not immediately make an essential qualitative difference to existing drug treatment practices in Dutch psychiatry.

Chlorpromazine in the Netherlands[49]

In the Netherlands, one of the first psychiatrists to test the newly introduced anti-emetic and anaesthetic drug chlorpromazine systematically (its wide range of pharmacological actions was expressed in its European trade name, Largactil, 'large action') was the psychiatrist and director of the psychiatric institution Maasoord, Frederik Tolsma.[50] He started this work in the summer of 1953. Nine months earlier, the French psychiatrists Jean Delay and Pierre Deniker had published the results of their pioneering study with the potent anti-histamine and so-called 'neuroplegic'(nerve-paralyzing) drug; they successfully applied chlorpromazine in the treatment of agitated psychiatric patients.[51] Tolsma was familiar with the sedative qualities of the chemically related anti-histamine drugs Antallergan (pyrilamine) and Phenergan (promethazine), which had been introduced in the 1940s by Barberot Specia, the Dutch subsidiary of the French company Specia Rhone Poulenc. Both had been licensed as anti-allergy medicines but had also proven useful as a psychiatric co-medication in the popular sleep therapy.[52] This form of somatic therapy involved keeping patients in a continuous sleep by the injection of sedative cocktails (e.g. Somnifen) for several days or even weeks with the rational of giving the nervous system a break and thereby a chance to stabilize.[53] In well-staffed institutional settings, this treatment, which required careful monitoring of the patients to prevent serious breathing problems, was being practised on a regular basis from the 1930s onwards. Despite frequent failures, it was claimed that sleep therapy achieved dramatic recoveries from psychiatric conditions:

> Agitated patients could turn quiet and orderly [...] boisterous manic patients could be cured of a manic episode, anxious melancholia patients could be freed from anxiety and restlessness.[54]

According to the Dutch historian Catharina Th. Bakker, Tolsma aimed to develop his institution into a centre of excellence for the research of somatic therapies and keenly followed the latest developments in the French and German literature.[55] As a result of his earlier research efforts, he had established close contacts with the Specia management. They were more than willing to provide him with free samples of Specia's latest therapeutic asset, Largactil, under the research label 4560 R.P. The initial idea was to reproduce the French 'artificial hibernation' method and stabilize the nervous system of patients by combining chlorpromazine with artificial cooling of the body.[56] Given the lack of expertise with the rather demanding cooling procedure, Tolsma reluctantly decided to administer chlorpromazine without further interventions. His small team of researchers started administering chlorpromazine alone or in combination with other sedatives as a form of sleep therapy to patients who had been unresponsive to other forms of therapy, regardless of their diagnosis. Although regarded as a sedative, chlorpromazine appeared to sedate patients in an unusual way. Did this drug essentially deliver an improved form of sleep therapy, or was there more to it?

Sedatives usually put patients to sleep or caused a lethargic drowsiness, but chlorpromazine appeared to be different in its actions. After a couple of days of mere drowsiness, this drug produced a strange but therapeutic form of detachment. This condition looked rather similar to the behaviour of patients who were leucotomised. Following their foreign colleagues, Tolsma and his associates considered this detachment part of a so-called 'pharmacological leucotomy'. They reported that the behaviour of severely disturbed patients, who had no prospect of recovery, improved in such a dramatic way that this 'last-ditch' surgical leucotomy procedure could be cancelled. If drug habituation might pose a problem in the future, chlorpromazine might at least be instrumental in the selection of patients for a surgical lobotomy. But there was more to report on chlorpromazine than this kind of association with a 'leucotomy'.[57]

In a rather spectacular way, some of the chlorpromazine-taking patients who had been hospitalised for several years with chronic psychiatric conditions opened up for communication and forms of social therapy ('actieve therapie'). A case in point is the following description of the therapeutic effect in a female patient:

> A forty-year-old woman was admitted in 1950. She was very aggressive, restless and impetuous [...] She could hardly be maintained as part of the wheelbarrow squad. She was initially given chlorpromazine by intramuscular injection (daily dose of 150 mg) followed by an oral regimen of 2 tablets three times a day (daily dose of 150 mg). Currently she is very calm. She has opened up for communication. She works on a regular basis in the laundry.[58]

One of the nurses working at the 'chronic disturbance' pavilion noted how within a period of about six weeks after the introduction of chlorpromazine, the unpleasant and aggressive atmosphere changed into the peace of a sanatorium.[59] In effectively calming the most agitated and unruly patients, 'the terror cases of the institution', the use of chlorpromazine was also reported to reduce significantly the overall consumption of hypnotics and sedatives at the institution.[60]

However positive in its clinical assessment, Tolsma's research group did add some critical remarks. Chlorpromazine did not have a lasting therapeutic effect. In most cases, the symptoms returned as soon as the patients stopped using the medication. Apparently, a maintenance dosage was required, but it was far from clear whether the medication should be maintained for an indefinite period, and what amount sufficed to control symptoms. Despite the fact that no 'consistently serious' problems seemed to ensue from the use of the drug, the medical staff observed unwelcome side-effects. Beside allergic reactions, problematic distortions in the blood picture and sudden drops in blood pressure were reported. The Tolsma group emphasized that Largactil should be handled with caution.[61] However cautionary, the message of promise and hope prevailed.

This did not necessarily mean that the new drug therapy was adopted overnight in Dutch psychiatry. Chlorpromazine had yet to prove itself.[62] Quite often, the stimulus of Specia's special force of salesmen was needed to persuade psychiatrists to test the free samples of what was advertised as an 'ideal medication to achieve peace and quiet by stabilizing the nerve system'.[63] The proof of the pudding was in the eating. Once the free samples of chlorpromazine had made their way into the clinic, the initial restraint would subside. As in the case of Tolsma, most psychiatrists would start giving chlorpromazine to their unruly patients in order to judge its qualities as an improved form of sleep therapy. It was the combination of the speed of the sedative effect, the rather swift recovery to a conscious state of peace and quiet, and the frequent opening up of schizophrenic patients to communication and forms of social therapy that invested chlorpromazine, and in its wake the cheaper alternative the *Rauwolfia* preparation reserpine (Serpasil), with an aura of therapeutic success.[64]

The nursing staff, in particular, was impressed by the effectiveness of chlorpromazine. In offering both an effective means of chemical restraint and a therapeutic tool that could produce visible recoveries in even the most desperate cases, chlorpromazine boosted the morale of the staff. The fact that chlorpromazine could also produce problematic side-effects did not seriously affect their enthusiasm. Nurses were already familiar with the occurrence of the side-effects of the conventional somatic therapies in general use in Dutch psychiatric practice, such as insulin coma therapy and electroshock therapy. They considered the management of side-effects as something that came with the job.[65]

Dutch nurses were going to play a central role in establishing everyday chlorpromazine treatment routines inside the mental hospitals. For instance, due to the shortage of nursing staff at the 'Duin en Bosch' hospital, the French procedure of providing chlorpromazine treatment in combination with bed nursing was simplified to drug therapy only.[66] Subsequently, after experiencing difficulties with the distribution of the badly tasting tablets to patients and taking a dislike to handling the increasing number of pills, which often left them with severe dermatological reactions, nurses promoted a change to the use of orange-coated tablets from 1955 onwards.[67] In another institution, 'Endegeest' mental hospital, the nursing staff played a seminal role in the change from the painful and necrosis-producing injections to the administration of chlorpromazine tablets.[68] The nursing staff in yet another mental hospital, 'Santpoort', initiated a fashion of wearing wide-brimmed hats among chlorpromazine-taking patients as a means to protect their photosensitive skin against the sun.[69]

The advance of chlorpromazine on the daily institutional drug regime manifested itself also in changes in the nursing routines. Using chlorpromazine on a large scale required new monitoring procedures to check the daily intake of the medication and to contain side-effects such as jaundice, cardiac problems, fever, hypotension or parkinsonian symptoms. In addition, nurses had to schedule time to shave the female patients who developed a chlorpromazine-induced growth of beard and to satisfy those patients who did not use chlorpromazine but had opened up for communication and therapy, relieved of the terror regime of fellow patients.[70]

As far as the medical staff was concerned, the emphasis was on integrating chlorpromazine into existing therapeutic practices.[71] Instead of immediately replacing conventional somatic treatments such as electroshock and sleep therapy, chlorpromazine was welcomed as a valuable asset to the *existing* armoury of 'somatic treatments'.[72] Chlorpromazine was added to insulin therapy, and combinations with electroconvulsive therapy and other sedatives were tested.[73] The dose was measured on a case by case basis, and both drugs were basically applied as an improved form of sleep therapy, which did not just produce sedation but also a special form of liberation or relaxation of the disturbed mind. Depending on the local culture of treatment and rehabilitation, chlorpromazine earned a reputation as either a most humane form of chemical restraint or an important aid to existing social and psychotherapeutic treatment programmes. In neither case was it regarded as a new form of chemotherapy of the mind, but as a state-of-the-art form of sedation for the individual patient.[74] Tolsma regarded chlorpromazine as an important catalytic agent in the recovery process. But like most of his Dutch colleagues, he was convinced that there was an essential interplay between the social climate of the setting in which the drug was provided and the effectiveness of this treatment. He even set up a buddy-system in his institution as a means to stimulate therapeutic optimism and to sustain chlorpromazine's favourable therapeutic effects.[75]

From the very beginning, Dutch doctors peppered their testimonies of the benefits of chlorpromazine with critical assessments of some of the problems associated with its use: from the social problems associated with the unexpected return of psychiatric patients to their families, to the high frequency of relapses and side-effects.[76] The sometimes rather severe side effects did not, however, prevent some psychiatrists from prescribing chlorpromazine in doses that went up to 2000 milligrams daily (average adult dosage 200-400 mg daily).[77] On the contrary, in a number of Dutch mental hospitals, psychiatrists began to use the neuromuscular reactions closely resembling parkinsonism induced by chlor-promazine as a clinical indicator of treatment at the optimum level.[78]

The growing support for the idea that the therapeutic effects and neurological side-effects went together played an important role in the growing acceptance of the concept of specifically effective psychotropic agents. Moreover, this stimulated efforts to differentiate drugs like chlorpromazine from conventional sedatives. At the end of the 1950s, new categories of psychotropic drugs were introduced – first the tranquillizers and subsequently the minor and major tranquillizers or neuroleptics.[79]

The Dutch enthusiasm for chlorpromazine may not have been as hyperbolic as in France, the UK and the USA, but the 'Seige cycle' of promise, hope, therapeutic optimism, and subsequent re-evaluation and disappointment manifested itself correspondingly.[80] At the end of the 1950s, a growing number of reports were published assessing the long-term therapeutic benefits of the growing list of chlorpromazine-like drugs in asylum psychiatry. The initial enthusiasm made way for a critical reassessment of the use of neuroleptics. The Dutch asylum psychiatrist Henk van Andel, for instance, raised questions about the fact that despite impressive improvements in the daily condition of chronic psychiatric inpatients, the new drug treatment programmes failed to lower the number of chronic patients in mental hospitals. On the basis of his experiences at the 'Dennenoord' mental hospital, Van Andel suggested that the new drug treatment in itself did not suffice to overcome the immense social and cultural gap between the worlds inside and outside the institution.[81] His colleague, Cees van Rhijn, who had studied the neuroleptics-related morbidity and mortality statistics at the Brinkgreven Mental Hospital, argued that by inducing a morbid awareness of the 'diseased self' vis-à-vis this very same social and cultural gap, the new drugs most likely contributed to a significant rise in suicide rates.[82] In order to improve the long-term therapeutic benefits of neuroleptics, both psychiatrists made a strong plea for social reforms in the mental hospitals.

A more radical voice could be heard from the director of the mental hospital at Zeist ('het Christelijk Sanatorium'), Adriaan Lit. In comparing the symptoms of Parkinsonism with the neuromuscular side-effects of the neuroleptics, he raised the question of whether the new medical direction in psychiatry was little short of a chemical mask. However important they were in terms of a technical innovation, Lit argued that the neuroleptics had a symptomatic and repressive effect in common with shock therapy, sleep therapy and leucotomy.[83] He set the tone for a growing public debate in the 1960s on the pros and cons of psychotropic drug use in the treatment of mental disorders.[84] In 1961, at the height of what would turn out to be a first wave of public concern about psychotropic drug use, the popular Dutch newspaper *De Telegraaf* published a leading article on the hazardous consequences of tranquilizer use, entitled 'A threat to mankind'.[85]

Right from the beginning, the pharmaceutical industry had been most helpful in emphasizing the new qualities of chlorpromazine (Largactil) and reserpine (Serpasil) and differentiating them from conventional sedatives. This is nicely reflected in the drug advertisements from the 1950s. Whereas in the case of chlorpromazine, Van Gogh's painting *The round of the prisoners* was used to promote its special relief-producing effect, in the case of reserpine, the image of a pill superimposed on a brain with the caption 'different from the barbiturates' served to underline the new combination between sedation and mental recovery.[86] To capture this new therapeutic profile and distinguish it from sedation proper, Dutch scientists began to label chlorpromazine and reserpine as 'tranquillizers' from 1956 onwards.[87]

The differentiation of the 'new' tranquillizers was given impetus by studies claiming that both chlorpromazine and reserpine counteracted the 'psychosis' induced by the hallucinogenic drug LSD.[88] LSD was regarded as a drug compound that could be used to artificially produce pathological states of mind. This was part of a flourishing international field of research studying the biochemical basis of psychiatric disorders. Within this context, LSD was regarded as a promising new laboratory tool. Following research by D.W. Woolley and E. Shaw and by J. Gaddum, schizophrenic states of consciousness were compared with an 'experimental psychosis' triggered by LSD. According to the Dutch founder of biological psychiatry, Herman van Praag, the resulting hypothesis that changes in behaviour might be related to changes in the chemistry of the brain (possibly because of disruptions in the production of the neurotransmitter serotonin) helped to stimulate biological psychiatric research.[89]

In suggesting a relationship between chemical and clinical psychosis, LSD research opened up a new scientific and public horizon: what in 1957 was still described by the neurologist Johan Booij as 'pharmaco-psychiatry' would become publicly known in the Netherlands as the 'chemistry of madness' by the end of the 1960s.[90] It was the experimental tool par excellence, LSD, and not chlorpromazine that paved the way for a productive alliance between neuropsychopharmacology and clinical psychiatry. LSD research helped to turn the 'neurotransmitter revolution in medicine' into an attractive form of neurological mythology: the chemically transformable mind.[91]

However, the promise of a psychoactive magic bullet, with a controllable and specific effect on the chemistry of the brain, was not kept by any of the new psychotropic drugs. On the contrary, the chemical effects of these drugs on the mind turned out to be remarkably *non*-specific. Medical and public profiles of the new drugs took different directions. Whereas LSD, after its failure as a therapeutic drug in medicine, received a magical mind-expanding drug aureole under street names as Purple Haze and Orange Sunshine, chlorpromazine was transformed into the 'mind-killing' icon of the Dutch anti-psychiatry movement of the 1970s.[92] At the time of the second wave of professional and public unrest about psychiatric drug use, however, chlorpromazine was already in the latter days of its psychiatric career, eclipsed by an armoury of new major tranquillizers.[93]

In 1968, on the occasion of the fifteenth anniversary of the introduction of chlorpromazine in the Netherlands, the pioneer Tolsma pointed out that like any improvement in psychiatric practice, the new drug regime was subject to a gradual process of 'habituation' in patients as well as in medical and nursing staff. In his view, the long-term use of neuroleptics was closely connected with a reduction of social tolerance regarding agitated behaviour in mental hospitals. Tolsma was seriously concerned that what he in the early 1950s had coined 'a Copernican revolution in psychiatry' was about to get bogged down to a mere continuation of the conventional practice of maintaining order and quiet in mental hospitals.[94]

Conclusion

On the basis of a comparison of the career paths of hyoscine and chlorpromazine, we argue that as far as drug treatment practices are concerned, talking in terms of evolution is far more productive than a Kuhnian construct of a 'Copernican revolution'. It is indeed rather tempting to read the enthusiastic acclaim for the therapeutic wonders of a new drug as a departure from the past. However, in the case of both hyoscine and chlorpromazine, we see an intriguing tango between old and new treatment features which produces gradual instead of abrupt developments and transformations. Marketed as new and innovative remedies, both chlorpromazine and hyoscine made their way into the medicine cabinet in an ad-hoc and pragmatic way as a helpful neighbour of existing psychotropic drug therapies. We showed that over time, as part of a trade-off process between old and new (continuities and discontinuities), the new successful neighbour helps to reconfigure the meanings and uses of psychotropic drugs as part of evolving treatment regimes in psychiatry.

The career paths of both hyoscine and chlorpromazine show similar cyclical dynamics. Expanding use of the drugs and high expectations of their effects after their introduction are followed by rising criticism and disappointments, a gradual easing of the demand, and subsequently by declining use and limited application. Since the German psychiatrist Max Seige was first in pointing out the

Mental Ills and the 'Hidden History' of Drug Treatment Practices cyclical nature of the careers of psychotropic drugs, we have named this kind of dynamics a 'Seige cycle'. These cycles sometimes end with the disappearance of the drug from mental health care, only to be replaced by new drugs with new profiles of promise and hope.

Seige cycles, however, are not static essences or ahistorical categories that unchangingly determine the careers of drugs or other therapeutic innovations. On the contrary, historical transformations that take shape over the course of cyclical career paths illuminate transformations in our ways of handling therapeutic innovations in psychiatry.[95] The specific details of the dynamics of a Seige cycle may, for instance, differ from one therapeutic drug to the other. In the case of both hyoscine and chlorpromazine, the duration and heights of the peaks and valleys of the phases of the cycle are clearly different. In the former they seem much 'flatter' than in the latter. More research into the details of these cycles and their meanings is necessary. There are indications that Seige cycles show phase differences when we look at the different regions of mental health care: asylums, extramural psychiatry, general practice, and the large but often neglected field of 'self-medication'. Neither can we neglect the differences in national settings and contexts. By taking a comparative approach of the courses and contexts of different Seige cycles, we can establish the importance of various factors involved: scientific, political, economic and cultural. The concept of the Seige cycle will connect a history of psychopharmacology in the long term with case histories of the medium and short term.

Notes

1.   G.H. Savage, 'Hyoscyamine, and Its Uses', *The Journal of Mental Science*, 25 (1880), 177-84: 184.
2.   E. de Windt, 'Het bezwaar van psychopharmaca bij de ambulante patiënt', *Nederlands Tijdschrift voor Geneeskunde*, 105 (1961), 2515.
3.   S. Snelders, 'LSD and the Dualism Between Medical and Social Theories of Mental Illness', in M. Gijswijt-Hofstra and R. Porter (eds), *Cultures of Psychiatry and Mental Health Care in Postwar Britain and the Netherlands* (Amsterdam: Rodopi, 1998), 103-20.
4.   This seems to correspond with an overwhelming increase in the number of psychiatric patients. For this increase see E. Shorter, *A History of Psychiatry: From the Era of the Asylum to the Age of Prozac* (New York: John Wiley, 1997) 46-8.
5.   A. Scull, 'Somatic Treatments and the Historiography of Psychiatry', *History of Psychiatry*, 5 (1994), 1-12. Favourable exceptions are D. Healy, *The Antidepressant Era* (Cambridge: Harvard University Press, 1997); *Idem, The Creation of Psychopharmacology* (Cambridge: Harvard University Press, 2002); A. Maehle, *Drugs on Trial: Experimental Pharmacology and Therapeutic Innovation in the Eighteenth Century* (Amsterdam: Rodopi, 1999); M. Weber, *Die Entwicklung der Psychopharmakologie im*

Zeitalter der naturwissenschaftlichen Medizin. Ideeengeschichte eines psychiatrischen Therapiesystems (München: Urban & Vogel, 1999).

6.　Cf. M. Gijswijt-Hofstra and H. Oosterhuis, 'Psychiatrische geschiedenissen', *Bijdragen en Mededelingen betreffende de Geschiedenis der Nederlanden*, 116 (2001), 162-97. And H. Oosterhuis, 'Insanity and Other Discomforts: A Century of Extra-mural Psychiatry and Mental Health Care in the Netherlands 1900-2000', paper presented at the workshop *Cultures of Psychiatry and Mental Health Care in the Twentieth Century: Comparisons and Approaches* (Amsterdam, 18-20 September 2003).

7.　We have discussed this subject in a few publications, e.g. S. Snelders and Ch. Kaplan, 'LSD Therapy in Dutch Psychiatry: Changing Socio-political Settings and Medical Sets', *Medical History*, 46 (2002), 221-40; T. Pieters, M. te Hennepe and M. de Lange, *Pillen & psyche. Culturele eb- en vloedbewegingen. Medicamenteus ingrijpen in de psyche* (Den Haag: Rathenau Instituut, 2002).

8.　In the 1970s Andrew Scull pointed out a similar problem in the conventional one-sided explanations for decarceration (the social versus the medical fix): A.T. Scull, *Decarceration* (Englewood Cliffs (NJ): Prentice Hall, 1977), 77-8.

9.　We have elaborated the concept of the careers of psychotropic drugs in: S. Snelders, C. Kaplan, T. Pieters, 'Psychotropic Drug Treatment in the 19th Century: On Cannabis, Chloral Hydrate, and Drug Career Cycles', paper at the International Conference of Drugs and Alcohol in History, Huron University College, London, Ontario (Canada), May 14, 2004. And T. Pieters, *Historische trajecten in de farmacie, medicijnen tussen maatwerk en confectie* (Hilversum: Verloren, 2004).

10.　G. Grob, *The Mad Among Us: A History of the Care of America's Mentally Ill* (Cambridge: Harvard University Press, 1994), 226-31; Healy, *op. cit.* (note 5), 2; Shorter, *op. cit.* (note 4), 239-62.

11.　Research on hyoscine was partly funded by a Wellcome Travel Grant awarded to one of the authors (Snelders). For a critical analysis of the introduction of these drugs in medical practice, see S. Snelders, 'Getemde heksenplant levert sedativum. Merck en de metamorfose van scopolamine', *Pharmaceutisch Weekblad*, 139 (2004), 120-3.

12.　H. Roessingh, 'Inlandse tabak. Expansie en contractie van een handelsgewas in de 17e en 18e eeuw in Nederland', *A.A.G. Bijdragen*, 20 (1976), 73-85.

13.　J. Starobinski, *Geschichte der Melancholiebehandlung von den Anfängen bis 1900* (Basel: J.R. Geigy S.A., 1960) B. Schwamm, *Atropa belladonna. Eine antike Heilpflanze* (Stuttgart: Deutscher Apotheker Verlag, 1988); A. Rutten, *Ondergang in bedwelming. Drugs en giften in het West-Romeinse rijk* (Rotterdam: Erasmus Publishing, 1997); C. Rätsch, *Enzyklopädie der psychoaktiven Pflanzen* (Aarau: AT Verlag, 1998).

14.　Rob Ellis, personal communications. Dr Ellis has made a comparative study of West Riding and North Riding Asylum at York.

15.　R. Lawson, 'A Contribution to the Investigation of the Therapeutic Action of Hyoscyamine', *The Practitioner*, 17 (July-December 1876), 7-19.

16.　R. Kobert, 'Ueber die Wirkungen des salzsauren Hyoscins. Nach den Versuchen des Herrn A. Sohrt', *Archiv für experimentelle Pathologie und Pharmakologie*, 22 (1887), 396-429; Shorter, *op. cit.* (note 4), 197.

17.　Kobert, *op. cit.* (note 16).

18. *Ibid.*

19. *Ibid.*

20. B. Issekutz, *Die Geschichte der Arzneimittelforschung* (Budapest: Akadémiai Kiadó, 1971); I. Käbin, *Die medizinische Forschung an der Universität Dorpat/Tartu 1802-1940. Ergebnisse und Bedeutung für die Entwicklung der Medizin* (Lüneburg, Verlag Nordostdeutsches Kulturwerk, 1986); H. Dumitriu, 'Die wissenschaftliche Entwicklung der Alkaloid-Chemie am Beispiel der Firma Merck in den Jahren 1886-1920' (Ph.D.-thesis, University of Heidelberg, 1993); I. Possehl, *Modern aus Tradition. Geschichte der Chemisch-pharmazeutischen Fabrik E. Merck* (Darmstadt: E. Merck, 1995); Weber, *op. cit.* (note 5); T. Rinsema, *De natuur voorbij. Het begin van de productie van synthetische geneesmiddelen* (PhD thesis, University of Leiden, 2000).

21. See *E. Merck's Jahresberichte über Neuerungen auf den Gebieten der Pharmakotherapie und Pharmazie* 1887-1902.

22. H. Pinkhof, 'Behandeling der slapeloosheid', *Nederlandsch Tijdschrift voor Geneeskunde*, 35-I (1899), 1056-64; L. Bouman, 'Krankzinnigengesticht en ziekenhuis', *Geneeskundige Bladen uit Kliniek en Laboratorium voor de praktijk*, 9 (1902), 269-300: 277.

23. Reported in *Geneeskundige Courant voor het Koninkrijk der Nederlanden* 25 March 1888.

24. M.H.J. Ruland, 'Over hydrochloras hyoscini in de psychiatrische therapie', *Psychiatrische Bladen*, 6 (1988), 236-43.

25. *Merck's Jahresberichte*, 1895, 119.

26. J. Braslow, *Mental Ills and Bodily Cures: Psychiatric Treatment in the First Half of the Twentieth Century* (Berkeley: University of California Press, 1997).

27. Wellcome Witness Seminar *Medicijnen en psychiatrie (1950-1985)* at the Free University Medical Centre, Amsterdam, 9 June 2001; H. van Praag, *Psychofarmaca. Een leidraad voor de praktiserend medicus* (Assen: Van Gorcum, 1966), 29.

28. E.g. Issekutz, *op. cit.* (note 20), 131-3.

29. Shorter, *op. cit.* (note 4), 197.

30. *Ibid.*, 30.

31. Weber, *op. cit.* (note 5). See also *Idem*, 'Die "Opiumkur" in der Psychiatrie. Ein Beitrag zur Geschichte der Psychopharmakotherapie', *Sudhoffs Archiv*, 71 (1987), 31-61.

32. Issekutz, *op. cit.* (note 20), 132.

33. Maehle, *op. cit.* (note 5), 186.

34. Weber, *op. cit.* (note 5), 75.

35. Schwamm, *op. cit.* (note 13).

36. Weber, *op. cit.* (note 5), 40-2.

37. J. Moreau (de Tours), 'Mémoire sur le traitement des hallucinations par le Datura Stramonium', *Gazette Médicale de Paris*, 9 (1841), 641-7, 673-80; *Idem*, *Du hachisch et de l'aliénation mentale. Etudes psychologiques* (Paris: Fortin, Masson et Cie., 1845); Carl D. Ritter von Schroff, *Lehrbuch der Pharmacologie*, 3rd. ed. (Vienna: Wilhelm Braumüller, 1868).

38. Shorter, *op. cit.* (note 4).

39.   E. Mendel, 'Die therapeutische Anwendung des Hyoscyamin bei Psychosen', *Allgemeine Zeitschrift für Psychiatrie und psychisch-gerichtliche Medizin*, 36 (1880), 366-72; Kobert, *op. cit.* (note 16).

40.   Kobert, *op. cit.* (note 16).

41.   This argument is further developed in Snelders, *op. cit.* (note 11).

42.   See Lawson, *op. cit.* (note 15), 11-15; L. Lewin, *Nebenwirkungen der Arzneimittel. Pharmakologisch-klinisches Handbuch*, 3rd ed. (Berlin, 1899), 184-90.

43.   Savage, *op. cit.* (note 1), 184.

44.   Bouman, *op. cit.* (note 22), 277.

45.   M. Seige, 'Klinische Erfahrungen mit Neuronal', *Deutsche Medizinische Wochenschrift*, 38 (1912), 1828.

46.   Weber, *op. cit.* (note 5), 101-9.

47.   F. Hall, *Psychopharmaka – Ihre Entwicklung und klinische Erprobung. Zur Geschichte der deutsche Pharmakopsychiatrie von 1844 bis 1952* (Hamburg: Verlag Dr. Kovac, 1997), 45; C. Hamer and J. Haverkate, *Leerboek bij het verplegen van geestes- en zenuwzieken* (Amsterdam: Van Mantgem & Does, 1950); J. Scheffer and A. Oort, *De verpleging van zenuwzieken en krankzinnigen* (Haarlem: Erven Bohn, 1924); A. Timmer, *Leerboek voor verplegenden van zenuwzieken en krankzinnigen* (Haarlem: Erven F. Bohn, 1947).

48.   In the early 1950s hypnotics and sedatives were used on a large scale in the Netherlands to treat nervousness in adults as well as children. This was not seen as problematic. B. Rypkema, 'Een onderzoek naar het geneesmiddelgebruik in Nederland' (PhD thesis, 1954); J. Uttien, T. Pieters and F. Meijman, 'Margriet weet raad op nervositeit', *Gewina* 25 (2002), 260-74.

49.   Largely based on the results of the Dutch Witness Seminar *Medicijnen en psychiatrie 1950-1985* at the Free University Medical Centre, Amsterdam, 9 June 2001. See T. Pieters, S. Snelders and E. Houwaart (eds), *Medicijnen en psychiatrie 1950-1985* (in preparation).

50.   The first Dutch chlorpromazine trial was performed by the female physician N.M. van de Wardt-Kikkert at Provinciaal Ziekenhuis Duinenbosch in Bakkum in the fall of 1952. N. van de Wardt-Kikkert and J. Rentmeester, 'Het largactil en zijn toepassing in de psychiatrie', *Geneeskundige Gids*, 24 (1953), 499-507.

51.   See for an extensive account of the testing of chlorpromazine in psychiatry: Healy, *op. cit.* (note 5), 76-101.

52.   C. Bakker, G. Blok and J. Vijselaar (eds), *Delta. Negentig jaar psychiatrie aan de oude Maas* (Utrecht: Trimbos, 1999), 91.

53.   C. Hamer and F. Tolsma, *Algemeen leerboek voor het verplegen van geestes- en zenuwzieken* (Leiden: Van Mantgem & De Does, 1956), 562-3.

54.   H. Schim van der Loeff and J. Barnhoorn, *Zielszieken en hunne verpleging* (Roermond: JJ Romen & Zonen, 1947), 396.

55.   Bakker et al., *op. cit.* (note 52), 91.

56.   Cohen Stuart at the Dutch Witness Seminar *Medicijnen en psychiatrie, op. cit.* (note 49).

57.   F. Tolsma, G. Jedeloo and J. van Kemenade, 'De betekenis van 4560 R.P. (Largactil) in de psychiatrie', *Nederlands Tijdschrift voor Geneeskunde*, 98 (1954), 997-1001: 998.

58.   *Ibid.*, 1000. A similar anecdotal report of the therapeutic of chlorpromazine can be found in: Van de Wardt-Kikkert and Rentmeester, *op. cit.* (note 50).

59.   Cohen Stuart at the Dutch Witness Seminar *Medicijnen en psychiatrie, op. cit.* (note 49).

60.   Tolsma et al., *op. cit.* (note 57), 1000.

61.   *Ibid.*

62.   In general, Dutch psychiatrists did not regard the introduction of chlorpromazine as an event to rank with the introduction of penicillin: Pieters et al., *op. cit.* (note 49).

63.   Dutch Largactil sales brochure, 1955. Interviews with D. Cannoo and Frits Busser, Special sales representatives, 7 and 10 September 2000.

64.   A. Boon, 'Largactil en verwante middelen in de psychiatrie en neurologie', *Nederlands Tijdschrift voor Geneeskunde*, 99 (1955), 2735-41.

65.   Pieters et al., *op. cit.* (note 49).

66.   Van de Wardt-Kikkert and Rentmeester, *op. cit.* (note 50), 505. Interview with N. van de Wardt-Kikkert, 13 December 2003.

67.   N.M. van de Wardt-Kikkert, 'Quelques aspects de l'application de la chlorpromazine dans un hôpital psychiatrique hollandais', in J. Delay (ed.), *Colloque internationale sur la chlorpromazine* (Paris: G. Doin & C, 1956), 400-4. However relief bringing, the medication practice of crushing and breaking up tablets still posed a problem to the nursing staff: 'Huidafwijkingen door chlorpromazine', *Nederlands Tijdschrift voor Geneeskunde*, 102 (1958), 2191.

68.   Interview with Dr. Marianne van der Plas, 25 April 2001.

69.   Interview with Dr. Thomas Bernard Kraft, 7 May 2001.

70.   Pieters et al., *op. cit.* (note 49); G. Blok, 'Onze kleine wereld', in J. Vijselaar (ed.), *Gesticht in de duinen* (Hilversum: Verloren, 1997), 166-91: 179-82. Interview with Mrs. and Mr. Pals (nurses at Zon & Schild), 15 May 2001. Interview with nurse Piet Rooijackers, 16 May 2001.

71.   'De betekenis van Largactil in de psychiatrie', *Pharmaceutisch Weekblad*, 89 (1954), 378; D. Westerink, 'De farmacologie en toepassing der fenothiazinederivaten', *Pharmaceutisch Weekblad* (1956), 113-44; A. Timmer, *Leerboek voor verplegenden van zenuwzieken en krankzinnigen* (Haarlem: Erven F. Bohn, 1957), 297-301; C. Hamer and F. Tolsma, *Algemeen Leerboek voor het verplegen van geestes en zenuwzieken* (Leiden: Van Mantgem & De Does, 1964), 207-14, 535-67; 'Largactil', *Verslagen der Provinciale Ziekenhuizen van Noord-Holland over het jaar 1955*, 1. Pieters et al., *op. cit.* (note 49).

72.   C. van Rhijn, 'De invloed van reserpine (Serpasil) op acute en chronische geesteszieken', *Nederlands Tijdschrift voor Geneeskunde*, 100 (1956), 1775-90.

73.   Interviews with the physician (internal medicine) Dr W. Gaulhofer, 3 May 2001 and the psychiatrists Dr P.J. Stolk, 9 May 2001; Dr A.C. Lit, 14 May 2001; Dr A.L. Kroft, 11 May 2001; Dr T.B. Kraft, 7 May 2001; and Dr C.H. Van Rhijn, 12 June 2001.

74.   Even in a biochemically oriented 1956 Dutch article on the pharmacology and uses of phenothiazine type of antihistamines, chlorpromazine is claimed to produce its therapeutic effects in mental disorders as a result of its sedative properties: E.G. van Proosdij-Hartzema, 'De farmacologie van chloorpromazine', *Nederlands Tijdschrift voor Geneeskunde*, 100 (1956) 833-42. According to the Dutch professor in neurobiochemistry Johannes Booij it was not before the end of the 1950s that the new drugs in psychiatry became regarded as a separate pharmacotherapeutic group of substances: J. Booij, 'Zon en schaduw der psychofarmaca. "Sudden falls" bij de behandeling met imipramine', *Nederlands Tijdschrift voor Geneeskunde*, 105 (1961), 158-61.

75.   F.J. Tolsma, 'Les neuroleptiques et le problème de l'adaptation humaine', in Delay (ed.), *op. cit.* (note 67), 841-49; C.H. van Rhijn, 'Beschouwingen over de factoren, die het resultaat van de kuren met tranquillizers bepalen', *Voordrachtenreeks van de Nederlandse Vereniging van Psychiaters in Dienstverband*, 2 (1960), 18-45.

76.   Van de Wardt-Kikkert, *op. cit.* (note 50), 403; F. Schwarz and H. van Marken Lichtenbelt, 'Icterus veroorzaakt door Largactil', *Nederlands Tijdschrift voor Geneeskunde*, 99 (1955), 3026-31; 'Afsluitings-icterus als gevolg van chloorpromazinegebruik', *Pharmaceutisch Weekblad*, 90 (1955), 634; W. Gaulhofer, J. Schaank and A. Vali, 'Galactorroe veroorzaakt door chloorpromazine', *Nederlands Tijdschrift voor Geneeskunde*, 101 (1957), 264-6; W. van Ketel, J. Morriën and H. Lenstra, 'Huidafwijkingen door chloorpromazine', *Nederlands Tijdschrift voor Geneeskunde*, 102 (1958), 1799-804; J. Garthier, 'Extra-piramidale stoornissen bij het gebruik van chloorpromazine en reserpine', *Nederlands Tijdschrift voor Geneeskunde*, 102 (1958), 1982; M. Fuldauer, 'Oogkrampen bij gebruik van reserpine', *Nederlands Tijdschrift voor Geneeskunde*, 103 (1959), 110; Van Rhijn, *op. cit.* (note 72); Booij, *op. cit.* (note 74); W. Gaulhofer and H. van der Helm, 'Icterus veroorzaakt door chloorpromazine', *Nederlands Tijdschrift voor Geneeskunde*, 105 (1961), 477-81.

77.   H.M. van Praag, *Psychofarmaca: Een leidraad voor de praktiserend medicus* (Assen: Van Gorkum, 1966), 47-52; S.J. Nijdam, *Ervaringen met moderne psychofarmaca* (Den Haag, Mouton & Co, 1966), 56-9, 122.

78.   B. van Paassen, H.J. Ronner, 'Langdurige behandeling van geesteszieken met hoge doses fenothiazine', *Nederlands Tijdschrift voor Geneeskunde*, 103 (1959), 2201-3. This view was promoted by French psychiatrists.

79.   M. Wertenbroek, 'De klinische ervaringen met de nieuwere psychofarmaca', *Voordrachtenreeks van de Nederlandse Vereniging van Psychiaters in Dienstverband*, 2 (1960), 3-17; Van Praag, *op. cit.* (note 77); Nijdam, *op. cit.* (note 77).

80.   Healy, *op. cit.* (note 5), 93-100.

81.   H. van Andel., 'Wijzigingen en verschuivingen in structuur en werkmethoden in de psychiatrische inrichting', *Maandblad voor de Geestelijke Volksgezondheid*, 15 (1960), 5-14.

82.   Van Rhijn, *op. cit.* (note 72).

83.   A.C. Lit, 'De betekenis van het parkinsonoïd bij de behandeling met neuroleptica', *Nederlands Tijdschrift voor Geneeskunde*, 103 (1959), 1294-6: 1296.

84.   P. Sorgdrager, 'Een proef met vijf "tranquilizers" bij psychoneurose', *Pharmaceutisch Weekblad*, 93 (1958), 733; 'De handel in "kalmte"', *ibid.*, 1085-86; Editorial,

'Psychopharmaca', *Nederlands Tijdschrift voor Geneeskunde*, 105 (1961), 2217; A.C. Regensburg, 'Tranquilizers', *Nederlands Tijdschrift voor Geneeskunde*, 105 (1961), 2217-24; J.G.Y. de Jong and H.J. Kreutzkamp, 'Psychopharmaca', *Nederlands Tijdschrift voor Geneeskunde*, 105 (1961) 2224-29.

85.   G. Bell, 'Bedreiging van de mensheid', *De Telegraaf*, 21-1-1961.

86.   Series of Largactil adds dating from 1957 provided by Dr T. Schok; *Medische Documentatie CIBA*, no. 1 (1956), 3.

87.   Van Proosdij-Hartzema, *op. cit.* (note 74).

88.   J. Booij, 'Farmaco-psychiatrie', *Nederlands Tijdschrift voor Geneeskunde*, 101 (1957), 1869-72.

89.   Snelders, *op. cit.* (note 3), 109-10.

90.   Booij, *op. cit.* (note 88). R. Campbell, 'The chemistry of madness', *Life*, 26 November 1971, 66-86.

91.   Healy, *op. cit.* (note 5), 106-109; C. Regan, *Intoxicating Minds* (London: Orion, 2000), 121-2; A. Solomon, *TheNnoonday Demon: An Atlas of Depression* (New York: Scribner, 2001), 22-6; J. Frantzen, *The Corrections* (London: Fourth Estate, 2001), 364-74; E. Wurtzel, *More, Now, Again* (New York: Simon & Schuster, 2002).

92.   Based on an extensive study of the *Gekkenkrant* in the period November 1973 – Februari 1980. S. Snelders, *LSD-therapie in Nederland. De experimenteel-psychiatrische benadering van J. Bastiaans, G.W. Arendsen Hein en C.H. van Rhijn* (Amsterdam: Candide, 2000); G. Blok, '"Messiah of the Schizophrenics". Jan Foudraine and Anti-Psychiatry in Holland', in Gijswijt-Hofstra and Porter (eds), *op. cit.* (note 3), 151-67; *idem, Baas in eigen brein. 'Antipsychiatrie' in Nederland, 1965-1985* (Amsterdam: Uitgeverij Nieuwezijds, 2004), 141-7.

93.   Interview with the internist, Hans Fabius, 25 April 2001. Annual reports of the Department of Internal Medicine of St Willibrord Mental Hospital, 1960-1970, Fabius personal archive.

94.   F.J. Tolsma, 'Largactil (chlorpromazine): Enkele herinneringen en feiten', *Acta Psychopharmacologica Specia*, 2 (1968), 118-21: 120.

95.   In 1966, at the 122nd annual meeting of the American Psychiatric Association, Garfield Tourney called for attention to the versatile historical phenomenon of the life cycle of new treatment methods in psychiatry. G. Tourney, 'A History of Therapeutic Fashions in Psychiatry', *American Journal of Psychiatry*, 124 (1967), 92-104.

Reflections

CHAPTER 17

From Exploration to Synthesis
Making New Sense of Psychiatry and Mental Health Care in the Twentieth Century

Frank Huisman

The essays in this volume are part of a major effort: rethinking and rewriting the history of psychiatry and mental health care in the twentieth century. It has often been reiterated that traditionally, the history of psychiatry was written by psychiatrists and for institutions. Hence, most publications were about psychiatric theory or were placing the asylum in the centre of attention. During the last two decades, however, there have been many calls to change the focus from theory to therapy, from blueprints to actual practice, and from doctors to patients. After having gone through a mild version of the Science Wars, the 'new' historians of psychiatry realize that their ambition should not be to replace the 'old' historiography – psychiatrists and asylums will always remain important to the mental health care system – but rather to integrate their findings into a story that is more complete, doing greater justice to the complexities of the social responses to mental illness.

In 1999, the Dutch editors of this volume – Marijke Gijswijt-Hofstra, Harry Oosterhuis, and Joost Vijselaar – decided to answer the calls by setting up an ambitious research programme, mainly funded by the Netherlands Organisation for Scientific Research (NWO). Ten researchers were involved in the project, called 'The disturbed mind. Theory and practice in the Netherlands in the twentieth century'. Each of them was assigned a specific topic, which included the psychiatric profession, psychiatric nursing, the patient, medication, the asylum, the mental health care system, state funding, and anti-psychiatry. Every researcher was expected to write a monograph on his or her particular topic, while the new research findings would be integrated into a synthetic volume by two of the initiators of the project. Over the past six years, many new sources on many new dimensions have been studied, and several theoretical perspectives tested. Collectively, the team of scholars has filled many lacunae, empirically as well as conceptually. In order to make sense of the abundance and the bewildering diversity of the available data, it was decided to organise an international conference in Amsterdam. The aim of the conference was twofold. First, it was an opportunity to present the many new research findings. Secondly, the organisers hoped to gain information and inspiration for the daunting task they were facing: writing a synthesis that is to be the crown on the project. Many distinguished historians of psychiatry from other countries were invited to the conference, to facilitate international comparison and put the Dutch findings into perspective.

I was invited to reflect on the methodological and historiographical merits of the essays brought together in this volume and would like to do so while bearing the aims of the research project in mind. My essay will be divided in two parts: in the first, I will be looking at the present volume, whereas in the second, my focus will be on the book that intends to offer a new synthesis. One could argue that there is a Dutch bias in this volume. Although that may be true, focusing on a specific national context would seem to be a logical choice, given the ambitious nature of the project as a whole. The goal is to analyse the theories and therapies of psychiatry and the organisation of mental health care in their mutual relationship and their cultural, social and institutional context. Establishing international differences and similarities (as is done by Oosterhuis in chapter 10) may help to shed light on what is 'universal' and what is distinctly local in the history of mental health care. In this sense, an analysis of the struggle of Dutch historians to move from the exploration of new data to a new synthesis may have an added – or even exemplary – value.

Psychiatric Cultures Compared

There is every reason to start by taking a close look at the essays by Marijke Gijswijt-Hofstra and Harry Oosterhuis, considering the fact that they tentatively present a start for a national (Dutch) synthesis. While Gijswijt-Hofstra offers an overview of institutional care between 1884 and 2000, Oosterhuis does the same for extramural care (1900-2000). Gijswijt-Hofstra starts by establishing the fact that the number of Dutch asylums increased from 14 in 1884 to 45 a little more than a century later. She adds that these figures mean relatively little, since psychiatric care profoundly changed in the intervening years. While the number of beds decreased, the number of admissions witnessed a sharp increase as a result of the introduction of the phenomenon of the 'revolving-door patient'. In its turn, the policy of admission changed as a consequence of changes in the system of psychiatric classification. An important phenomenon to which Gijswijt-Hofstra points our attention concerns the discrepancy between public attention and actual financing in psychiatric care. While it is well-known to historians that intramural care is far more expensive than extramural, it is on developments in the latter domain that public attention is focused. This need not surprise us, because it is here that most therapeutic gain (and therefore social recognition for psychiatrists) is to be accomplished. However, it is important to bear this in mind, since it can lead to serious historiographical bias. Finally, Gijswijt-

Hofstra makes it clear that mental health care is a supply-driven domain: building or expanding asylums always tended to create a 'need' for them. In other words: the dimensions of the market for mental health care were never determined by psychological needs or medical indications, but rather by social factors like the availability of financial means and clinics. Thus, she argues: 'As long as the economic situation had permitted this, the growing supply of asylum beds had more or less created its own demand. Once there was less money available, this mechanism no longer worked.'

In his rich overview, Oosterhuis has dealt with the institutional organisation of outpatient mental health care, with the many actors on both the supply and demand sides of the market, and with the various approaches to mental well-being during the twentieth century. He argues that the simultaneity of the emergence of the psychiatric profession and the first form of outpatient psychiatry was no coincidence. At the end of the nineteenth century, a new group of patients and new nervous afflictions were 'invented' by psychiatrists looking for a niche in the market outside the asylum. From then onwards, they steadily increased their working domain by stressing the moral character of their contribution to the nation-building process, culminating in the 'psy-network' of the mental hygiene movement of the 1920s. Their advice and measures related to family life, sexuality, education, crime and many other topics that were geared to achieving good citizenship. The success of their crusade led to a split in the 1930s between institutional psychiatry and extramural mental health care. The extramural domain became autonomous and, after the war, professionalised to such an extent that members of the clergy began to feel threatened in their position as mental counselors. Psychotherapy reached its zenith during the 1970s, when both clients and therapists began to consider themselves as members of a cultural avant-garde, who should be held capable of sensing what was wrong with modern society. However, after the relative decline of the welfare state in the 1980s, both domains were integrated again into 'multifunctional units' a decade later. From the 1950s onwards, Oosterhuis argues, a symbiotic system of public welfare developed that had religious as well as secular-scientific characteristics: 'the psychotherapeutic frame of mind has permeated both private and public spheres'.

Oosterhuis is trying to contextualise developments within extramural care as much as possible, presenting the mental health care system as the barometer of culture and society. Or to put it differently: the mental health care system and Dutch society are presented as each other's mirror image. Here, there is a danger of tautology. In his story, the tendency towards consensus is presented both as a historical fact (the Dutch are inclined to seek consensus through debate, negotiation and accommodation; social problems in the Netherlands are often pacified by medicalising or psychologising them) and as a heuristic instrument. Oosterhuis is clearly inspired by the theory of figuration developed by Norbert Elias, which was propagated in the Netherlands by, among others, Abram de

Swaan. The 'Elian' notions of chains of interdependence, of the proto-professionalisation of clients, and of the mutual embrace of psy-experts and their clients all fit very well with the social historical perspective that Oosterhuis wants to employ for himself and for the project as a whole. It is illuminating to see how the system of mental health care expanded when the *Fremdzwang* (outward coercion by church and government) gradually evolved into *Selbstzwang* (psy-experts helping the public with the internalisation of social norms and values in an autonomous self). When the certainties of law and bible were replaced by negotiations about what is desirable and attainable in life, there were great opportunities for a further psychologisation of society and an expansion of the domain of mental health care. Like Gijswijt-Hofstra, Oosterhuis presents an image of the domain as supply-driven; like her, he concludes that the dynamics of the care system were a function of professional concerns rather than of humanitarian needs. I will return to this crucial fact later on.

In their stories about the twentieth century, these two authors are using different caesuras. Although their criteria are not very clear, the former divides the century into six periods, while the latter organises it into four. Whoever wants to write an overview cannot ignore periodisation, which is the explicit topic of Volker Roelcke. It is an important matter, since the criteria for it reveal much about the author's perspective, method, and agenda. Although any periodisation may be criticized and any caesura replaced by continuity, it is the organising potential that counts. Roelcke establishes that the history of twentieth-century German psychiatry is often divided into three periods, which run parallel to political eras. They are the Empire and the Weimar Republic (characterised by the success of founding fathers like Kraepelin and Alzheimer); the Nazi era (stained by racial ideologies, eugenics and systematic 'euthanasia') and the Federal Republic of Germany (when German psychiatry was 'normalised'). Roelcke argues that this periodisation was created by post-war psychiatrists, for obvious reasons. He informs us that there had hardly been a de-nazification of psychiatry after the Second World War: the majority of the psychiatric professionals who had been active during the Nazi period continued working. Feeling a need to create a good self-image in which there was no place for eugenic atrocities, they distanced themselves from their past by presenting the Nazi era as an exception to German history. Roelcke argues that this periodisation is unsatisfactory because it suggests 'wrong' caesuras, thus hiding much continuity from view. Although it is ironic to see that his essay is organised along the lines of the conventional periodisation, what he wants to argue is clear. A new generation of historians of psychiatry can afford (without denying or downplaying cruelties committed during the Nazi-era) to point out that there has been much more continuity in the history of German psychiatry and mental health care than is suggested by the conventional periodisation, and that developments in Germany have been much more in line with those elsewhere.

The other 'overviews' do not cover all of the twentieth century but limit themselves to the post-war era. Like Roelcke, Franz-Werner Kersting shows how the Nazi past corrupted post-war German historiography. Unlike Roelcke, however, Kersting considers the Nazi era as a demonic exception to German history, with the late 1950s and 1960s as the 'take-off' period of German psychiatry. His is a story with strong ethical overtones. After the Nazi programme of racial hygiene, forced sterilisation and outright murder, de-nazification failed to materialise. Instead, there was a general atmosphere of social silence. In the early 1960s, the National Socialist past returned to haunt collective memory, including that of the psychiatric profession. This ranged from confronting the past to exposing continuities between the Third Reich and the Federal Republic and outright calls for reform. As elsewhere, these included the introduction of new psychotropic drugs and of group therapy. The difference with other countries, however, was the fierceness of German anti-authoritarian protest in the late 1960s, fuelled by feelings of guilt and shame about crimes committed by psychiatrists during the Nazi era. As elsewhere, German critics were calling for a radical change of the structures of psychiatric care. Combined with a strong awareness of the past, however, the newly developing political consciousness led to deeper differences of opinion than elsewhere. In Germany, the *Vergangenheitsbewältigung* (coming to terms with the Nazi past) went hand in hand with Marxist criticism of capitalism and anti-psychiatry, arguing that humanitarianism was the only solid motivation for care. In this context, Kersting points to the synergy that existed between the 'Socialist patient collective' in Heidelberg and the *Rote Armee Fraktion* (Red Army Party).

The American historian Greg Eghigian takes one step further in debunking the older historiography (and, I would add, common lay perceptions). It has often been assumed that psychiatry was abused for ideological purposes in countries with totalitarian regimes like Nazi Germany or Eastern Europe during the Cold War, whereas in liberal countries, it only served individual humanitarian goals. However, through an analysis of psychiatry in the former German Democratic Republic, Eghigian argues that there are no fundamental differences between the state of psychiatry in liberal, fascist and communist countries. In all of them, psychiatry played a similar role, which was related primarily to the process of modernisation, of which the development of mass society – with all its problems and challenges – was an integral part. In all of them, the psy-disciplines were used – quite regardless of nationality or ideology – in efforts to invent and re-invent society according to the challenges of the times. They were part of a comprehensive reflection on the organisation of state and society. Eghigian argues that everywhere in twentieth-century Europe, there was an ongoing process of social engineering in which modern society was shaped and transformed by policymakers and psy-workers in symbiotic co-operation. While psychiatry supplied the state with a language to frame new policies, the state in its turn rendered legitimacy to psychiatry. Because Eghigian is extending Roelcke's suggestion of continuity from the temporal to the spatial dimension, his paper may be read as an invitation to rethink the relationship between politics and psychiatry from the perspective of shaping citizenship and building the modern nation.

Whereas the chapters by Roelcke, Kersting and Eghigian give abundant proof for the observation that modern psychiatry is thoroughly political, Hugh Freeman shows that the political dimension is not limited to *German* psychiatry – and this applies to the historical as well as to the historiographical dimension of his story. As an historian, he gives us a long-term analysis of British psychiatry from 1601 onwards; as a psychiatrist, he is launching an attack on the demise of the National Health Service through the doings of Margaret Thatcher. The bottom line of his historical account – that runs from the Poor Law enacted by Elizabeth 1 in 1601 up to the conservative Thatcher government – is one of progress. Freeman is suggesting a trend from utilitarianism and local charity via moral treatment to a comprehensive system of free psychiatric care. During the 1950s, the system witnessed an enormous growth. By the mid-1960s, total admissions to mental hospitals had increased nearly ten times compared with 1945, while first admissions had tripled in number. The problems of expenditure and overcrowding in asylums were addressed by the Thatcher government, whose start in 1979 represents another political watershed to Freeman. Inspired by a monetarist ideology, the new government replaced doctors by managers and strongly reduced the number of beds. To Freeman, the introduction of market forces is a moral outrage: he argues that when Thatcher handed over psychiatric care to the forces of the market – claiming that 'there is no such thing as society' – the expertise and professional pride of British psychiatrists were squandered, together with their ideals of public service. It was traded for endless bureaucracy and cold calculation, to the detriment of the patient. As such, his chapter reads like a call for a return to pre-1979 conditions. However, there is also an awareness that 'psychiatry has had to accommodate to this changed world as well as it can'. In this concluding line, Freeman's understanding of the mental health care system seems to be in accordance with Eghigian's claim about the role psychiatrists play in any process of modernisation.

Jean-Christophe Coffin focuses on the discursive side of this co-operation. In his chapter, he does not deal with psychiatric practice, but rather with the debates and the blueprints of a French psychiatric think-tank organised around the journal *L'Information psychiatrique* (*IP*). In post-war France, as elsewhere, mental health care was in need of adaptation to the demands of the times. Many psychiatrists agreed that the asylum system – as it was defined in the late nineteenth century – had become obsolete. Asylums were giving psychiatry a bad reputation because they were overcrowded, the quality of care was low, and they were associated with poor relief rather than health care. They needed to become more permeable and to be integrated into a larger mental health network. Therefore, the IP-group propagated a radical break with pre-war psychiatry, conceptually as well as institutionally. Its members were keen on extending care beyond the walls of the institution, establishing an integrated mental health system, centralising state authority, and enlarging the competence of psychiatrists. However, the hospital maintained its predominant role within the mental health network. On the other hand, psychiatrists were quite successful in furthering their professional interests. All good intentions of the IP-group notwithstanding, the system had become very costly. In the early 1980s, 'the increasing difficulty to curtail health expenses [...] made it less and less legitimate to maintain the welfare state'. Although French community care did fairly well, all governments were forced to respond to the turning of the economic tide in the 1980s.

The remaining essays in this volume are either complementary to the reviews discussed above or offer important counterpoints to them. They concern themselves with therapeutic skepticism in psychiatry, critical or anti-psychiatry, de-institutionalisation and – last but not least – patients. One could be tempted to qualify their *microstorie* as a form of debunking. Because they challenge the history of ideas and institutions, these samples of micro-research are an important correction of the 'Big Picture' in the history of psychiatry. Methodologically, they offer important arguments against finalism.

In her chapter on standards for psychiatric nursing, Cecile aan de Stegge focuses on developments in views on restraint and isolation in asylums, using nine different nursing handbooks written by ten asylum doctors as her source. At first sight, the decision to use handbooks as a source would seem to be an obvious one: they were written with the explicit goal to educate students to become skilled nurses, who were the pillars of psychiatric care. When we know what they were taught, we know what they thought and did during their professional lives. Still: the source is not unproblematic, because it is prescriptive rather than descriptive; it is characteristically Janus-faced, for it is supposed to be both reflecting and creating standards for nursing practice. Therefore, it is too easy to take the handbooks at face value and presume that the twentieth century witnessed a trend from restraint to non-restraint to active therapy and finally to responsibility, reflection and self-realization. However, it is interesting to see what happens when we turn the 'weakness' of this source into a strength, by focusing on the agenda of its authors, who were nearly all psychiatrists. When looking at the handbooks more closely, it becomes clear that they not only had a humanitarian and a didactic purpose, but a professional agenda as well. Their authors show great concern about the negative public image of asylums and the psychiatric discipline in general. B. van Delden, for example, was quite explicit about this. Writing in 1897, he considered mechanical restraint as one of the most important hindrances to the public's acceptance of the asylum as a 'psychiatric hospital'. Emphasizing the (therapeutic) use of restraint and isolation would not have contributed to the image of psychiatry as a humanitarian, academic discipline. On top of that, handbooks had a hierarchical effect within the psychiatric domain. As a genre, a symbol, they were the expression of the teacher/student relationship between psychiatrists and nurses as academic men and non-academic women. In short: handbooks were instrumental in creating social acceptance for the asylum, as well as in reinforcing hierarchical structures within the asylum.

The chapter on Sweden by Gunnel Svedberg is very much in line with this. As elsewhere, psychiatry in Sweden was exposed to criticism and public distrust by the beginning of the twentieth century. The discipline felt a strong need to professionalise, and an important way to achieve this goal was through the professionalisation of nursing, which would have important repercussions for the public image of the asylum and psychiatry as a whole. Svedberg points out that the people involved – psychiatrists, male attendants and female nurses – were staging an interesting class and gender conflict. Considering that the stakes were high – public acceptance of the psychiatric hospital – it is not surprising that the training of mental health care personnel was by no means a technical didactic matter, but rather a power struggle. In their fight for priority, nurses had the best cards. In order to be accepted by the male academic establishment, women with the ambition to become a nurse had to steer a strategic middle course between the labour movement and the women's rights movement. As many attendants were members of local trade unions, they were associated with social unrest and strikes. Realizing that a course of confrontation would be counter-productive, the Swedish nursing association had liberal, middle-class leanings. For medical directors and asylum boards, the choice was clear: male, potentially rebellious attendants lost out, while female, co-operative, bourgeois nurses won. For the boards and directors, it was the best way to ensure a good public image for the asylum.

Toine Pieters and Stephen Snelders do not deal with the asylum or a profession, but with the 'hidden history' of drugs. They establish that the historiography of psychiatry has paid relatively little attention to psychotropic drugs. They think this is a major flaw, because "there can be no history of psychiatry without a history of psychopharmacology". By tracing the cultural identities and careers of two drugs – hyoscine and chlorpromazine – they undermine two notions derived from the history of ideas. First, that knowledge production is unproblematic and autonomous, and second, that there is progress in therapeutic practice. They argue that there was no such thing as a 'therapeutic revolution' in psychiatry in the 1950s. Quite the contrary: when compared to the end of the nineteenth century, psychiatric practice had very much remained the same. In this context, they point to the cyclical career pattern of psychiatric therapy, biomedical as well as psycho-social. The key concept of their essay is the 'Seige cycle', named after the German psychiatrist Max Seige. In 1912, he published an article in which he indicated the great constant in the history of psychiatric therapy: the cycle of promise and therapeutic optimism via scepticism and growing criticism to disillusionment and even fatalism. When a drug had entered the last phase, the pharmaceutical industry tried to bring new hope by either introducing a new generation of drugs or by offering new rationalizations for drugs that were already in use. After that, the cycle repeated itself – *ad infinitum*. The cycle was kept going by the hope for a 'magic bullet'.

That the magic bullet need not be a drug but can be any therapy is shown by Gemma Blok. After a decade or so, the psychotropic drugs that had been introduced in the 1950s entered the third phase of the Seige cycle: doubts and criticism grew, because it was 'killing the mind' and because of other unwelcome side-effects. The interesting thing is that this was no external criticism of psychiatry but rather self-criticism of certain psychiatrists who resented the 'medical model' and presented the 'social model' as the new magic bullet. Blok is turning the evaluation of anti-psychiatry upside down by arguing that it was not a product of the counter-culture of the 1960s and 1970s, but instead a plea for the psychologisation of culture with a strong secular moral agenda (which corroborates the claim made by Eghigian and Oosterhuis that psychiatrists are functional in accompanying profound social changes; citizenship has to be readjusted continually to the needs of the times). Psychiatry was not to be abolished, but rather reformed and extended. The goal was physical and mental well-being in a 'post-materialist' culture; the road leading to it nothing less than the moral re-education of the citizen. Because of the enormous possibilities for expansion this offered, it was considered strategic if psychiatry would dispose of anything that reminded people of its biomedical past. Therefore, Dutch psychiatrists decided in 1974 to separate from the neurologists, with whom they had been united in a professional association for many decades. With some exaggeration, one could argue that anti-psychiatry considered all society to be a lunatic asylum, which of course implied an enormous expansion of the working domain for the psy-sector. In retrospect, this movement can be considered as the biggest effort to 'medicalise' (or maybe rather 'psychiatrise') society in the history of psychiatry. If the asylum reform at the beginning of the twentieth century was an attempt to create legitimacy for psychiatry, anti-psychiatry can be seen as outright professional imperialism. However, it would seem that the most important sources of inspiration for anti-psychiatry were instrumental in taking it to the third phase of the Seige cycle. On the one hand, there was the notion of autonomy and personal responsibility, derived from Sartrian existentialism. On the other, there was the Freudian notion that psychological symptoms are functional, considering turning neurotic or psychotic as a defense mechanism or a valve mechanism. Combined, they led to the endless expansion of the domain, to exponentially rising costs, and ultimately to the fall of the social model as it had been conceived by anti-psychiatry.

When the asylum – once regarded as the symbol of an enlightened nation – entered the third phase of the Seige cycle (partly influenced by anti-psychiatry), the time had come to introduce a new remedy. Gerald Grob deals with the paradoxical consequences of de-institutionalisation in the USA. By the way he contextualises his story, Grob succeeds in showing that the experiment was more about a rearrangement of political relations between federal, state and local levels of government than about new views on mental health. American de-institutionalisation was not about the quality of care, but rather about the balance of power between the state governments and Washington, and about the distribution of financial means. Grob makes it clear that from the beginning there was an ambivalence in the system that necessarily caused the experiment of de-institutionalisation to fail. Community care was conceptualised, regulated and financed at the federal level but was expected to take shape at the local level. Thus, while the *National* Institute of Mental Health wanted to replace psychiatric hospitals with community-based care, at the level of the *Community* Mental Health Centers, the lack of psychiatrists was painfully felt. Federal officials and policy-makers who thought they knew it all considered state governments to be the biggest obstacles on the road to realizing their goals. The final result: embittered state officials, frustrated psychiatrists working in the CMHCS, and the total neglect of de-institutionalised chronic patients, who more often than not criminalised and ended up in jail or homeless in the streets. It proves to be an illusion to think that local integrated therapeutic centres can be realised from the capital of the country. Grob evaluates the experiment in terms of a victory of ideology over reality. In the process, the people who were most vulnerable were victimised. De-institutionalisation did not lead to integrated care but to fragmentation and disorganisation. Because the mental health system became anonymous, nobody really felt responsible for anything anymore. Those who were expected to profit most from the experiment became its biggest victims. As such, Grob's chapter reads like an indictment against (American) de-institutionalisation.

Most of the chapters included in this volume demarcate their research object by focusing on mental health activities involving psychiatrists. Even radical movements like anti-psychiatry and de-institutionalisation were led by psychiatrists, so that it need not surprise us that the stories about them focus on psychiatrists and asylums. Unintentionally, they confirm the traditional image that psychiatry and the asylum were one and the same thing. To be sure, psychiatrists and asylums *were* an important part of the mental health care system. However, by taking a 'psychiatrist-centred' perspective, there is the danger of hiding much relevant activity from view. In this context, we can think of social workers and psychologists working in community centres, factories and schools as well as ministers, pastoral workers and other 'psy-experts'. A similar 'bias' may be avoided by adopting a bottom-up perspective instead of 'confining' oneself in the profession or the institution. In other words: by taking the conceptualisation of mental suffering and the needs of (the family of) the insane as the point of departure. The chapters by Vijselaar, Suzuki and Guarnieri do exactly this. Their bottom-up research opens up new horizons, suggesting new directions for research. Their most important conclusion would seem to be that the mental health system is actually a 'network' of which asylums were only a part – although an important one. Much more research like this is needed to obtain a comprehensive view of the social response to mental illness.

Joost Vijselaar's research of the patterns of admission, stay and discharge in three Dutch psychiatric institutions during the first half of the twentieth century is an important contribution to the renewal of the historiography of psychiatry and mental health care, if only because of the type of sources he is using. His analysis of psychiatric patient records has proven very worthwhile, in that it renders possible a new image of the 'system' of mental health care. His conclusions are twofold: they concern the position of asylums in the broader social and cultural context and the therapeutic regime in asylums (or maybe rather the lack of it). Vijselaar argues that the traditional image of the asylum as a closed, static institution used to put away people showing deviant behaviour is in need of serious revision. A social-historical analysis of individualised source material – rather than aggregated ones – leads him to conclude that the asylum was a much more open and dynamic institution than has always been presumed. It was hardly a unique instrument of repression, but rather a link in a chain of care, in which the family played the most prominent role. Other alternatives for care included admission to a guesthouse or a workhouse, to a sanatorium, or to a somatic general hospital. Very often, the initiative lay with the relatives of the person showing aberrant behaviour, not with the psychiatric expert. Matters of admission and discharge were decided in an interactive process of consultation and negotiation. Also, admission was hardly ever for life. From his discharge data, Vijselaar concludes that approximately one-third left the asylum 'cured' or at least 'improved'. In short: families had a high tolerance for extreme behaviour, and the walls of the asylum were much more permeable than has been suggested. Secondly, Vijselaar deconstructs traditional views concerning the relationship between scientific ideas and everyday practice, giving a rather sobering image of continuity in care practice despite all rhetoric. Paradigmatic and comprehensive change was, to a high degree, limited to congress and lecture halls; they seldom reached the asylum. Academic psychiatry and daily care in the 'periphery' were two separate circuits. Vijselaar concludes that 'Therapeutic or medical interventions [...] did not stamp life on the wards. Therapy, if it was used at all, was marginal and incidental [...] (The asylum) was characterised by a culture of care, not of cure [...] At the level of everyday life and routine, changes were slow, almost imperceptible, and continuities strong'. Taken together, research findings like those of Vijselaar – that the asylum was part of a much broader social network and that there were major differences between scientific rhetoric and daily life on the wards – should have profound implications for the history of psychiatry.

Like Vijselaar, Akihito Suzuki is convinced of the need to examine the role of the family, both as a care unit complementary to the asylum and as an important actor in psychiatric institutionalisation in the early twentieth century. As in Europe, the family and the asylum were complementary parts of the Japanese system of care. Yet there was an important difference, compared with Europe (Germany), as Suzuki shows by differentiating between male and female admissions, and by having a keen eye for differences in Japanese perceptions of the public and the private domain. Focusing on one particular kind of diagnosis – schizophrenia – Suzuki establishes that there was a striking male excess in Japanese asylums, whereas in Europe, no real differences between the sexes were to be seen. At the time, the differences were in fact noted by Japanese psychiatrists, but they did not try to account for them. To Suzuki, they are intriguing enough to invite him to speculate on what caused them. Although he admits that his hypothesis is sustained only by circumstantial evidence, it sounds interesting enough to explore further. Presuming that the prevalence of mental disorder in Japan and Europe was the same, Suzuki argues that the differences must have been caused by variations in hospitalisation policies, suggesting a hidden pattern of home care for women and asylum care for men. It was caused by a different perception of the danger that men and women posed to public order. Since men – considered to be more aggressive – dominated the public domain, it was they who most qualified for admission to an asylum. Women – associated with the private domain – were at most a danger to themselves; because they were deemed less aggressive, they could be looked after by their relatives. In short: the Japanese gender asymmetry in the meaning of symptoms caused families to negotiate differently when admission to an asylum was at stake. Because the Japanese man was more aggressive than his European counterpart – or because he had a stronger public presence – Japanese asylums were forced to focus more on custody than on care (as European institutions could afford to do). Thus, the most interesting conclusion of Suzuki's chapter would seem to be that the cultural context (i.e. perceptions concerning the role of men and women in both the public and private domain) is an important determining factor of the identity of the asylum in the interest of public order.

Like Vijselaar and Suzuki, Patrizia Guarnieri has the ambition of 'doing psychiatric history from below' in an attempt to remove the traditional historiographic bias. Like them, she argues that historians have always been too selective, only looking for their research object in the psychiatric hospital. Guarnieri makes it clear that care for mentally ill people did not just include asylums, but families as well; not just psychiatrists, but lay-people; not just men, but women. By looking outside the asylum, she discovers forms of care that have hitherto been neglected. Like Vijselaar, she claims that the asylum was no dumping ground for families who wanted to get rid of their disturbed relatives. As in the Netherlands, Italian inmates could – and in fact did – leave the asylum. Unlike the Dutch case, however, in Tuscany this was not because the person involved was 'cured'. As Guarnieri points out, discharge was the result of professional politics of psychiatrists and budgetary policies on behalf of the Province. Like elsewhere, the asylum of Florence was overcrowded, and like elsewhere, this gave psychiatry a bad image. It was decided that the problem of overcrowding should be addressed by 'creaming off' inmates to the surrounding countryside, where non-related farmers took pity on them. Given the fact that asylum care was three times as expensive as family care, the transfer of inmates represented a considerable budgetary advantage to the Province. Thus, (paid) home care in Italy was not complementary, but rather a way to cut the costs of the asylum. However, the policy had unintended effects when families who took care of their own mentally ill also applied for a provincial subsidy. Therefore, Guarnieri argues that in order to do justice to the 'system', the history of psychiatry needs to be a combination of social history and family history.

Towards a 'Braudelian Model'?

Reviewing the many diverse sources, perspectives and stories, we have to wonder how a synthetic overview of twentieth-century psychiatry and mental health care could be organised. We might consider – as has often been done – a linear perspective, using concepts like humanization and progress. It would benefit the composition and readability of the narrative if we could start with an indefinite and uncertain group of psychiatrists around 1900, to end with the 'closure' of a self-confident, highly regarded profession a century later. Gijswijt-Hofstra signals a trend from forced confinement in closed asylums to voluntary or informed admission to open mental institutions. Can we call this progress? Certainly not without qualification, for in her essay, she also signals an awkward paradox taking place in our own times. On the one hand, the therapeutic function of the mental institution has been strengthened, whereas on the other, we have to establish that the number of patients who are 'cured' has not grown proportionally. She informs us that medical aspirations for treating and curing the insane have been frustrated repeatedly, adding that it is no simple matter to assess the quality of institutional or other types of care of the mentally ill as it developed in the course of the twentieth century. At the same time, there is a sense of loss of public morals at the end of that century. The recent emphasis on personal freedom and self-determination has had the tragic, unintended effect that growing numbers of chronic patients no longer receive the care they need, while the affluent, narcissistic elite continues to work on its 'self-realization'. These findings are more or less in accordance with the neglect of chronic Dutch patients signaled by Oosterhuis and the tragic fate of de-institutionalised American patients described by Grob. And finally, we have to establish that movements that would seem to have had the noblest intentions – like the humanisation and socialisation of care and the de-institutionalisation of hospital residents – had painful unintended effects like increased bureaucracy, increased costs and the criminalisation of the de-institutionalised.

Over the course of the twentieth century, psychiatry has expanded enormously. While around 1900 there was only limited institutional care, a century later, psychiatry is involved with all domains of life, from the cradle to the grave. In 2005, psy-expertise is omnipresent: it is not only to be found in psychiatric clinics, but also in general hospitals, in universities, in many diverse institutions of ambulatory care, and even in schools, factories and courts of law. There is a universal inclination to conceptualise problems of life and matters of conduct in medical and psychiatric terms. Everybody has become a patient, if not *de facto*, then at least potentially. This may be truly called a great success for the psychiatric lobby, which made its first uncertain moves to recognition and professionalisation only a century ago. But what is the wider meaning of this enormous expansion? A similar question should be asked with regard to the exponential cost increase. In addition to the professional success of psychiatrists, managerial considerations and commercial motives gained importance in mental health care. The twentieth century witnessed a trend from the state to the entrepreneur as the prime mover of mental health care. One may deplore the recent commercialisation of care, but it would seem to be the logical consequence of the fact that mental health care is a supply-driven domain. More often than not, the system is treating patients that it first helped to create by defining and classifying mental illness. Thus, psychiatric care not only has therapeutic effects, but pathogenic ones as well. Over the course of the century, the number of 'patients' increased not despite but rather because of the system. In particular, the growth of the welfare state led to increasing possibilities for care. This in turn caused families to define their disturbed relatives as 'untenable' or 'unmanageable', so that admission to an asylum or other treatment 'could no longer be avoided'.

Because psychiatric standards tend to be subjective and very much a product of their time, we do not have any criteria in hand to measure linear development. It remains to be seen whether this represents a loss to the history of psychiatry. It is true that value judgements are part of history writing, and this especially applies to the history of psychiatry. But exactly because this is the case, a certain degree of irony and distance should be welcomed. They prevent the historian from taking the perspective and rhetorics of the historical actors he is studying at face value. A certain degree of aloofness would seem to be a precondition to understand the unintended effects of the thoughts and actions of historical actors. To put it in an exaggerated way: the historian does not want to celebrate (like psychiatrists) or to criticize (like social scientists); he wants to analyse.

From Exploration to Synthesis

Precisely because historians are not involved in mental health care – and hence do not feel any professional loyalty towards psychiatric workers or personal loyalty towards psychiatric patients – they can afford the luxury of taking a distanced stance. And because of this distance, they may be thought capable of analysing mental health systems of the past in such a way that it leads to an understanding of their complex dynamics. It may even contribute to the political and social reflection of the system in the present, inspiring policy-makers to certain actions. A linear perspective does not satisfy the historian, because it does not do justice to the paradoxes and frictions that are part and parcel of the system. Every system has its absurdities and frictions, and a linear perspective would hide these from view.

The research object of the 'new' history of psychiatry is not the discipline or the profession of psychiatry, but rather the market for mental health care. This market is conceived of as a more or less coherent whole, where ideas about health and illness (c.q. normality and abnormality) are considered to be the result of an interactive process of giving meaning to the challenges of life. The 'new' historians no longer think of psychiatry as a discipline – scientific, and thus superior – that is above all other parties involved, but rather as one way among many to respond to different behaviour. Whoever wants to study psychiatry in its social and cultural context needs to be aware of the fact that culture, state and society cannot be understood teleologically and as isolated phenomena, but only functionally and in their mutual relationship. Therefore, I think a synthetic overview would profit most from a systematic perspective. I would like to argue that a functional system approach is able to shed more light on developments in psychiatry and mental health care than an isolated linear perspective, because it does not have an exclusive focus. Rather, it addresses the broader question of how society at large deals with deviant behaviour, including cultural notions about the desirability and organisation of care, financial considerations about its feasibility, and available scientific instruments for intervention.

If the market for mental health is considered as a coherent system, how should we conceptualise its constituent parts? To answer this question, I would like to suggest taking a closer look at the classic written by the French historian Fernand Braudel many years ago, *La méditerranée et le monde méditerranéen à l'époque de Philippe II*. For his magnum opus, Braudel had collected much material of varying character. When he was facing the compositional problem of how to order this enormous pile of disparate material, he opted for an original solution. Because he felt the need to do justice to the spatial as well as the temporal, and because he wanted to combine a diachronic with a synchronic approach, he developed a tripartite architecture for his book, organising it along the lines of geographical, social and individual time. He devoted the first part of his book to man in his natural environment. In it, he supplied the almost unchanging background of his *dramatis personae* by writing about the geography of the Mediterranean. To Braudel, this was the level of *l'histoire quasi-immobile*, and of the *longue durée*; it was the level where the climate and the landscape defined the margins for human action in an almost inescapable way. In the second volume, he writes about the social-economic dimensions of the Mediterranean. Contrary to the first level, change did take place here, be it in a gradual, cyclical way. This was the level of the organisation of cultural habits and social institutions, that only gradually changed. His third volume was devoted to the relatively ephemereal events of *l'histoire événementielle*. It dealt with politics, diplomacy and warfare.

It would be worth the effort to transpose this tripartite analytical division of structure, cycles and events to the history of psychiatry and mental health care, in an attempt to do justice to scientific theory and therapeutic practice; to the question of care as a public or a private matter; to prevention, care and cure; to collective and individual arrangements; to the biological and the psycho-social discourse. Many authors in this volume argue – but perhaps Eghigian, Oosterhuis and Blok most explicitly – that psychiatry has always been instrumental in instilling contemporary ideals and values of citizenship, ranging from moderation and self-control in the common interest (in the early phases of modern nation-building) to autonomy and personal responsibility in the interest of the individual (when the welfare state was firmly established). When looked at in this way, it is possible to evaluate the Seige cycle positively. A drug has not become flat and dead during the third phase; rather, the cultural meaning ascribed to it no longer meets the needs of a changed world. Another drug or other connotations for the same drug are required to offer renewed therapeutic hope that is considered meaningful in the new era.

How could we translate the above in a way that makes sense for the history of psychiatry? The first 'Braudelian level' – that of the *longue durée* – is the level of the human condition and of the psychiatric patient. It is the level of repetition and regularity; of an almost immobile history; of a care practice that remains equal to itself. It is the level of continuity, of incurable psychiatric misery despite all rhetoric; of therapeutic hope followed by disillusion; it is the level of the Seige cycle. In this context, one is reminded of Blok's remark that 'On many wards, especially those for chronic patients, hospital life continued much as it was before'. It might be worth considering a distinction between chronic and curable insanity (or psychosis and neurosis): whereas the former would relate to congenital, universal mental disturbance, prevalence of the latter is more susceptible to impulses from the cultural environment. Whereas the size of the group of people belonging to the former category is more or less constant, the size of the latter group is a function of fluctuations of the second braudelian level.

The second level is the level of cycles, in other words: of slow change. It is the level of economics and politics; of financing and legislation: it is the level of actually existing care. The size and nature of intramural care is strongly dependent on the availability of public means and the political will to use them for this goal.

From Exploration to Synthesis

Guarnieri shows how the Tuscan government tried to keep the number of admissions paid by the state as minimal as possible. When the Florentine asylum became prohibitive, the government decided on an early form of de-institutionalisation: not for therapeutic but for financial reasons. Similarly, it would seem that the success of anti-psychiatry in the 1970s was as much the result of financial possibilities of the welfare state as it was of the humanitarian arguments behind it. Freeman shows that the availability of funds has always been of the utmost importance for the arrangement of the mental health system. His indignation about Thatcher notwithstanding, he makes it clear that the NHS was built on a misconception, because its architect – Sir William Beveridge – had estimated the costs of the NHS too low. They turned out to be prohibitive and to have 'unfortunate effects'. Contrary to what Beveridge had expected, the costs for the system did not decrease but rather increased.

The second level is also the level of legislation and governmental policies. To governments, the central question always remained the same: is the state responsible for individuals with psychiatric abnormalities? And if so, how far did that responsibility go? Therefore, it is also the level of political priorities; of the political will to spend the available means on psychiatric care. Although the legal and administrative framework may be qualified as prescriptive, it sets out the margins within which care takes shape. As Guarnieri argues, welfare and charity require choices and checks regarding the recipients that usually reveal a lot about benefactors as well as controllers. Oosterhuis and Eghigian both point to the increasing social integration of the psy-sector or, to put it differently, to the mutual penetration of the mental health sector and society. In a world that was secularising at a rapid pace, it was expected that the mental health sector would supply direction and meaning; the help that the sector offered could be afforded because of the new prosperity of the welfare state. A decade later, however, the situation had changed profoundly: the strongly increased demand for help necessitated cuts in the budget. The choice for particular political priorities was an important determinant factor for what would be the dominant care discourse. Classical values of the 1960s and 1970s like autonomy and self-realization were debated in the 1980s and 1990s, when the economic tide had turned. In short: at any given time, the organisation of the mental health system is the result of what is considered attainable and what can be afforded.

Finally, the third level is the level of events and rhetoric (or maybe rather: of the relationship between rhetoric and 'reality'). This includes, for example, rhetoric concerning the right of definition and intervention of psychiatry in mental health matters (e.g. what is normal? What is abnormal? What are the criteria of demarcation of the caring professions? What are criteria for admission to an asylum? How are psychiatric hospitals to be arranged?). But it includes political and administrative rhetorics as well (What is the relationship between state and society? What are the responsibilities of the state? How are the interests of public order and public morality to be served without harming the interests of the individual?). In other words: at this level, the Seige cycles in mental health care are being accompanied rhetorically. When a promising therapy is being introduced, its dynamics are being explained; similarly, when hope has turned into frustration, there are explanations as to why this was an anomaly, and why a new therapy is the answer. We may wonder why the cycle of therapeutic optimism – doubts – fatalism never led to the demise of psychiatry. But since it was the hope of the 'magic bullet' that kept the cycle going, the real merit of a new paradigm was relief from uncertainty. It was always a matter of rationalization with a two-fold goal: on the one hand, sanctioning actions in the present, on the other, offering hope for a better future with the help of science.

A few examples taken from the essay by Gijswijt-Hofstra (corroborated by Oosterhuis) may serve to illustrate the above. In the first three decades of the twentieth century, the enthusiasm for asylum building and current therapeutic ideas resulted in a rise of a 'social-psychiatric awareness' and an overcrowding of institutions. However, when the consequences of the Economic Depression began to be felt, the Dutch government promulgated a stop to building asylums, while the number of admissions to existing ones stagnated. Family care reached an all-time high, linking up to the discourse created by the psycho-hygienic movement. The affluence of the 1960s was accompanied by a discourse on the importance of human values like well-being, self-development, personal responsibility, and the right to psychiatric help for everybody, culminating in the Exceptional Medical Expenses Act (AWBZ). The state started to interfere actively, with the AWBZ as its most important steering instrument. Mental health care was democratised, becoming accessible to everyone. It led to an enormous increase in the intramural as well as the extramural sector in the 1970s. Criticism of hospitalisation and the calls for de-institutionalisation – which could be heard for quite some time – found a response when the economic tide was turning in the 1980s. The rhetoric of de-institutionalisation and socialisation fitted very well with the financial demands of the period, as Grob also points out: the rhetoric that accompanied de-institutionalisation in the USA claimed that the community, not the hospital, was psychiatry's natural habitat. It was said that ultimately, the asylum would become obsolete. In the Netherlands, the crisis of the welfare state led to a temporary moratorium on the building of psychiatric hospitals, while community care – considered to be cheaper than institutional care – was on the increase. The managerial revolution entered psychiatric care, and 'pragmatic' considerations (i.e. deregulation and leaving it to the market) gained importance.

Of course, this is not to suggest that there is a strict causal relationship between the three 'Braudelian levels', but it seems to me that the relationship between the prevalence of 'insanity', the financing and organisation of care, and legitimating rhetoric is too intriguing to ignore. Psychiatric care shows a cyclical

From Exploration to Synthesis

pattern: at certain times, the state considers it imperative to take care of insane, vulnerable, economically unproductive fellow citizens; at other times, it is much less inclined to do so. Psychiatry and the mental health system comply to the rhythm of the three levels. Grob wonders if history is capable of providing us with a narrative that offers policy guidance but has to admit that the answer to this ostensibly simple question is extraordinarily complex. Although there may not be a direct line between the past and the present, it is up to historians to examine critically the organisation of mental health care in the past. Their distanced stance can be an important contribution to understanding the complex dynamics of the past, enlightening contemporary policy-makers in the process.

CHAPTER 18

Progress, Patients, Professionals and the Psyche

Comments on Cultures of Psychiatry and Mental Health Care in the Twentieth Century

Ido de Haan and James Kennedy

Progress

There is no set standard for evaluating historical developments in psychiatric care, Marijke Gijswijt-Hofstra seems to conclude in her chapter in this volume. Not only is it difficult to find any consensus on the relative weight of criteria by which we should judge 'progress' (the presence of strong professional expertise, caring communities of solidarity, robust patients' rights, etc.), as she notes, 'it makes a significant difference whether the quality of care is judged by past or present standards'. At the same time, it is acknowledged that the history of psychiatry has been full of reformers and reform movements which have rejected the deficiencies of the past: 'Time and again, this has resulted in pointing out shortcomings that were formerly not recognised as such.'

Gijswijt-Hofstra's carefully worded assessment about the medical, social and moral relationship of psychiatry to its own past – including the question, implicit or explicit, of the place that progress figures in any assessment of that past – is indicative of a tension within the history of psychiatry, and within this volume as well. To what extent can one – should one – speak of an increasingly 'humane' psychiatric regime, at least in some parts of the world, over time?

On the one hand, there are few, if any, authors in this volume who have clearly answered this question in the affirmative. Many historians avoid making moral judgements of this kind, certainly in respect to something as triumphalist as 'progress', an idea that has generated more than its fair share of sceptics in recent decades. Among historians of psychiatry, this suspicion has been felt acutely, given the strong relationship between psychiatry and a frequently overblown confidence in scientific advance, in the ability of humanity to liberate itself, and in Enlightenment notions of progress. This great confidence in the future on the part of psychiatrists – and the felicitous effects of leaving the benighted past behind – figures prominently in several of the articles presented, not least in the rise and fall of psychiatric institutions as emblems of social progress. Developments *within* those institutions, too, were often tied to a strong sense of progress. Cecile aan de Stegge's account of early twentieth-century Dutch textbooks designed for training nurses at psychiatric hospitals shows how these texts emphasized the confinement and cruelty of the past as sharply anti-thetical to the evolving contemporary norm of 'non-restraint.' This view of the past was partially shaped by the influential Jacob van Deventer, who in 1907 interpreted the current policy of non-restraint as 'ratified' by history, which showed how chains and handcuffs had been replaced with vests and leather belts, then by the isolation cell, and now increasingly by a 'single room'. This persistent belief in the emancipatory benefits of new forms of psychiatric care figures prominently elsewhere in this volume. Nor were the high hopes for breakthroughs confined to a more remote past, as evidenced in the post-1945 hopes for a radically different organisation and approach in psychiatry (as exten-sively elucidated by Jean-Christophe Coffin), in the move toward anti-psychiatry in the 1960s (as sketched out by Gemma Blok and others). De-institutionalisa-tion, too, was hardly devoid of its therapeutic, progressivist promise, at least for a while. These articles underscore once again how important progress in psych-iatry was related to hopes of social and political progress, and how pharmacology and genetic and neurological research are held in almost as high esteem today as they were at the end of the nineteenth century.

But these hopes, all too often, brought too little of what they promised, or worse, generated regimes that brought, on balance, anything but better care to patients. Influential historians like Porter and Grob have, in varying ways, made us wary of the notion of progress in psychiatric and psychological care. And whether or not we share a radical Foucauldian suspicion of psychiatry and its purposes, it is perhaps more plausible for us to see irony or tragedy in the devel-opments within psychiatry. Instead of sketching an upward line, historians tend to show unintended consequences, poor co-ordination and, despite good inten-tions or at least pious talk, often regressive trends.

This tendency, too, is evident in the present volume, as evidenced by Gerald Grob's article on the move toward de-institutionalisation in the USA from the 1960s onwards. 'Whatever its meaning,' he writes, 'there is little doubt that out-comes have had relatively little to do with original intentions and expectations. Although not necessarily a complete failure, de-institutionalisation can hardly be characterised as a policy triumph.' Similarly, Patrizia Guarnieri's poignant account of state intervention in the Italian mental health sector from the 1860s to the 1930s, which was launched and maintained in part (and only in part) by progressive, humanitarian sentiment, suggests how financial and political fac-tors undermined whatever improvements there were for the mentally ill and their families. But the partial or wholesale failure of psy-policy in various coun-tries over time is, of course, not the only reason to avoid any reference to pro-gress. Another obvious reason is that the changes described in the chapters here are complex and refracted, seldom heading in a single direction. Moreover, there remains a lot we do not know, vital information missing from the statistical trends. For example, in his engrossing article Akihito Suzuki points out how much information we lack about the (disproportionately female) mentally ill who remained at home in pre-World War II Japan.

Furthermore, a number of contributions de-emphasize the significance and speed of change, showing how much stayed the same, and how contested and problematic change could be. The two articles on West German psychiatry emphasize these two points. Volker Roelcke challenges the facile periodisation within German psychiatry that interprets the years after 1945 as the time of 'normalisation'. This wrongly ignores, he writes, the lines of continuity, in both staffing and ideas, with either the Nazi or pre-1933 periods. Franz-Werner Kersting, though confirming the 'basically positive long-term trends' in psychiatric reform in post-war West Germany, also stresses the difficulties in this reform which by the 1960s included a marked period of radicalisation and politicisation. Reform, he concludes, came at a high price. But one need not look to institutions alone to see how lines of continuity with the past remained strong. Toine Pieters and Stephen Snelders show in their chapter on the Dutch situation that ostensibly new drugs of the 'psychopharmacological revolution' often had long histories – and not just within the confines of professional psychiatry, but within broader nineteenth-century developments.

All of this, then, is reason enough to doubt that psychiatric practice and insight within democratic societies necessarily improve over time. Furthermore, we ought to restrain ourselves, Greg Eghigian suggests, from readily assuming that psychiatry and psychology are only compatible 'with the modern liberal project of promoting more autonomous, intelligent, happy and enterprising citizens.' East Germany, too, developed a psychiatric regime that was partially driven by state security concerns and partially imitated models from west of the Iron Curtain, resulting in a hybrid (and contradictory) model of psychiatric care for 'the socialist citizen'. This chapter re-emphasizes an insight from recent historiography: that the relationship between 'good' government and 'good' science (or psychiatry) is not always predictable.

Despite these complexities, the history of psychiatry continues to raise, perhaps ineluctably, questions about progress over time. In asserting this, one should hasten to add that a sense of progress and regress in psychiatric care need not be based on an Enlightenment teleology at all. Concerns about improvement or the deterioration of mental health care, as sometimes expressed at the conference in which these papers were initially presented, are not by definition tied to an assumption that human rationality and compassion have increased in the last two centuries and will continue to do so. But it is hard to avoid a moral commitment to the notion that psychiatric care should improve over time, because the quality and accessibility of care and therapies offered by psy-communities remain essential benchmarks for the way that many people evaluate the moral

Progress, Patients, Professionals and the Psyche

condition of society as a whole. Evaluating the progress or decline in psychiatric regimes continues to serve as an important component in measuring the 'humane' character and, by implication, the democratic and egalitarian commitments of a given society. It is not a coincidence that Hugh Freeman – the author with perhaps the longest record of actual experience within the psychiatric sector – is most explicit in his article about progress and its impediments as he describes the British historical context, openly lamenting the return to the 'Trade in Lunacy'. In doing so, current British practice is *back* to the way it was two centuries ago, before the reforms of the Georgian Dissenters. Those who, like Freeman, are concerned with the weal and woes of psychiatric care will find it hard not to think in terms of some kind of progress, perhaps particularly if they possess a historical long-term view of the sector.

There is, moreover, another feature of this volume that generates reflection about progress, and that is its comparative approach. Only one article is systematically comparative: Harry Oosterhuis's balanced article on extramural psychiatry and mental health care in six countries, which shows both important historical similarities and persistent differences between France, Germany, Italy, the Netherlands, the UK and the USA. Oosterhuis scrupulously avoids making judgements about improved or worsened care in each of the countries; that is not the purpose of his contribution. Yet his article raises implicit questions about the desirability of far-reaching de-institutionalisation in Italy, the UK and the USA, in contrast to the moderate pace of a similar development in France, Germany and the Netherlands. Such explicit evaluations are largely left out of the chapters in this volume – though it should be added that such evaluations constituted a part of some of the initial papers of the Amsterdam conference from which these articles are drawn.

But one – admittedly very imperfect – indication of the relative progress achieved in various countries may be found in the ways various authors of this volume have framed their stories. The Anglo-American accounts have focused on policy shortcomings stemming from (among other factors) a lack of public funds and poor co-ordination. Specifically, Grob's work illustrates how mental illness in the USA gets defined to the advantage of the middle class and to the disadvantage of the chronically ill and the perennially poor. As for Italy, Guarnieri's account of the increasing accent on the patient's danger to others is another example of how mental illness is constructed on grounds far removed from medical and therapeutic motivations. Furthermore, the three narratives on Germany focus on the character of psychiatry as it stood, in various ways, under the shadow of totalitarian governments past and present. Very different in frame and tone, however, are the Swedish and most (not all) of the Dutch accounts, which tend to focus on incremental change over time, with relatively little emphasis on systemic crises or deficiencies. Given the historical contours of Dutch psychiatry, perhaps the authors from that country can be forgiven this rather benevolent approach: no authoritarian state making unsavoury use of psychiatric power, no eugenics movement, no insurmountable barriers to health care access, the presence of mostly benign sub-cultural institutions with strong ties to their grassroots, and a consensus culture sensitive to sensible reform. Perhaps a leading Dutch social scientist, Paul Schnabel, *was* right when he said (some twenty years ago now) the country has – or should we say: had – the best mental health care system in the world.[1]

All in all, these contributions can help stimulate a wider and vitally important set of questions about how 'progress' – however defined – might be measured. Is a quantitative increase (more patients, doctors, nurses, therapists) an indication of a better or worse mental health system? Is the degree of professionalisation an important measure? Gender balance? And what kinds of professional traits are most essential for a good mental health system – self-awareness, expertise, technological know-how, or other forms of expertise? In a word, what kinds of professional power constitute progress? Or have all of these questions lost sight of what *patients* would define as improved care? And which patients – the most seriously ill or the most numerous? Are self-reflection, self-development, self-searching and individual independence characteristics that characterise a kind of moral or social progress? Working through these questions more systematically would help us in our assessment of the diversity of international developments presented in this volume.

Patients

Let us start with the quantitative issues. Practically all of these papers identify a similar two-track development. On the one hand, they sketch a development between the end of the nineteenth century and the middle of the twentieth of an initial increase of patients confined for a long term in large-scale and often overcrowded asylums. This was followed by a fall in the numbers of patients confined for a long time in the second half of the twentieth century. In opposition to the Great Confinement, the historiography of mental health care now seems to be in the grip of the Great De-institutionalisation. On the other hand, mental health care seems to be democratised: more people with more and more varied mental problems are helped by more professionals in a more egalitarian and humanitarian way in more and more diverse mental care institutions that are less separated from the rest of society.

However, at a closer look, these general trends are more complex. To begin with, an increase during most of the twentieth century in the number of people staying for a long time in a closed asylum is not everywhere of the same magnitude and nature. In the case of the Netherlands in the first half of the twentieth century, a substantial proportion of the patients entering an asylum were first admitted to a general hospital, while an even more substantial proportion left at an earlier or later moment, sometimes against the doctor's advice, as Vijselaar has argued. Also in Japan, the asylum was not the only place where mentally disturbed people were put. In the beginning of the century, a majority was managed at home, while the increase of institutionalised people was to a large extent due to the increased number in private hospitals. Only the very poor stayed in public asylums. As Roelcke argues for the German case, the greatest increase in numbers had already taken place between 1870 and 1914, after which an initial shift to outpatient care facilities took place, at least until 1933.

Also, the fall in numbers of people staying for a longer period in closed facilities is not always self-evident. The figures for the USA which Grob has presented at first sight point clearly in the direction of de-institutionalisation: in 1950, 558,000 people were resident in public mental hospitals, declining to 65,000 in 2000, a decrease which is even more spectacular if one takes the population growth into account. Also, the length of stay declined from months and years to days. However, at the same time, Grob argues, 'de-institutionalisation is somewhat of a misnomer', since at least 200,000 if not more of these people were simply transferred to nursing homes. In the Netherlands, 'de-institutionalisation was late and also slow', as Marijke Gijswijt argues. She observes a decline in the number of beds from 27,000 beds in 1950 to 23,000 in 2000, yet then there were still 10,000 long-term patients.

This means that the experience of voluntary but also of forced stay within psychiatric institutions is still very much with us, and even more 'democratically' shared than ever before. For instance, in the Netherlands, the number of admissions increased from 10,000 in 1965 to 52,000 in 2000. While the number of asylums may have declined in the USA, the number of inpatient psychiatric units in general hospitals grew between 1963 and 1977 from 622 to 1056, while the number of admissions rose between 1955 and 1983 from 1.7 million to 7 million.

And a final consideration of these numbers: how many people leave psychiatric institutions, and how do they do so? As Vijselaar demonstrated for the Netherlands in the first half of the century, contrary to the image of life-time confinement, around 36 per cent of the cases he investigated left the asylum cured or improved, many within a year. It might be the case that the number of releases is currently much higher, but if we take into account that the rising number of admissions is probably to a great extent due to the increase in re-admissions, then we still have a steady group of people who spend much of their life within the walls of a mental care facility. Moreover, not all leave the asylum cured, to use an understatement: Vijselaar observed a mortality rate of 40 per cent. Since then, mortality rates have sharply declined in the Netherlands, partly because of a decline in mortality due to tuberculosis, partly because elderly patients were put in separate geriatric wards outside the psychiatric hospital.

However, it is not self-evident which normative conclusion one should draw from mortality rates: does a high value indicate that care is bad, or that only the worst patients stay in these institutions forever, that is, until their death?

Notwithstanding the problems of interpreting these figures, it is clear that there has been a shift in most of the countries discussed in this volume, from often forced confinement in closed facilities to voluntary engagement with a plethora of mental health care institutions. Again, the numbers and, even more importantly, the timing of this shift varied considerably between countries. As Oosterhuis makes clear in his international comparison of outpatient care, outpatient facilities were already being developed in the first decades of the twentieth century in the UK, Germany, France, the USA and the Netherlands, but not in Italy. Moreover, his comparison makes clear there is no simple zero-sum relationship between a decline of institutional confinement and the rise of ambulant facilities. Due to the refusal by central governments of the late 1970s to provide the necessary financial means, de-institutionalisation in the UK, the USA and Italy did not lead to a substantial growth of outpatient facilities. On the other hand, the Netherlands together with France, Germany and Belgium lagged behind, but soon became the vanguard of ambulant mental health care. As becomes clear in the papers of Gijswijt and Oosterhuis, mental health care in the Netherlands became a normal welfare state provision, providing services to around 800,000 clients.

How to explain this development? From the perspective of a Whig history of psychiatry, this development is presented as a natural process of psychiatric practices becoming more democratic and more humane due to the force of the underlying emancipatory ideology and against the forces of reaction that try to block the path of progress in the name of vested interests, be it the ruling class, religion or the pharmaceutical industrial complex. However, even if we assume that there indeed is an ideological force at work here, we still need to explain the different receptiveness for its blessings between countries.

We have already mentioned one factor explaining these differences: the financial means available largely dictate the possibilities of developing alternative mental health care institutions. However, public finance is a matter of political debate and priorities, and needs itself to be explained. In the various chapters, this political context of the development of mental health care is not always systematically addressed, and in the framework of this commentary it is impossible to do so in a satisfying way. However, it is perhaps useful to consider a few issues.

To begin with, the legal structure of mental health care provisions changed in most countries at two moments: around the turn of the century, and again in the first two decades after the Second World War. It appears that most of the laws enacted around 1900 were a codification of an already longer lasting practice, in which the care of mentally disturbed persons was part of the system of poor relief (like most other elements of health care). The kernel of these laws was

Progress, Patients, Professionals and the Psyche

to regulate the forced confinement of people who had not committed any crimes but were considered dangerous to themselves, to others or to public decency. As Guarneri argues, this kind of law was also expected to serve the rights of patients, but generally resulted in a criminalisation of mental illness.

The second wave of legislation might best be considered as a way to integrate the laws on mentally disturbed persons within the emergent systems of social security. In this context, care was no longer primarily a disciplining strategy to deal with people who were considered a nuisance, but first of all a social right. Many of these laws, like the Medicare and Medicaid Acts in the USA or the AWBZ in the Netherlands, regulated first and foremost the financial issues around (mental) health care, while later legislation in the 1980s and 1990s addressed first of all the cost of mental health care or how to keep this in check by way of protocols, evidence-based medicine and limitations on the duration of therapy.

The link with poor relief and social security systems might be an important factor to explain the development of mental health care institutions. To begin with, these shared some of the characteristics of poor relief: to police the poor and to take care of those who were unable to provide for their necessary means of living. People were generally confined because they were considered dangerous to themselves, a social annoyance to others or an affront to public decency, and almost never confined because it facilitated effective treatment. As Vijselaar states 'the asylum, [...] was a place to stay. It was characterised by a culture of care not of cure, regulating disturbed behaviour dominated its daily practice'.

This link might also explain something of the phenomen Grob and others have commented upon as a new and troublesome development since the 1960s. Community mental health care was based on the optimistic expectation that a decentralised and localised set of centres would guarantee effective and humane treatment, yet in the end proved unable to care for the hard cases of people with multiple disorders, often combined with substance abuse and homelessness. Consequently, these groups were again criminalised, while mental health professionals preferred to focus their attention on the relatively easy treatment of the 'yavis'-patients – young, attractive, verbal, intelligent and social. From the perspective of mental health as part of the whole system of social care, this is not at all surprising but is rather a continuation of a much older tendency.

The context of social welfare provision may also explain the different development of mental health care within the different nations in another way. There is a full library written on types and routes in the developments of social security systems, but what is important in this respect is the difference between the division of labour or competition between the state, voluntary associations and the local level or, in the case of the USA, the relationship between the federal level and the states.

For instance in the Dutch case, mental health provision was part of an extended sector of social care in which local authorities and denominational associations were responsible. Since the end of the nineteenth century, private schools, charity and health care associations were independently governed yet financed by the local public authorities, catering for a denominationally divided clientele, without the direct support of the central state. This changed after the 1960s, when most of the denominational institutions became fully subsidised by the state and therefore vulnerable to cuts in the national budget. Only then did the Netherlands come to resemble the USA, where community health care was mandated by the federal government.

Also in another way, the role of the state is crucial, as is clear from the German example: mental health care was easily integrated into the Nazi state and after its defeat seriously de-legitimised – but also then no less dependent on the state, now functioning as benevolent reformer. This might explain, at least in part, the strong politicisation of mental health care in the 1960s.

This leads to a final point about the political context of the development of mental health care, which is the role of war. As Freeman has argued for the UK after 1918 and Grob for the USA after 1945, the experience of treating soldiers with shell shock and war trauma added to the faith in short-term and ambulant mental health care. In another way, as Coffin has argued for the French case, the mood during the occupation and immediately after the liberation inspired mental health care professionals, who had a close relation to circles around De Gaulle and the liberation elite, to pursue reforms of the mental health care system energetically. The same can be said of the impulse the mental health care movement received in the Netherlands, as witnessed by the *Maandblad voor Geestelijke Volksgezondheid*, founded immediately after the liberation. Finally, both the German and the Dutch examples underline the importance of the psychiatry of victims of war and persecution. The work of Baeyer and others in Germany and of psychiatrists like De Wind and Tas in the Netherlands has not only contributed to the public recognition of these victims, but also introduced psychic suffering as a legitimate subject and vocabulary in the public arena.

With this, we are far removed from quantitative evaluation of the history of psychiatry. What these comments so far amount to is the relevance of national political contexts for the development of mental health care: even when we think there was progress, it was not the outcome of the triumphant march of reason and humanity, but of highly contextual and also not so humane social and political developments and experiences. Moreover, what these comments demonstrate is the fact that the impact of psychiatry cannot be measured only by numbers of patients.

Professionals

This brings us to a second issue by which to evaluate the tendencies discussed in this volume: the development of psychiatry and mental health care as a profession: did we get more, better, more humane, more effective professionals, or do their rising numbers indicate we are in ever greater trouble?

One thing is made abundantly clear: we obtained more of them. Grob estimated that their number in the USA rose from 28,000 in 1946 to 600,000 in 1992. In an unpublished paper at the preceding conference, the Dutch political scientist Ido Weijers demonstrated for the Netherlands that the number of doctors rose from 100 in 1900 to 1,900 in 1995 – of which psychiatrists/doctors working in psychiatric hospitals declined from two-thirds to one-third of the total number, while the number of women increased from zero to around one-third of all doctors. This percentage is much higher among other professionals, such as psychiatric nurses, the numbers of which rose even more dramatically, from 1,200 in 1900 to 30,000 a century later. These percentages are equal to those in the USA, and probably higher than those in other nations, although elsewhere, too, the trend appears to be going in the same direction.

This would be a blessing if all these professionals were good, effective and humane, and increasingly getting even better. But are they? This is of course difficult to tell, especially since these are rather subjective issues, based on perception and evaluation. In this respect, there is one thing that immediately strikes the eye: professionals have tried to influence this perception and to enhance their status by varying means.

As Roelcke has demonstrated, German psychiatrists sought to model their professions on the 'hard' science of biology, which put them on the track of eugenics and of denouncing the much vaguer psychoanalysis as a Jewish fraud. Also, the social face of the mental health movement was much weaker in Germany than, for instance, the Netherlands, where prevention of mental degeneration was not pursued by genetic engineering or genocide, but through social work. The legitimation of mental health care professionals by an appeal to science was even weaker in the UK where, according to Freeman, academic psychiatry never really got off the ground.

Next to science, mental health workers could improve their status by organising within professional organisations. About this side of the culture of mental health care we heard only scattered remarks, for instance in the paper of Svedberg on the unionisation of Swedish nurses, but the issue of titles and entitlements, both professionally and financially, seems crucial to understanding the perception of the whole sector.

However, it is clear that the performance of professionals cannot only be measured by how they appear to be but, more importantly, by what they do. Contrary to the technological optimism that characterises many parts of the medical profession, psychiatry does not appear to have become more effective. Around 1900, about a third of the patients could hope for a satisfactory level of recovery, and that number appears not to have risen. Also, the technological advance was modest, as Pieters and Snelders suggest: in the past hundred years doctors did not get more or fundamentally new drugs at their disposal. Nevertheless, therapies changed, in general terms, from hierarchical treatment to egalitarian encounter, or as Aan de Stegge states, 'a generally diminishing tolerance for unnecessary restriction in patients' freedom was translated into greater expectations of nurses' capability to negotiate with patients and to monitor symptoms of oncoming unrest or aggression. [...] Thus: the Dutch attitude towards non-restraint was finally translated into a clearly circumscribed need for reflective and professional nurses.' This shift was accompanied by the rise of an environmental aetiology after 1945, as a result of which the clinic had to change into a model of a non-pathogenic society or, according to some, disappear altogether, to make room for the struggle for an actual non-pathogenic society. The nature of professionals changed accordingly. The psychiatrist was now confronted with many other professionals, like psychologists and social workers. In some cases this led to serious power struggles, which were often fought out under the guise of anti-psychiatry, but as the paper of Gemma Blok demonstrates for the Dutch case, these were often conflicts between different sections of the professionals, not only about their internal hierarchy, but also about the best strategy to defend the profession against outside criticism and, more importantly, budget cuts.

As Svedberg makes clear, these conflicts also had an important gender dimension. Many of the old guard in Sweden consisted of female psychiatric nurses, with a very crucial place in the clinic. As Aan de Stegge demonstrates, nurses were expected to develop an ethos of both natural authority and patience, benevolence as well as self-reflection. Their position was threatened by the political radicalism that entered the clinic in the 1960s, which made nursing suddenly a much more combative and masculine job than before.

This example of gendered status conflict makes us aware of the fact that not all that happens in the clinic is always done in the best interest of the patient. Therefore, we would like to warn again that when there is an actual humanization of the relationship between patients and professionals, this should not be interpreted automatically as the dawning of a more humane ideology. It can also be construed as the unintended consequence of strategies and interactions, based on altogether different perspectives.

Moreover, even the humane encounter between professionals and patients is structured by the parameters of the mental health care system, constraining both. This is made clear by Aan de Stegge, who observes a return of the strict regulation of coercive means, which was part of the legislation around 1900, but which had gradually disappeared since. Seen from this perspective, mental health care has not made progress from restricted care to democratised cure, but developed by a temporary relaxation of the rules constraining professionals, enabling both benevolent and also malicious or even murderous therapeutical experiments, followed by a crisis over the limits of paternalism in the 1960s and a new strictness since the 1980s. Much dynamism, but is it progress?

Psyche

The idea of progress in psychiatry has been inextricably bound up in the idea of modernity, in which a new set of consciously 'modern' insights and practices came to supplant those of the pre-modern world. The rise of a consciously modern 'secular religion', or at least secular morality, is also evident in Blok's account, in which the moral values of 'critical psychiatry' came to fill the void left by a rapidly secularising society, as the Netherlands was, perhaps like no other, in the 1960s. Sweden's psychiatric regime, Svedberg tells us, was secular at its inception because of Sweden's early secularisation, although she notes the nonsectarian religious influence of Florence Nightingale on Swedish nursing in the nineteenth century, and the Lutheran deaconesses' emphasis on duty as historical factors in the development of the profession.

But it is not that the conflict between religion and psychiatry is emphasized in most of the chapters; on the contrary. Coffin makes note of the role of both Catholics and Protestants (as well as communists) in seeking psychiatric reform in post-war France, while Oosterhuis demonstrates that it was religious institutions (first in liberal Protestant circles, after the war in Catholic institutions) and a therapeutic elite that paved the way for the thorough 'psychologisation' of Dutch society, in which psychological concepts occupied an important place in everyday discourse. What is striking is that 'psychologisation' seems to have achieved the greatest success in culturally 'Protestant' countries with the highest church attendance rates in the Western world until the 1960s: Australia, Canada, the Netherlands and the USA. It is at least tempting to view psychologisation as a form of secularisation that ultimately 'transcended' the religious sensibilities that long had guided explorations into the psyche.

But interpreting psychiatry and psychology as the contemporary replacement of religion does not fully underscore the cultural interplay between the two, as is evident in the extensive 'psychologisation' of American religion, which seems as resilient as ever despite or perhaps because of this process. And it is not only that religion has been psychologised; psychiatry has itself been influenced by the spiritual. There is a tendency in some of the historiography to understand psychiatry as a largely rational, scientific, intrinsically secular (or secularising) and implicitly 'modern' enterprise, with all the accoutrements of modernity, such as rationalized organisation and a professionalised cadre. That psychiatric care often had its *origins* in religious sensibilities, at least in Great Britain, is noted by Freeman. But less attention has been paid to how religion and psychiatry continued to inform each other, and it is in this respect that several of the Dutch articles (Gijswijt-Hofstra, Aan de Stegge, Oosterhuis, Vijselaar) are particularly valuable, showing as they do the decades-long interplay between organised religion (often of an orthodox sort) and highly developed psychiatric regimes. This did not mean that religious denominations were successful in shaping psychiatry in accordance with their particular insights – if indeed they tried to do so at all – but that their role in creating and sustaining communities of psychiatric care is an important chapter in the history of psychiatry. The Netherlands, though certainly not the only country to confessionalise its psychiatric system in the twentieth century, is an important and fascinating international test case in the interface between 'soul' and 'mind'.

Organised religion, of course, is not the only cultural force in dialogue with psychiatry. The 1960s, for example, were a time when the dividing line between psychology and psychiatry on the one hand and arts, philosophy, literature and 'spirituality' (as consciously distinct from organised religion) on the other hand became more porous. The rise of anti-psychiatry and the (re)appreciation of humanistic psychology challenged the rationality of established practices. More than that, anti-psychiatry and other counter-cultural challenges (including the importance of drugs like LSD, as Pieters and Snelders inform us) tried to create room in an overly rationalized society for a consciously primitivist, 'gnostic', highly individualised spirituality which radically immanentised the divine. The psychologisation of society not only created a 'secular religion' or a secular morality but new forms of spirituality, which helped shape public understandings of the spiritual, and particularly for the spiritual potentiality of every individual. To speak about psychiatry and psychology chiefly within its clinical and laboratory settings is to make these practices more conventionally scientific and rational than either the ideological roots of psy-practice or its wider cultural impact would suggest. The notion of progress, here defined as secularisation, thus becomes harder to defend, even though the far-reaching individualisation of spirituality has clearly had important 'secularising' effects in the public sphere.

In the end, though, psychiatry as a form of spirituality foundered after 1980 in the face of pharmacology, genetics, biological psychiatry and evidence-based medicine approaches very frequently naturalistic and functionalistic in their assumptions. In this respect, there seems to be very little room in current psychiatric understanding for the 'spiritual' psyche. Nevertheless, Blok and Oosterhuis make the important observation that contemporary psychiatry comes with its own set of moral imperatives, its own understanding of human freedom, and ultimately its own understandings of what constitutes a good society. In particular, increasing self-awareness has been one of the key ways to define progress in the psychologisation of society. That this 'civilising' process, as Norbert Elias has outlined, does not invariably lead to greater human happiness is something that has been noted by Oosterhuis, among others. Especially in a country like the Netherlands, where much is expected of the individual and at the same time few hard and fast rules are articulated, people struggle to make a host of internal judgements that they, as autonomous individuals, are expected to make by themselves. But are 'protoprofessionalised' people (to cite a term from Abram de Swaan) happier, or more prone to sickness? The Dutch, together with the Icelanders, seem to be the happiest people among the nations polled, though such a collective profession of felicity may not tell us very much. Progress as increased self-awareness must remain mired in ambiguity.

Everywhere, there has been a marked trend toward self-reliance as an ideal, from self-help books to self-medication, de-institutionalisation, and even (and not just in the Netherlands) the trend toward assisted suicide, in cases where the patient is judged to be rational enough – and autonomous enough – to make an informed decision about the value of his or her life. Progress as self-reliance, a theme of the neo-liberal 1990s, is perhaps even more clearly evident as a social ideal than progress as self-awareness or self-actualisation had been in the 'spiritual' 1970s. That this ideal of autonomy is often ultimately unattainable seems clear enough, in part because self-reliance remains paradoxically dependent to a large extent on the assistance of psy-professionals, in part because the very concept of autonomy denies the fundamental reality of our social relationships. We die in the arms of others, Peter Filene has written in his book about the right-to-die in America, and we also live in the arms of others. Indeed, the social structure paradoxically required for self-reliance remains often one of the frustrating neglected components of mental health care.

Finally, to what extent can we speak of progress in the last decade, as we have witnessed the rise of an increasingly consumerist mental health care? To what extent can the new therapeutic discourses serve as a reliable guide to the human good? And to which critics should we turn for a helpful angle of critique, with the right measure of critical distance? Has 'psychologisation' – to the extent we can define and measure such a concept – obscured the social and political challenges we face, even, maybe especially, among its critics? Do societies having undergone a lesser degree of 'psychologisation', with less psychobabble, have a clearer view of social and political problems, or does it make little difference? The answers cannot be easy to give. But a sustained discussion on the relationship between human progress and the weal and woes of twentieth-century psychiatry cannot be the wrong place to start.

Note

1.   P. Schnabel, 'Bij ons is alles beter, maar we weten het niet', *Maandblad Geestelijke Volksgezondheid*, 36 (1981), 201-2.

About the Contributors

Gemma Blok (1970) is currently working at the History Department of the University of Amsterdam, where she teaches courses on the history of psychiatry and the history of drugs. She has co-written several books on the history of Dutch psychiatric hospitals. In 2004, her dissertation was published: *Baas in eigen brein. 'Antipsychiatrie' in Nederland, 1965-1985* ('Master of one's own mind. "Anti-psychiatry" in the Netherlands, 1965-1985').

Jean-Christophe Coffin (1961) is assistant professor at the Department of Medical Ethics and Legal Medicine of the University of Paris-René Descartes and he is associate researcher at the Institute for the History of Science A. Koyré (CNRS). He is the author of *La Transmission de la folie, 1850-1914* (2003) and co-editor of the two-volume *Le consentement en santé mentale* (2004) as well as of a number of papers on the history of French psychiatry in the nineteenth and twentieth centuries.

Greg Eghigian (1961) is Associate Professor of Modern European History at Pennsylvania State University in the USA. He is the author of *Making Security Social: Disability, Insurance, and the Birth of the Social Entitlement State in Germany* (2000) and co-editor of *Pain and Prosperity: Reconsidering Twentieth-Century German History* (2003). He is presently writing a book on the science and politics of deviance in Nazi, East and West Germany.

Hugh Freeman trained in medicine and psychology at Oxford and was then employed at the Maudsley Hospital, London. He was a consultant psychiatrist and head of a teaching unit in Manchester, until becoming editor of the *British Journal of Psychiatry*. He has worked extensively overseas as a consultant for the World Health Organisation. He has been the author or editor of numerous books, including *A Century of Psychiatry* (1999). His main historical interest is twentieth-century European psychiatry, and he is Secretary of the Section of Psychiatry of the World Psychiatric Association. He has been awarded the Honorary Fellowship of the Royal College of Psychiatrists, the Medal of Merit of Charles University Prague, and an Honorary Visiting Fellowship at Green College, Oxford.

Marijke Gijswijt-Hofstra (1940) is Professor of Social and Cultural History at the University of Amsterdam. She has published on the granting of asylum in the Dutch Republic, deviance and tolerance (16th-20th centuries), witchcraft and cultures of misfortune (16th-20th centuries), the reception of homoeopathy in the Netherlands (19th-20th centuries), and on women and alternative health care in the Netherlands (20th century). She is currently working on the history of psychiatry and mental health care in the Netherlands in the twentieth century. She has edited, with Roy Porter, *Cultures of Psychiatry and Mental Health Care in Postwar Britain and the Netherlands* (Amsterdam: Rodopi, 1998), and *Cultures of Neurasthenia. From Beard to the First World War* (Amsterdam: Rodopi, 2001).

Gerald N. Grob (1931). Henry E. Sigerist Professor of the History of Medicine, Emeritus, Institute for Health, Health Care Policy, and Aging Research, Rutgers University, New Brunswick, NJ. His general field of research is the history of medicine with a specialization in the history of mental health policy as well as the history of disease in the USA. Publications include *The Mad Among Us: A History of the Care of America's Mentally Ill* (Free Press, 1994) and *The Deadly Truth: A History of Disease in America* (Harvard U. Press, 2002).

Patrizia Guarnieri (1954) is Professor of History, and was Fulbright Scholar at Harvard University, CNR-NATO Fellow at the Wellcome Trust Centre for the History of Medicine in London, Jean Monnet Fellow at the European University Institute. She currently teaches at the Faculty of Psychology in the University of Florence, and she is the editor of *Medicina & Storia*. Among her publications are *A Case of a Child Murder* (Polity Press, 1993), *Bambini e salute in Europa/Children and Health in Europe 1750-2000* (Polistampa, 2004).

Ido de Haan (1963) is Professor of Political History at Utrecht University. He has published, among other topics, on the history of the welfare state, the history of youth health, and the psychiatry of victims of persecution. His main fields of interest are the political history of the Netherlands, the history of citizenship and state formation, and the political and cultural consequences of war and violence. On the last topic he is currently leading a comparative project involving France and the Netherlands around 1600, 1815 and 1945. Publications include: 'The Construction of a National Trauma. The Memory of the Persecution of the Jews in the Netherlands', *Netherlands Journal for Social Science*, 34/2 (1998), 196-217. 'Vigorous, Pure and Vulnerable: Child Health and Citizenship in the Netherlands since the End of the Nineteenth Century', in: Marijke Gijswijt-Hofstra & Hilary Marland (eds), *Cultures of Child Health in Britain and the Netherlands in the Twentieth Century* (Amsterdam: Rodopi, 2003), 25-54. 'Paths of Normalization after the Persecution of the Jews. The Netherlands, France, and West-Germany in the 1950s', in: Richard J. Bessel & Dirk Schumann (eds), *Life after Death. Approaches to a Cultural and Social History of Europe During the 1940s and 1950s* (Cambridge: Cambridge University Press, 2003), 65-92.

Frank Huisman (1956) teaches at the Department of History of the University of Maastricht. He is the author of *Stadsbelang en standsbesef. Gezondheidszorg en medisch beroep in Groningen, 1500-1730* (1992), a local case study of early modern Dutch health care, and co-editor with John Harley Warner of *Locating Medical History. The Stories and their Meanings* (2004), a volume on medical historiography in the nineteenth and twentieth centuries. He has published on the cultural authority of medicine, quackery and historiography. Currently, he is working on a book exploring the transformation of the Dutch health care system between 1880 and 1940.

James Kennedy (1963) is Professor of Contemporary History at the Free University of Amsterdam. He has published books on the Netherlands during the 1960s, on the history of euthanasia in the Netherlands, and on the history of higher education in the USA. His interests lie in, among other things, the intersection of political culture, public policy and religion in contemporary Europe.

Franz-Werner Kersting (1955), Dr. phil. habil., Research Associate at the Westfälisches Institut für Regionalgeschichte (Westphalian Institute for Regional History), Münster, and Extraordinary Professor for Modern and Contemporary History at the University of Siegen. Main areas of research and fields of teaching (chiefly in the 19th and 20th centuries): history of youth; history of psychiatry; Federal Republic of Germany, International Relations. Most recent publication: Editor, in conjunction with Hans-Walter Schmuhl: *Quellen zur Geschichte der Anstaltspsychiatrie in Westfalen* (Sources from the History of Institutional Mental Care in Westphalia), vol. 2: 1914-1955 (Paderborn: Schöningh, 2004).

Harry Oosterhuis (1958) teaches history at the Faculty of Arts and Culture of the University of Maastricht. His current research focuses on the cultural and social history of mental disorders and psychiatry as well as of sexuality and gender. His publications include *Homoseksualiteit in katholiek Nederland: Een sociale geschiedenis 1900-1970* (Amsterdam: Sua, 1992); *Homosexuality and Male Bonding in Pre-Nazi Germany: The Youth Movement, the Gay Movement and Male Bonding Before Hitler's Rise* (New York and London: The Haworth Press and Harrington Park Press, 1992) and *Stepchildren of Nature: Krafft-Ebing, Psychiatry, and the Making of Sexual Identity* (Chicago and London: The University of Chicago Press, 2000). He was co-editor (with Michael Neve) of *Social Psychiatry and Psychotherpay in the Twentieth Century: Anglo-Dutch-German Perspectives*, special issue *Medical History* 48, 4 (October 2004).

Toine Pieters (1960), Senior Lecturer in the History of Medicine, VU Amsterdam Medical Centre, Department of Medical Humanities and Professor of the History of Pharmacy at Groningen University. Fields of research: psychotropic and cardiovascular drugs, cancer, genetics and heredity. Author of *Interferon: The Science and Selling of a Miracle Drug* (Routledge, 2005).

Volker Roelcke (1958), Institute for the History of Medicine, University of Giessen, Germany. His main research interests are nineteenth- and twentieth-century German psychiatry, interrelations between eugenics and medical genetics, history and ethics of human subjects research. His current research is on the history of psychiatric genetics in Germany, the UK and the USA. Publications include: *Krankheit und Kulturkritik: Psychiatrische Gesellschaftsdeutungen im bürgerlichen Zeitalter, 1790-1914* (Frankfurt, 1999); *Psychiatrie im 19. Jahrhundert: Forschungen zur Geschichte von psychiatrischen Institutionen, Debatten und Praktiken im deutschen Sprachraum* (ed. with E. Engstrom; Basel, 2003); *Twentieth Century Ethics of Human Subjects Research: Historical Perspectives on Values, Practices, and Regulations* (ed. with G. Maio; Stuttgart, 2004).

Stephen Snelders (1963), Senior Researcher in the History of Medicine, vu Amsterdam Medical Centre, Department of Medical Humanities. Fields of research: psychotropic drugs, genetics and heredity. Author of *LSD therapy in the Netherlands* (Candide/Wrede Veldt, 2000).

Cecile aan de Stegge (1957) is a psychiatric nurse with a master's degree in Western Philosophy. She is a PhD student at the Department of History of the University of Maastricht. She works at her private address: Zuster Spinhovenlaan 11, 3981 CR Bunnik, the Netherlands.

Akihito Suzuki (1963) is a Professor of History at the School of Economics, Keio University in Tokyo. His book, *Madness at Home: The Psychiatrist, the Patient, and the Family in England 1820-1860*, is forthcoming from University of California Press. He is now preparing a book on a private mental hospital in Tokyo in the early twentieth century.

Gunnel Svedberg (1937). Reg. Nurse, Licenced Psychotherapist, PhD. Senior lecturer at Department of Nursing, Karolinska Institutet, Huddinge, Sweden. Research topic: The history of psychiatric nursing, using narratives as main sources. Main publication: *Omvårdnadstraditioner inom svensk psykiatrisk vård under 1900-talets första hälft* (Nursing traditions in Swedish psychiatric care during the first half of the twentieth century. Summary in English.) (Stockholm: Department of Neuroscience, Karolinska Institutet, 2002).

Joost Vijselaar (1957) is Professor in the History of Psychiatry at Utrecht University and staff-member of Het Dolhuys, museum for the history of psychiatry in Haarlem. He is currently working on a study on the Dutch psychiatric hospital in the twentieth century, based on patient records. Among others he published *De magnetische geest. Het dierlijk magnetisme 1770-1830* ('The magnetic spirit. Animal magnetism 1770-1830') (2001).

Index

by Anne Hilde van Baal

London 121, 125-26, 130, 135, 137, 251
lower classes, see working/lower classes
LSD 381-82, 393-94
Lübbe, Hermann 206
Luminal, see barbiturates
lunatics 118, 295, 299
Lundborg, Herman 360-61

M

Maasoord, Rotterdam mental institution
see also Delta mental hospital 51, 68-9,
388
MacDonald, Michael 278
MacKenzie, Charlotte 277
Malade mental dans la société (The insane
within society), le 235
malaria 284
malaria fever therapy, malaria fever treatment, malarial treatment 45, 120, 145
malnourishment 174, 203
Manchester 120, 128-29
Royal Infirmary 117
Mannheim Circle 164, 211, 260
Marx(ism) 133, 194, 215
Massachusetts 143, 146
Mathijsen, Joost 104
Matsuzawa Hospital 302, 304
Maudsley Hospital (London) 126, 132, 165,
251
Medicaid 20, 148, 151-52, 160, 259, 431
medical model 17, 54, 85, 104-06, 108-10,
266, 413
medical records see also patients' records;
case histories 22
Medicare 20, 151, 259, 431
medication, see specific medicines; drugs;
psychopharmaceuticals
Medico-Psychological Association, Royal
126
Meerenberg asylum see also Provincial
Hospital near Santpoort 35, 39, 43, 46,
331, 333, 360
Meijers, F.S. 75
Meiji Restoration 296
Meinecke, Friedrich 206
men/males
see also gender

Japan (and Japanese)
over-representation of patients 22,
295-311
nurses 23, 48, 370-71
Sweden
masculinity 370-71
meningitis 323-24
Menninger, Karl 146
Menninger, William 146
Mental After-Care Association 121, 251
Mental Health Act
Britain (and British) 128, 136, 259
Japan (and Japanese) 297
United States (and American) 146, 255
Mental Hygiene, American National
Committee for 145, 249, 255
mental hygiene (movement) see also
psycho-hygiene; specific countries 14,
17, 28, 80
mental illness, chronic 9, 86, 135-36, 142,
147, 153-54
mentally deficient 44, 127, 234
mental retardation 16, 132, 280, 285
methodical bedside nursing 338-39
Meyer, A. 249, 255
Micale, Mark 295
middle classes 268, 412
Netherlands (and Dutch) 87
United States (and American) 149, 255,
427
Sweden (and Swedish) nurses 360
Mielke, Fred 201, 207
Milbank Memorial Fund 147
milieu therapy 148
Miller, J. 119
Millerand, Alexandre 227
Mitscherlich, Alexander 201, 207
Minkowski, Eugène 230, 235
modernity 15, 435
monoamine 110
mood disorders, see specific conditions
moral treatment 35, 46, 112, 118, 410
morphine 381, 383, 385
Morrison, Herbert 125
movement therapy 49
Muller, Carel 53
Müller, Max 201

Weimar period (and Republic) *20, 162-63, 166, 169-70, 174, 178, 250, 408*
    welfare state *166*
Weizsäcker, Viktor von *201, 208*
welfare state *13-4, 25, 418, 420-21*
    Britain (and British) *122-23, 267*
    France (and French) *241, 411*
    Netherlands (and Dutch) *27, 36, 50, 86, 89, 95, 266, 270, 407, 422, 430*
    United States (and American) *259*
Welterhof, psychiatric centre (Heerlen) *54*
Wendeburg, F. *250*
Westphalian Euthanasia Trials *206*
West Riding Pauper Lunatic Asylum (Yorkshire) *384*
wet packs *338, 340, 348, 354*
Whitaker, Carl *105*
Wieser, Stefan *210*
Winkler, Walter Theodor *209-10*
Winter Veterans Administration Hospital *146*
Wolfheze, mental institution *48, 51, 279, 285, 343*

women/female *see also* gender
    emancipation of *52, 87, 111, 211, 322*
    caretakers
        Italy (and Italian) *321-323*
    nurses, *see* nursing Sweden (and Swedish); Netherlands (and Dutch)
    patients *22, 54, 186, 295, 302, 307, 309, 340, 391*
        Japan (and Japanese) *22, 302-303*
        schizophrenic *300, 302, 307*
    personnel *367-69, 373*
Woolley, D.W. *393*
Worcester State Hospital (Massachusetts) *146*
working/lower classes
    Italy (and Italian) *322*
    Netherlands (and Dutch) *78, 87, 332*
work therapy, *see* occupational therapy
World Health Organization (WHO) *9*
World Psychiatric Association *192, 208*
World War I, *see* First World War
World War II, *see* Second World War

Y

youth, at-risk (*gefährdete*) *189*